Fetus and Neonate is a series of practical, focused texts which concentrate on that critical period of human development, from late fetal to neonatal life. Each volume in the series examines a particular body system, looking at the physiological mechanisms which underlie the transition from intrauterine to extrauterine life, the pathophysiological processes which may occur, and the application of new basic scientific knowledge to the clinical situation.

This, the second in the *Fetus and Neonate* series, concentrates on breathing. This book is divided into sections on physiology, pathophysiology and clinical applications. Recent research and concepts about fetal breathing, the transitions at birth and the control of postnatal breathing are reviewed. The role of pathophysiological processes in the aetiology of respiratory diseases is discussed and important new developments in diagnosis and treatment are reviewed. The book is written by international authorities in the field, who are active researchers in clinical and basic science as well as practitioners in this area of medicine. It will serve as a valuable source of information for those involved in research in perinatal breathing, or training in paediatrics, neonatology and obstetrics. It will also stimulate the interest of a wider range of health care professionals concerned with keeping abreast of new ideas in this important area of medicine.

BREATHING

Fetus and Neonate: Physiology and Clinical Applications

Volume 1: The Circulation
Volume 2: Breathing

BREATHING

Edited by
MARK A. HANSON
JOHN A. D. SPENCER
CHARLES H. RODECK

Department of Obstetrics and Gynaecology, University College London Medical School

Guest editor
DAFYDD WALTERS

Department of Child Health, St George's Hospital Medical School, London

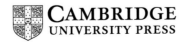

CAMBRIDGE
UNIVERSITY PRESS

Published by the Press Syndicate of the University of Cambridge
The Pitt Building, Trumpington Street, Cambridge CB2 1RP
40 West 20th Street, New York, NY 10011-4211, USA
10 Stamford Road, Oakleigh, Melbourne 3166, Australia

First published 1994

Printed in Great Britain at the University Press, Cambridge

A catalogue record for this book is available from the British Library

Library of Congress cataloguing in publication data

Breathing/edited by Mark A. Hanson, John A. D. Spencer,
Charles H. Rodeck; guest editor, Dafydd Walters.
p. cm. – (Fetus and neonate; v. 2)
Includes index.
Includes bibliographical references and index.
ISBN 0-521-41765-1 (hardback):
1. Fetus – Respiration and cry. 2. Respiration – Regulation.
3. Lungs – Physiology. 4. Respiratory insufficiency in children.
5. Infants (Newborn) – Physiology. I. Hanson, Mark A. II. Spencer,
John A. D. III. Rodeck, C. H. IV. Series.
[DNLM: 1. Fetus – physiology. 2. Infant, Newborn – physiology.
3. Respiratory System – physiology. 4. Respiration – physiology.
WQ210.5 B828 1994]
RG620.B74 1994
612.2 – dc20
DNLM/DLC
for Library of Congress   93-31377   CIP

ISBN 0 521 41765 1 hardback

PN

Contents

Preface to the series

The factual burden of a science varies inversely with its degree of maturity,
P. Medawar 'Two Conceptions of Science': 'Anglo-Saxon Attitudes', Henry
Tizard Memorial Lecture, Encounter 143, August 1965

The idea for a series on the applications of fetal and neonatal physiology
to clinical medicine came from the need of our students for something
intermediate between a textbook and review articles. Textbooks provide
breadth of coverage but tend to lack critical discussion. Reviews can
provide such discussion but represent the view of one authority and may
need a balance. For the student, such reviews are not a substitute for
original papers and are better taken after consumption of a full course of
such papers rather than as an hors d'oeuvres to them.

We envisage the readership of the series as 'students' of the subject in
the widest sense, from undergraduates learning about fetal and neonatal
physiology as part of a basic science degree or preclinical medical
students, to postgraduate and postdoctoral scientists and clinicians spe-
cializing in obstetrics, neonatology or paediatrics. We decided that all
needs would best be met by producing a series of multiauthored volumes.
This will allow rapid production of short texts that will keep the material
focused whilst still allowing the subject to be reviewed from several points
of view. None the less, we have decided to adopt a 'systems' approach
because it has the advantages of simplicity and conformity to textbooks of
physiology.

The chapters in each volume of the series are arranged in sections:
Physiology, Pathophysiology and Clinical Applications. They are not
intended to be all-inclusive but rather to demonstrate the applications of
basic scientific research to clinical medicine via improved understanding
of pathophysiological processes.

ix

The series concentrates on late fetal and neonatal life (the perinatal period). In late gestation the fetus must have established the mechanisms which will permit it to make the transition to becoming a neonate, whilst still being highly adapted to the peculiar intrauterine environment in which it remains. The importance of making the transition successfully is underlined by the fact that this is one of the most dangerous periods of human life. In the course of it, some physiological processes continue, whilst others cease to function, undergo drastic change, or are initiated. The understanding of the underlying controlling processes constitutes one of the greatest challenges in physiology.

Our feeling that such a series is necessary has been reinforced by the increasing number of students who are keen to learn more about this fascinating area. They are aware of the possibility of obtaining biological information from the human fetus using non-invasive methods, but as they see the difficulties of interpreting such information in clinical practice, they perceive the need for a greater understanding of fundamental physiological processes. We hope that this series will stimulate some of them to take up research in this field.

Finally, the series stands for two things which seem temporarily out of fashion. First, by illustrating the clinical applications of basic research, it demonstrates how advances in modern medicine are based on animal research. We cannot, in setting out to improve the care of the human fetus or neonate, have one without the other. Secondly, we believe and teach that the knowledge gained using techniques from a range of disciplines (biochemistry, molecular biology, physics etc.) must ultimately be integrated into concepts of how the body works as a whole. Such integration is precisely the realm of physiology; nowhere is the power of the method more clearly evident than in the fetus and neonate. This synthesis into a whole is not to generalize, but to push our understanding to greater depths.

Mark Hanson
John Spencer
Charles Rodeck

University College London

Acknowledgements

We would like to thank our Guest Editor Dafydd Walters for all his help in putting this volume together. MAH is indebted to the Wellcome Trust who have supported his research in fetal and neonatal physiology through some lean years for science in the UK. Dr Richard Barling encouraged us to develop the series and both he and Peter Silver at Cambridge University Press have been extremely helpful and considerate. Finally we are indebted to Jinette Newns for all her help in preparing the manuscript of this volume.

Contributors

David C. Andrews
Nuffield Department of Obstetrics and Gynaecology, John Radcliffe Hospital, Maternity Department, Headington, Oxford OX3 9DU, UK.

Philip L. Ballard
Children's Hospital of Philadelphia, Philadelphia, PA 19104-4399, USA.

Carlos E. Blanco
Department of Neonatology, State University of Limburg, University Hospital Maastricht, Maastricht, The Netherlands.

Monique Bonora
Laboratoire de Physiologie Respiratoire, Faculté de Médecine Saint-Antoine, 75012 Paris, France.

Michèle Boulé
Laboratoire de Physiologie Respiratoire, Faculté de Médecine Saint-Antoine, 75012 Paris, France.

Peter H. Burri
Department of Developmental Biology, Institute of Anatomy, University of Berne, Berne, Switzerland.

Nicholas M. Fisk
Institute of Obstetrics and Gynaecology, Royal Postgraduate Medical School, Queen Charlotte's and Chelsea Hospital, London W6 0XG, UK.

Stephen J. Gould
Paediatric Pathology, Maternity Department, John Radcliffe Hospital, Headington, Oxford OX3 9DU, UK.

Henry L. Halliday
Neonatal Intensive Care Unit, Royal Maternity Hospital, Belfast, Northern Ireland.

Mark A. Hanson
Department of Obstetrics and Gynaecology, University College London Medical School, 86–96 Chenies Mews, London WC1E 6HX, UK.

Richard Harding
Department of Physiology, Monash University, Melbourne, Victoria 3168, Australia.

Heather Jeffrey
Dept of Perinatal Medicine, King George V Hospital, Royal Prince Alfred Hospital, Missenden Road, Camperdown, NSW 2050, Australia.

Paul Johnson
Nuffield Department of Obstetrics and Gynaecology, John Radcliffe Hospital, Maternity Department, Headington, Oxford OX3 9DU, UK.

Peter J. Moore
Department of Obstetrics and Gynaecology, University College London Medical School, 86–96 Chenies Mews, London WC1E 6HX, UK.

Jacopo P. Mortola
Department of Physiology, McGill University, 3655 Drummond Street, Montreal, Canada.

Christian F. Poets
Department of Paediatric Pulmonology, Children's Hospital, Hannover Medical School, Hannover, Germany.

C. Andrew Ramsden
Department of Paediatrics, Monash Medical Centre, 246 Clayton Road, Clayton 3168, Victoria, Australia.

Bengt Robertson
Research Unit for Experimental Perinatal Pathology, St Goran's Hospital, Stockholm, Sweden.

Michael Silverman
Department of Paediatrics and Neonatal Medicine, Royal Postgraduate Medical School, Hammersmith Hospital, London W12 0NN, UK.

David P. Southall
Academic Department of Paediatrics, North Staffordshire Hospital Centre, Newcastle Road, Stoke-on-Trent, Staffordshire ST4 6QG, UK.

Vugranam C. Venkatesh
Children's Hospital of Philadelphia, Philadelphia, PA 19104-4399, USA.

Dafydd V. Walters
Department of Child Health, St George's Hospital Medical School, London SW17 0RE, UK.

Physiology

1

Structural development of the lung in the fetus and neonate

PETER H. BURRI

Introduction

The primary function of the lung is to provide the organism with a continuous supply of oxygen. Although the lung has other functions too, its structural design and its developmental history are governed by the task of gas exchange. The lung comprises three compartments: air, blood and tissue, with the latter building an uninterrupted and, over wide areas, an extremely thin barrier between air and blood. In this remarkable construction, the tissue represents a delicate and compliant, but at the same time resistant and stable framework, while the air and blood phases are continuously exchanged.

Structural and functional design of the mature lung

The functional organization of the lung can also be defined with respect to the hierarchical structure of the airways and blood vessels. The organ can then be subdivided into three functional zones (Fig. 1.1): a zone of conduction responsible for the mass transport of air and blood, a respiratory zone where gas exchange takes place between the two media, and an intermediate or transitional zone, where the airway structures still contain purely conductive sections but also allow gas exchange.

The respiratory region contains the gas exchanging generations of the airway tree, i.e. several generations of alveolar ducts terminating in the blind-ending alveolar sacs. Both these structures have no solid wall proper; rather they are lined by the alveoli which, in fully inflated lungs, resemble the cells of a honeycomb. The interalveolar septum forms the wall between neighbouring alveoli. Typically, it consists of a central, single-layered network of densely packed capillaries, interwoven with a

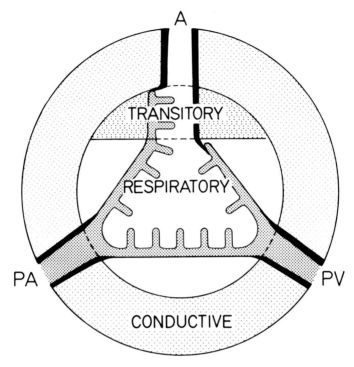

Fig. 1.1. Functional zones of the lung. A = airways, PA = pulmonary artery, PV = pulmonary vein. (Reproduced with permission from Burri, Gil & Weibel, 1989.)

fibrous skeleton made of collagen and elastic fibres and sandwiched between two leaflets of alveolar epithelium (Fig. 1.2). The fibre system is particularly reinforced around the alveolar openings or mouths, a region which may contain smooth muscle cells in addition to the myofibroblasts found elsewhere in the interstitium. The interstitium with its fibrous network forms a continuum that extends from the pleura to the hilum and hence assures transmission of chest wall and diaphragm movements to the central regions of the lung. It contributes to a small degree to the retractive forces of the lung parenchyma (Weibel & Bachofen, 1979), the major part being brought about by surface forces of the air–liquid interface. The epithelial cover of the respiratory region comprises three cell types: type I, type II and type III pneumocytes. The type I pneumocytes represent squamous cells that cover about 93% of the alveolar surface (Zeltner et al., 1987). They are specialized cells forming the air–blood barrier, which in its thinnest portions reaches a mere thickness of

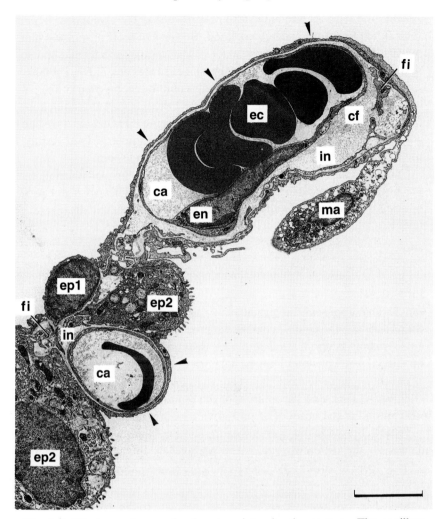

Fig. 1.2. Electron micrograph of mature interalveolar septum. The capillary network (ca) forms a single layer with the typically thin air–blood barrier on one side (arrowheads) and a slightly thicker barrier containing elements of the interstitium (in) on the opposite side. ma = macrophage, ep 1 = type I pneumocyte, ep 2 = type II pneumocyte, en = endothelial cell, ec = erythrocyte, fi = cell processes of fibroblasts, cf = collagen fibrils. Magnification: 3800×; Bar = 5 μm.

0.1–0.3 μm. The type II pneumocytes covering the remaining 7% of the alveolar surface are cuboidal cells, often located within niches between two capillaries. They contain characteristic lamellar bodies representing the storage form of the surfactant material secreted by these cells.

Finally, the type III pneumocytes are rare cells in the alveolar wall and their function has not yet been defined. Because of their short and squat microvilli projecting from their top surface toward the alveolar space, they have also been called alveolar brush cells (Meyrick & Reid, 1968).

Between 80 and 85% of the total lung volume is composed of the so-called pulmonary parenchyma, which bears the gas exchange function. The remainder of the lung volume consists of non-gas exchange tissue and comprises the conducting bronchial tree, the non-capillary blood vessels, the lymphatics and the connective tissue sheaths and sheets.

Lung development is directed towards creating this gas exchanging machinery and preparing for its function at birth. The structural processes involved in this endeavour are to be discussed in the present review.

Lung development: the stages and their timing

Lung development starts in the fourth week after fertilization with a simple and minuscule diverticulum of the foregut, and ends early in childhood with the complex and mature organ. It is thus evident that lung development is subdivided into two distinct phases, a prenatal non-functional and a postnatal functional period. Birth represents an important event in the developmental process, although the effects on the lung structure of the rapid substitution of the liquid contained in the airways with air and of the onset of respiration are poorly understood.

Table 1.1 provides an overview of the stages of lung development. The names for the different periods are purely descriptive and are mainly derived from the morphological aspects of the airspaces.

Embryonic period

The embryonic period corresponds to the phase of organ formation and is not specific to the lung. The lung arises as an outpouching of the foregut, which is cleaved distally from the oesophagus by the deepening and merging of the bilateral laryngotracheal grooves. Proximally, the lung primordium and the foregut remain connected, forming later the entrance to the larynx. The lung bud rapidly divides into two branches that grow into the surrounding mesenchyme. Each branch soon undergoes further divisions. At the end of the seventh week, the future airway tree is preformed down to the subsegmental bronchi.

Table 1.1. *Staging and timetable of lung development*

Periods	Stages	Timing	Developmental processes
I Embryonic period		4–7 weeks	Appearance of ventral bud in foregut Epithelial tube sprouts, divides and grows into surrounding mesenchyme Vascular connections
II Fetal period	Pseudoglandular stage	5–17 weeks	Development of conductive airway tree, paralleled by formation of vascular tree Periphery contains parenchymal precursors
	Canalicular stage	16–26 weeks	Addition of further generations of airways and of vascular tree Differentiation of type I and type II cells Formation of thin air–blood barriers Start of surfactant production
	Saccular stage	25 weeks–birth	Formation of additional airway generations Dilatation of prospective gas exchanging airspaces Maturation of surfactant system
	(Alveolar stage)	36 weeks–birth	Start of alveolar formation
III Postnatal period	Alveolar stage	birth–18 months	Formation of alveoli by outgrowth of secondary septa
	Stage of microvascular maturation	birth–3 years	Reduction of double capillary network to single-layered network Reduction of interstitial tissue mass, fusions of capillaries, preferential growth of single-layered capillary network areas

There is evidence that growth and branching of the epithelial tubes are controlled or at least modulated by interactions between the mesodermally derived mesenchyme and the endodermally derived epithelial buds (Alescio & Cassini, 1962; Spooner & Wessells, 1970).

During this early period, the vascular connections to and from the lungs are also established. The pulmonary arteries branch off from the sixth pair of aortic arches and reach the pulmonary mesenchyme, while the venous connection arises from the left sinoatrial portion of the heart as a single evagination.

By day 50 the embryonic period terminates and is superseded by the fetal stages proper, the first of which is called pseudoglandular, because the lung resembles a primitive compound gland.

Fetal period

Pseudoglandular stage

The morphological alterations manifest during this stage, which lasts from the 5th to the 17th week of gestation, are very unspectacular. Nevertheless, the lung increases in volume, and the number of airway generations increases markedly so that, by the end of this stage, the complete adult conductive bronchial tree is preformed. In rats and mice, immunofluorescent (Ten Have-Opbroek, 1981; Ten Have-Opbroek, Dubbeldam & Otto-Verberne, 1988) and morphological studies (Burri & Moschopulos, 1992) yield evidence that precursor cells of the future alveolar lining epithelium are present at the extreme periphery of the epithelial tubes. This means that the tips of the conductive airways contain cells of the prospective gas exchange tissue (Burri & Moschopulos, 1992). These findings are in agreement with the observation made by Boyden (1977) that the boundaries of the future acinus, (defined by him as the airway spray peripheral to the terminal bronchiole), become visible at the transition of the pseudoglandular to the canalicular stage.

Differentiation of both airway epithelium and mesenchymally derived airway wall elements proceeds in a centrifugal direction, i.e. ciliated and goblet cells, smooth muscle cells and cartilage appear first in the most central airways and extend peripherally with development.

Canalicular stage

This period lasts from the 16th to the 26th week of gestation and can be designated as the period of parenchymal development, i.e. of formation of the prospective gas exchange region. Indeed, as in the earlier stage, lung volume is still increasing markedly, but now due to the formation of airway generations belonging to the future respiratory region. For the first time during lung development, some characteristic features of the gas exchange tissue can be made out as a consequence of the differentiation of the cuboidal airspace epithelium into type 1 and type 2 pneumocytes. This event results in the formation of the typically thin air–blood barrier and in the initiation of the synthesis and secretion of alveolar surfactant.

Simultaneously with the addition of airway generations, the airways distal to the conductive zone grow in length and widen, pushing into the surrounding mesenchyme which contains a three-dimensional capillary network. This process provides each airway segment with a sleeve of capillaries, becoming in a way a kind of local proprietary network, that expands with the growth of its airway. The capillary sheath around each canalicule is, nevertheless, continuous with those of the proximal and distal airway generations, and has also multiple interconnections with those of the neighbouring airways. The structural changes in the capillary network occurring during this stage represent the clue to the understanding of the origin of the capillary bilayer present later in the intersaccular walls and the key to the mode of alveolar formation (Fig. 1.3).

Saccular stage

At the end of the canalicular stage, the airway generations down to the last prospective respiratory bronchioles are present and, attached to them are a bunch of irregularly shaped saccules. According to Boyden (1977), these saccules (or terminal sacs) are connected to the respiratory bronchiole by a transitional duct, which is a kind of short straight tubule lined by a flat epithelium. From week 25 to birth, further airway generations, i.e. the future alveolar ducts and alveolar sacs, are produced by growth and irregular dichotomous divisions from the cluster of saccules. This means that any given saccule will become with time (as it divides peripherally) a tube or duct, until the last airway generation has been formed. Because of the ever-changing morphology of these channels and saccules till the end of the branching process, we have proposed to term these structures transitory ducts and transitory saccules, respectively (Burri, 1985). In microscopy, it would even be preferable to speak of transitory airways, since it often cannot be safely determined on sections, whether one is dealing with a duct or a saccule. With alveolization, the transitory ducts and saccules will finally turn into alveolar ducts

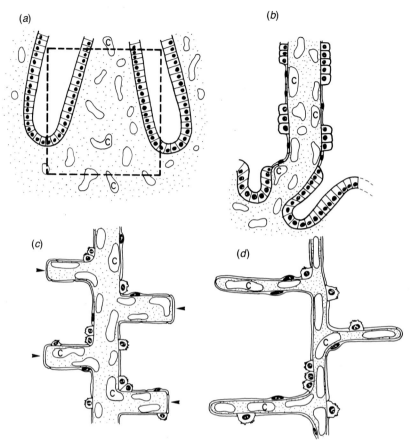

Fig. 1.3. Development of parenchymal structures and in particular of parenchymal microvasculature. (*a*) Pseudoglandular stage: epithelial tubes invade the mesenchyme containing a loose three-dimensional capillary network (*c*). (Figs. (*b*), (*c*) and (*d*) illustrate the further development of the structures contained in the frame of Fig. 1.3(*a*).) (*b*) Canalicular stage: differentiation of airspace epithelium and expansion of peripheral airspaces at the expense of the intervening mesenchyme; the capillaries are rearranged around the epithelial tubes, so that the interairspace walls finally contain a 'capillary bilayer'. (*c*) Alveolar stage: secondary septa (arrowheads) arise from primary septa. All septa are of the primitive type with a double capillary network and a central layer of connective tissue. (*d*) Mature lung. Interalveolar walls contain a single capillary network. (Reproduced with permission from the *Annual Review of Physiology*, **46**, 1984 by Annual Reviews Inc.)

and alveolar sacs. During the saccular stage the peripheral airway generations further increase in width, sandwiching between them the highly cellular interstitium with its capillary networks. By this process, the capillary sheath around each airway approaches laterally those of the adjacent airways. As a consequence, the transitory airways of this stage show a typical wall structure consisting of a central sheet of connective tissue flanked on both sides by a layer of capillaries, that are laterally covered by the alveolar epithelium. During this stage, elastic tissue starts to appear in the interductal and intersaccular walls, an important preparative step for alveolar formation.

Postnatal period

Stage of alveolar formation

Boyden (1977) stated that the newborn lung contained no alveoli and that all alveoli were formed postnatally. More recent work, however, reports that alveolar formation starts as early as week 36 of gestation and that the first alveoli can sometimes even be detected as early as week 32 or 34 (Langston et al., 1984). These latter authors counted on average about 50 million alveoli at birth. Because the adult lung contains 300 million alveoli or more (Weibel, 1963; Angus & Thurlbeck, 1972), over 80% of all alveoli are formed after birth, i.e. the process of alveolization is mainly a postnatal event. The structural details of postnatal lung development have been analysed in small rodents, where alveolar formation starts during the first week of life (Burri, Dbaly & Weibel, 1974; Burri, 1974; Kauffman, Burri & Weibel, 1974; Amy et al., 1977). According to these investigations, alveoli are formed by a septation of the transitory ducts and saccules. The new septa, called secondary septa, represent the prospective interalveolar walls. They arise from the interductal and intersaccular walls (called primary septa) by a lifting off from one of the two capillary layers present in those walls. This usually takes place where elastic fibres have been deposited during the saccular stage (Dubreuil, Lacoste & Raymond, 1936). This mechanism seems to be no different in the human lung (Zeltner & Burri, 1987). We have therefore postulated that the presence of a double capillary network in the airway wall is a prerequisite for alveolar formation – no double capillary layer – no alveolar formation.

The question of the duration of the stage of alveolar formation has been much debated in the past and still cannot be answered definitively. Within the last 30 years, the endpoint of alveolization has been systematically lowered from puberty (Emery & Mithal, 1960) to the age of 8 years (Dunnill, 1962), and then to about 2 years (Langston et al., 1984; Zeltner & Burri, 1987) and there are several reasons for this. First, the methodology of alveolar counting has not always been adequate and, so far, no bias-free stereological approach has been applied to this particular problem, although such methods have been available since 1984 (Sterio, 1984; Cruz-Orive, 1986). Secondly, the definition of what represents an alveolus on a section, and even more an alveolus in statu nascendi, is a delicate and tricky matter and subject to erroneous interpretation. Thirdly, alveolization is not likely to stop abruptly, and biological variation between individuals and topographical variations within a single organ may further add to the difficulty of assessing the end of this stage. Based on the morphological investigation of the rat lung (Burri, 1974) and of the human lung (Zeltner & Burri, 1987), it is evident, on the one hand, that what can be called 'bulk alveolar formation' is a relatively rapid process, accompanied by a typical morphology (Fig. 1.4(a)). In the rat lung, it happens mainly during the second postnatal week, and in the human, it starts at about one month before birth (Langston et al., 1984) and lasts into the postnatal period. At the postnatal age of 1 month, the process is still blooming, but by 6 months the intensity of alveolar formation has much decreased. On the other hand, the limit of 2 years generally agreed on today does not preclude the addition of a limited number of alveoli at a slow pace after that age. In the rat there is evidence that this indeed happens after the age of two to three weeks (Massaro et al., 1985; Blanco, Massaro & Massaro, 1989, 1991).

Stage of microvascular maturation

As has been explained above, alveolization can only occur on inter-airspace walls which contain a double capillary network. Such walls have been called 'primitive', in contrast to the mature interalveolar septa containing a single capillary layer. The origin of the capillary bilayer in the primary septa has been discussed in the sections on the canalicular and saccular stage. Bearing in mind the mode of formation of secondary septa (see Fig. 1.3), it is evident that the latter are of the primitive type, too. Indeed, most of the newly formed interalveolar walls exhibit, in the electron microscope, a capillary bilayer, as exemplified in Fig. 1.4(b) for the human and in Fig. 1.5(a) for the rat lung. The adult lungs of both species, however, have thin interalveolar walls that contain a single capillary network (Fig. 1.2 & Fig. 1.5(b)).

As a consequence of these facts, the alveolar stage cannot be the last stage in lung development. Alveolization must be followed by a stage of microvascular maturation, during which the septal structure, the capillary network which is its key element, has to be completely remodelled (Burri, 1991).

Years ago, we had hypothetized that this microvascular maturation could be achieved by a process of multiple focal fusions between the capillary layers, followed by a preferential growth of the fused areas (Fig. 1.6) (Zeltner & Burri, 1987). In the rat, the amount of interstitial tissue within the interalveolar septa decreases during the third week, while the septa actually grow in height and the alveoli deepen. This coincides with the reduction of the capillary bilayer to a single layer and a slimming of the interalveolar septa. We have recently succeeded in demonstrating by electron microscopical investigation of serial sections of interalveolar walls that fusions between the two capillary layers do actually occur during this phase of rat lung development (Burri & Tarek, unpublished observations). In several instances, a merging of two capillaries could be observed, their lumina being separated only by one or two thin leaflets of an endothelial cell. In a single case, a tiny circular luminal interconnection of about 0.5 μm was found between two closely apposed capillaries. These observations strongly support the concept of a reduction in the double capillary network by a process involving focally distributed intercapillary fusions followed by the preferential expansion of the fused areas. The latter mechanism is relevant for the spreading of the maturation over the whole lung. Various paces of growth for different elements or different areas of an organ are a well established principle in embryology. By such mechanisms, for example, the developing heart is transformed (while it is already working) from a simple tube to a complex pumping device with four chambers and feeding two distinct circulatory systems. Preferential growth of areas where the two capillary networks are interconnected may therefore represent a reasonable explanation for the profound septal transformation.

It may be of interest in this context to indicate that expansion of the capillary system probably does not occur by sprouting of capillaries, but by intussusceptive capillary growth, i.e. by formation of new transcapillary tissue pillars which, by growth, will become new intercapillary meshes (Fig. 1.6). This concept of capillary network growth, first mentioned by Short (1950), was rediscovered while investigating the capillary fusion process in methacrylate casts of rat lungs (Caduff, Fischer & Burri, 1986). Its existence could be further assessed by electron microscopy of serial sections through interalveolar walls (Burri & Tarek, 1990). There is also evidence that intussusceptive capillary growth may occur in other organ systems too (Patan et al., 1992).

After the structural transformations of the pulmonary microvascular system, the interalveolar wall of the rat lung looks practically mature at

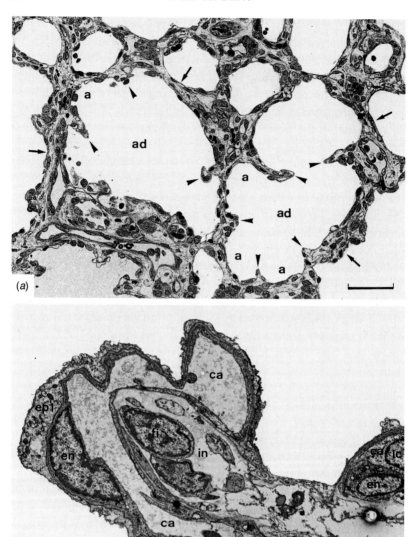

the age of three weeks. In man, microvascular maturation starts during alveolization and proceeds rapidly: at six months numerous interalveolar walls, and by $1\frac{1}{2}$ years most septa, are at least partially of the mature type.

As with alveolization, the endpoint of this stage cannot be determined precisely, because some isolated immature septal portions can be detected even in adult lungs. Some indications can, however, be derived from indirect evidence: on the one hand, we know from morphometric data that the growth of lung compartments, and in particular capillary growth rates, are very different between the first 18 months of life and the period afterwards (Zeltner et al., 1987); on the other hand, the lung was found to correspond morphologically to a miniaturized adult lung at 5 years of age. These observations led us to suggest that the transition between lung development and normal lung growth may occur somewhere between the age of $1\frac{1}{2}$ and 5 years, most likely during the third year of life. From there onwards, the lung compartments grow (with exception of the interstitium) in a proportion to each other and to body weight. This steady phase of lung growth is likely to continue as long as body growth goes on. Then, following a period of relative structural stability, the lung compartments may start again to shift their volume proportions in processes related to the aging of the lung.

Conclusion

The gas exchange tissues are derived from two germ layers: the epithelial elements of the airway tree (from the trachea to the subpleural airspaces) stem from the endoderm, the remaining tissues have their origin in the mesoderm. All along the developmental stages, interactions between the two components play a role in tissue and cell differentiation. Following the embryonic period of organ formation, the lung traverses five partially overlapping phases of development, i.e. the pseudoglandular, the canalicular, the saccular, the alveolar stage and the stage of microvascular

---

Fig. 1.4. (*a*) Light micrograph of human lung aged 26 days. Notice typical immature aspect with thick primary septa (arrows) and new secondary septa (arrowheads). All septa contain at least partly a double capillary network. a = alveoli, ad = alveolar duct. Magnification: 250×; Bar: 50 μm. (*b*) Electron micrograph of human lung aged 26 days. Secondary septum with capillary loop (ca) and central layer of interstitium (in). ep 1 = type I pneumocyte, en = endothelial cell, fi = fibroblast, ec = erythrocyte. Magnification: 3000×; Bar: 5 μm.

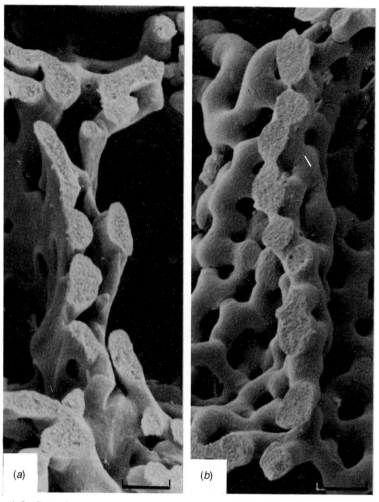

Fig. 1.5. Scanning electron micrographs of methylmethacrylate casts of rat pulmonary microvasculature. (*a*) Rat aged 7 days: immature aspect with capillary bilayer. (*b*) rat aged 139 days: mature aspect with one capillary layer in inter-airspace wall. Magnification: 1300×; Bar: 10 μm.

maturation. In man, the time of birth falls into the early alveolar stage with more than 80% of the alveoli being formed postnatally. Morphological and quantitative findings suggest that lung development is completed during the third year of life, when it merges imperceptively into the phase of normal growth.

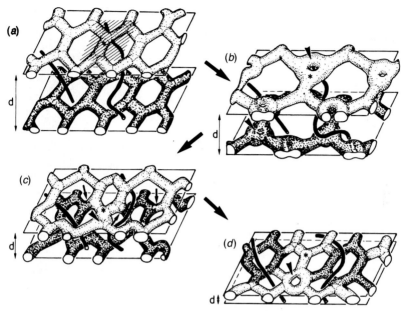

Fig. 1.6. Current model of the transformation of the septal capillary system during the stage of microvascular maturation. In all four panels the lower capillary system (or portions derived from it) are shown in a darker shade. The distance (d) illustrates the thickness of the interstitial layer. The two dark strands symbolize the position and course of the interstitial fibre network. For orientation the asterisks mark the same spot in all four panels. The shaded area in panel (*a*) delineates the frame of panel (*d*). (*a*) At birth, two separate capillary networks lie on both sides of a broad interstitial layer. (*b*) Within each capillary network, new meshes (arrowheads) are formed by intussusceptive growth, i.e. by formation of new meshes within expanded sheet-like areas of the capillary bed. (*c*) The reduction in thickness of the interstitial layer favours the punctuate fusion (arrows) of the two capillary systems. Furthermore, preferentially grown areas of either capillary system slide into widened meshes of the other system. Arrowhead marks the site of appearance of a new mesh (see panel (*d*). This occurs by intussusceptive growth. (*d*) By means of reduction in thickness of the interstitial layer, capillary fusion and eventually also obliteration of some capillary segments, a strictly single capillary system could theoretically represent the end of the microvascular maturation. Practically, this idealized end stage may not be achieved even in a mature lung. Arrowhead marks new capillary mesh formed by intussusception.

Acknowledgements

This work was supported by grant No. 3100.27775.89 of the Swiss National Science Foundation. I thank Mrs E. de Peyer, Mrs B. Krieger, Mr B. Haenni and Mr K. Babl for their excellent technical collaboration.

References

Alescio, T. & Cassini, A. (1962). Induction in vitro of tracheal buds by pulmonary mesenchyme grafted on tracheal epithelium. *Journal of Experimental Zoology*, **150**, 83–94.

Amy, R. W. M., Bowes, D., Burri, P. H., Haines, J. & Thurlbeck, W. M. (1977). Postnatal growth of the mouse lung. *Journal of Anatomy*, **124**, 131–51.

Angus, G. E. & Thurlbeck, W. M. (1972). Number of alveoli in the human lung. *Journal of Applied Physiology*, **32**, 483–5.

Blanco, L. N., Massaro, G. D. & Massaro, D. (1989). Alveolar dimensions and number: developmental and hormonal regulation. *American Journal of Physiology*, **257**, L240–7.

Blanco, L. N., Massaro, G. D. & Massaro, D. (1991). Alveolar size, number, and surface area: developmentally dependent response to 13% O_2. *American Journal of Physiology*, **261**, L370–7.

Boyden, E. A. (1977). Development and growth of the airways. In *Lung Biology in Health and Disease. Development of the Lung,* ed. W. A. Hodson. Vol 6. pp. 3–35. M Dekker, New York.

Burri, P. H. (1974). The postnatal growth of the rat lung. III. Morphology. *Anatomical Record*, **180**, 77–98.

Burri, P. H. (1985). Development and growth of the human lung. In *Handbook of Physiology: Section 3, The Respiratory System*, ed. A. P. Fishman & B. Fisher. pp. 1–46. American Physiological Society: Bethesda.

Burri, P. H. (1991). Postnatal development and growth of the pulmonary microvasculature. In *Scanning Electron Microscopy of Vascular Casts: Methods and Applications*, ed. P. M. Motta, T. Murakami & H. Fujita. pp. 139–56. Kluwer Academic Publishers, The Hague.

Burri, P. H. & Moschopulos, M. (1992). Structural analysis of fetal rat lung development. *Anatomical Record*, **234**, 399–418.

Burri, P. H. & Tarek, M. R. (1990). A novel mechanism of capillary growth in the rat pulmonary microcirculation. *Anatomical Record*, **228**, 35–45.

Burri, P. H., Dbaly, J. & Weibel, E. R. (1974). The postnatal growth of the rat lung. I. Morphometry. *Anatomical Record*, **178**, 711–30.

Burri, P. H., Gil, J. & Weibel, E. R. (1989). Ultrastructure and morphometry of the human lung. In *General Thoracic Surgery*, 3rd edn, ed. T. W. Shields. pp. 16–38. Lea & Febinger: Philadelphia, London.

Caduff, J. H., Fischer, L. C. & Burri, P. H. (1986). Scanning electron microscopic study of the developing microvasculature in the postnatal rat lung. *Anatomical Record*, **216**, 154–64.

Cruz-Orive, L. M. (1986). Arbitrary particles can be counted using a disector of unknown thickness: the selector. *Journal of Microscopy*, **145**, 121–42.

Dubreuil, G., Lacoste, A. & Raymond, R. (1936). Observations sur le développement du poumon humain. *Bulletin d'Histologie et de Technique Microscopique*, **13**, 235–45.

Dunnill, M. S. (1962). Postnatal growth of the lung. *Thorax*, **17**, 329–33.

Emery, J. L. & Mithal, A. (1960). The number of alveoli in the terminal respiratory unit of man during late intrauterine life and childhood. *Archives of Disease in Childhood*, **35**, 544–47.

Kauffman, S. L., Burri, P. H. & Weibel, E. R. (1974). The postnatal growth of the rat lung. II. Autoradiography. *Anatomical Record*, **180**, 63–76.

Langston, C., Kida, K., Reed, M. & Thurlbeck, W. M. (1984). Human lung growth in late gestation and in the neonate. *American Review of Respiratory Disease*, **129**, 607–13.

Massaro, D., Teich, N., Maxwell, S., Massaro, G. D. & Whitney, P. (1985). Postnatal development of alveoli. Regulation and evidence for a critical period in rats. *Journal of Clinical Investigation*, **76**, 1297–305.

Meyrick, B. & Reid, L. (1968). The alveolar brush cell in rat lung – a third pneumonocyte. *Journal of Ultrastructure Research*, **23**, 71–80.

Patan, S., Alvarez, M. J., Schittny, J. C. & Burri, P. H. (1992). Intusussceptive microvascular growth: A common alternative to capillary sprouting. *Archives of Histology and Cytology*, **55**, Suppl., 65–75.

Short, R. H. D. (1950). Alveolar epithelium in relation to growth of the lung. *Philosophical Transactions of The Royal Society of London. Series B: Biological Sciences*, **235**, 35–87.

Spooner, B. S. & Wessells, N. K. (1970). Mammalian lung development: interactions in primordium formation and bronchial morphogenesis. *Journal of Experimental Zoology*, **175**, 445–54.

Sterio, D. C. (1984). The unbiased estimation of number and sizes of arbitrary particles using the disector. *Journal of Microscopy*, **134**, 127–36.

Ten Have-Opbroek, A. A. W. (1981). The development of the lung in mammals: an analysis of concepts and findings. *American Journal of Anatomy*, **162**, 201–19.

Ten Have-Opbroek, A. A., Dubbeldam, J. A. & Otto-Verberne, C. J. (1988). Ultrastructural features of type II alveolar epithelial cells in early embryonic mouse lung. *Anatomical Record*, **221**, 846–53.

Weibel, E. R. (1963). *Morphometry of the Human Lung*. Springer Verlag, Heidelberg.

Weibel, E. R. & Bachofen, H. (1979). Structural design of alveolar septum and fluid exchange. In *Pulmonary Edema*, ed. A. P. Fishman & E. M. Renkin, pp. 1–20. American Physiological Society, Maryland.

Zeltner, T. B. & Burri, P. H. (1987). The postnatal development and growth of the human lung. II Morphology, *Respiration Physiology*, **67**, 269–82.

Zeltner, T. B., Caduff, J. H., Gehr, P., Pfenninger, J. & Burri, P. H. (1987). The postnatal development and growth of the human lung. I. Morphometry. *Respiration Physiology*, **67**, 247–67.

2

Surfactant: ontogeny, hormonal control and function

PHILIP L. BALLARD and VUGRANAM C. VENKATESH

Introduction

The history of the discovery of pulmonary surfactant is relatively short. The first definite description of the importance of surface tension on lung mechanics is attributed to von Neergaard (1929), who found that inflation of degassed lungs with air required more pressure than if a liquid was used. Other key contributors included Gruenwald (1947), Pattle (1955) and Clements (1956). The link between surfactant deficiency and clinical hyaline membrane disease was made in 1959 by Avery & Mead. Since then, there has been an exponential growth in our knowledge of the subject. This short chapter provides an overview of the surfactant system with a focus on more recently elucidated information regarding regulation. A very detailed discussion of all aspects of pulmonary surfactant is given in a book edited by Robertson, van Golde & Batenberg (1992).

Composition

Pulmonary surfactant, a complex mixture of lipids and proteins, is synthesized by alveolar type II epithelial cells and secreted into peripheral air spaces. Surfactant is composed mainly of lipids (~90%), and its ability to lower alveolar surface tension is due primarily to dipalmitoyl phosphatidylcholine (DPPC, ~45% by weight). Phosphatidylglycerol (PG), which is present in uniquely high concentrations in type II cells, comprises about 5% of surfactant. A variety of other lipids, including neutral lipids, are present in surfactant but their physiological relevance is unknown (Fig. 2.1).

Proteins comprise 5–10% of isolated surfactant and are mainly serum proteins which are likely to be a contaminate of bronchoalveolar lavage.

20

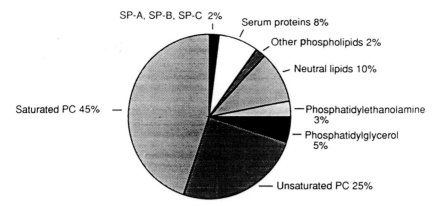

Fig. 2.1. Composition by weight of surfactant isolated from lung lavage. SP, surfactant protein.

Four non-serum surfactant-associated proteins have been identified and the cDNAs and genes cloned (Hawgood & Benson, 1989; Weaver & Whitsett, 1991). The properties and in vitro functions of the proteins are summarized in Table 2.1. The largest and most abundant is SP-A, a water soluble glycoprotein of MW 28 000 –36 000 D which, in its native state, forms an 18 subunit oligomer. The monomers consist of 248 amino acids composed of a 20 amino acid amino-terminal signal peptide followed by 24 repeats of a glycine-X-hydroxyproline type collagenous domain. A stretch of 120 amino acids in the carboxy end has structural and functional similarities to C-type lectins which bind carbohydrate moieties in a divalent cation-dependent fashion.

SP-B (8000 D) is a 79 amino acid peptide resulting from the proteolytic processing of a 39 kD pre-pro-protein. It is rich in hydrophobic amino acids (leucine, isoleucine and valine) and two amphipathic helices have been predicted in its secondary structure which would interact with the phospholipid membrane. Mature SP-C (5000 D) is a 32–35 amino acid polypeptide generated by proteolytic processing of a 22 kD precursor. The two cysteine residues in the mature peptide are palmitoylated. The secondary structure of SP-C is predicted to have a single membrane spanning helix. Because of their lipophilic nature, both SP-B and SP-C co-isolate with surfactant lipids and are present in replacement surfactant preparations derived from natural sources.

SP-D is a hydrophilic protein that is less well characterized than the other surfactant proteins. It has structural similarities to SP-A with a 59

Table 2.1. *Surfactant associated proteins*

	MW (kD)	Properties	Functions
SP-A	28–36 (monomer) ~650 (native)	Hydrophilic Collagen region Ca^{2+} binding Lipid binding Carbohydrate binding	Regulate surfactant secretion and recycling Influence surfactant structure Immune defence
SP-B	39 → 8	Hydrophobic Membrane spanning domain	Enhance film formation and spreading Reduce surface tension
SP-C	22 → 5	Hydrophobic Contains two palmitic acids	Enhance film formation
SP-D	43	Hydrophilic Collagen region Ca^{2+} binding Carbohydrate binding	Immune defence ? surfactant metabolism

Known surfactant-associated proteins are listed and are reviewed in detail in references cited in the text. All the proteins have been purified (from broncho-alveolar fluid) and the cDNAs and genes cloned. Processing of the proteins is indicated by changes in molecular weight (SP-B and -C). The identified functions are from in vitro experiments.

amino acid collagenous region and a carboxy terminus with divalent cation-dependent carbohydrate binding properties. Under reducing conditions it migrates at ~43 kD and under non-reducing conditions as disulfide-bonded trimers. Other post-translational modifications, including hydroxylation and N-linked glycosylation have been described.

Life cycle of surfactant

There is considerable information available regarding the metabolic life cycle of surfactant lipids (for review see Batenburg, 1992; Wright & Hawgood, 1989) but relatively little data for surfactant proteins. All the lipid and protein components of surfactant (except serum proteins) are synthesized in alveolar type II cells. SP-A and SP-B are also synthesized in bronchiolar Clara cells where they have as yet unknown functions.

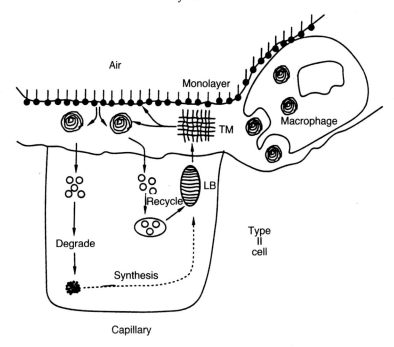

Fig. 2.2. Model of the life cycle of surfactant. Newly synthesized lipids plus SP-B, SP-C and possibly other proteins combine with recycled phospholipid and SP-A in multivesicular bodies to form lamellar bodies (LB). These organelles fuse with the cell membrane and the contents are secreted into the aqueous alveolar lining layer where the lipids rearrange into tubular myelin (TM) under the influence of SP-A and SP-B. A lipid monolayer forms and is enriched in DPPC during compression to provide alveolar stability at low volume. Phospholipid is continually lost from the monolayer and either degraded by macrophages or recycled into type II cells. (Reprinted by permission from Wright & Hawgood, 1989.)

According to current concepts, the lipid components along with newly synthesized SP-B, SP-C and some recycled SP-A are packaged into lamellar bodies which have a unique macro-organization of concentrically arranged phospholipid bilayers (Fig. 2.2). Lamellar bodies are secreted into the alveolar space by membrane fusion and exocytosis, a process influenced by a variety of stimuli (see Table 2.2). Most, if not all newly synthesized SP-A is secreted separately from lamellar bodies and interacts with the unravelling lamellar bodies to promote formation of a highly organized lattice-like structure termed tubular myelin. This structure is composed of long tubules with intersecting lipid bilayer membranes containing SP-A and SP-B molecules (Williams, Hawgood & Hamilton, 1991). Subsequently, the phospholipids are adsorbed into a monomolecular film at the alveolar air–liquid interface. The monolayer is

Table 2.2. *Agents affecting surfactant in fetal lung*

Increased synthesis	*Increased secretion*
Glucocorticoids	Beta-sympathomimetics/cAMP
ACTH	ATP and adenosine
Thyroid hormones	Calcium ionophores
Thyrotropin releasing hormone	Phorbol esters
Beta-sympathomimetics	Leukotrienes
Prostaglandins	
cAMP	*Decreased synthesis*
Estradiol	Glucocorticoids
Epidermal growth factor	Insulin
Fibroblast pneumonocyte factor	Dihydrotestosterone
Interferon-γ	Transforming growth factor-β
(Prolactin)	Tumor necrosis factor-α
	Phorbol esters

Listing of hormones, growth factors, cytokines and other agents that have been shown to stimulate or inhibit synthesis of one or more components of surfactant or to stimulate secretion. Only glucocorticoids increase production of all components of surfactant. Prolactin appears to act permissively in the fetal sheep and its effect in organ culture is controversial. Experimental results are reviewed in Ballard (1986), Weaver and Whitsett (1991), Ballard (1986).

enriched in DPPC by a process of selective removal of non-DPPC lipids during expansion and contraction produced by the breathing cycle and receives continuous replenishment of components.

Lipids not utilized in monolayer formation and those removed from the monolayer are collected into uni- and multivesicular structures for reuptake or degradation. Most vesicles are endocytosed by type II cells, apparently via a membrane receptor for SP-A, and are incorporated into newly developing lamellar bodies. Up to 85% of alveolar surfactant is recycled in 3 day-old rabbits and less in the adult. Alveolar macrophages also take up the lipids for degradation.

Functions of surfactant components

Lipids

Experiments in vitro have demonstrated that a monolayer of DPPC is capable of reducing the surface tension to nearly zero during compression of the film. This is consistent with observed properties of high compliance and stability on deflation of the surfactant replete lung. PG and possibly other surfactant lipids are probably involved in adsorption, spreading and enrichment of the DPPC monolayer film.

This property of altering surface tension in response to compression is important in maintaining lung volumes during the breathing cycle. During expiration when alveolar volume decreases, the monolayer is compressed and surface tension decreases, preventing smaller alveoli from emptying into the larger ones. This stabilizes the alveoli and maintains lung compliance. A deficiency in surfactant leads to alveolar collapse and decreased lung compliance and is the major cause of infant respiratory distress syndrome (RDS).

Surfactant lipids also play an important role in lung fluid absorption and maintenance of lung liquid balance. The oscillation of alveolar surface tension during breathing probably contributes to the turnover of alveolar fluid and the low surface tension promotes fluid reabsorption by the alveolar capillaries. In surfactant deficiency, the extra-alveolar interstitial pressure decreases (becomes more negative) causing capillary leak. It has been suggested that without surfactant, the respiratory bronchioles would fill up with a column of liquid and hinder airflow (Liu et al., 1991) (see Chapter 3).

SP-A

Although the physiological role of SP-A in intact animals is not yet well defined, in vitro data suggest a number of important functions. SP-A along with SP-B and calcium is required for formation of tubular myelin in reconstitution experiments. Since tubular myelin is apparently a requisite intermediate between lamellar bodies and the monolayer, it is likely that SP-A is necessary for efficient monolayer formation. DeMello et al., (1987) have reported an absence of tubular myelin but not lamellar bodies in air spaces of infants dying of RDS and suggest that RDS may be a disease of SP-A deficiency.

In isolated type II cells, purified SP-A inhibits both basal and induced surfactant lipid secretion, including that in response to mechanical stretch. This inhibition, acting as a feedback mechanism, is apparently mediated by binding of SP-A to a receptor (not yet isolated) on type II cells. In vitro, SP-A increases the uptake of DPPC by type II cells and alveolar macrophages. Studies with alveolar surfactant subfractions suggest that this effect also occurs in vivo and the properties of this process are consistent with mediation by the putative SP-A receptor. The observations that SP-A enhances lipid re-uptake and inhibits secretion has led to the speculation that SP-A plays a major role in the regulation of surfactant pool sizes in vivo.

Evidence is accruing for an important role for SP-A in lung immune defence mechanisms (Weaver & Whitsett, 1991; van Iwaarden, 1992). SP-A has collagenous and carbohydrate binding domains similar to complement factor C1q and mannose binding proteins which play important roles in macrophage phagocytosis. In vitro, SP-A has been shown to stimulate chemotaxis of alveolar macrophages and phagocytosis of serum-opsonized *Staphylococcus aureus* and complement-coated erythrocytes. SP-A also promotes intracellular killing of pathogens by stimulating the respiratory burst and production of oxygen radicals. In addition there is evidence that SP-A itself functions as an opsonin to promote internalization of both bacteria and viruses by the alveolar macrophages. These effects of SP-A are mediated through interaction with the membrane binding site for C1q and possibly via a separate high affinity SP-A binding site similar to that on type II cells. The content of SP-A in surfactant may be modulated as part of the immune response to lung infection. In cultured lung explants synthesis of SP-A mRNA is markedly stimulated by interferon-γ whereas another cytokine, TNF-α, is inhibitory (Ballard et al., 1989; Dulkerian & Ballard unpublished data.) At present there is no information regarding in vivo effects of pathogens or cytokines on SP-A synthesis.

SP-B

The recent availability of purified preparations of natural and recombinant SP-B and various synthetic peptide domains of SP-B has helped to delineate various functions of this protein. SP-B, either alone or in combination with other surfactant proteins, markedly increases the rate of adsorption of phospholipid to the air–liquid interface in vitro. Experiments using the pulsating bubble and the Wilhelmy balance techniques have demonstrated that SP-B significantly enhances the surface tension lowering properties of various phospholipid mixtures in response to compression. Other experiments indicate a role for SP-B in tubular myelin formation and possibly in phospholipid recycling (Hawgood & Benson, 1989; Williams et al., 1991; Whitsett & Baatz, 1992).

Instillation of SP-B/phospholipid mixtures into the trachea of animals with experimental RDS markedly improves lung compliance and alveolar stability, mimicking the response to native surfactant. Tracheal instillation of monoclonal antibodies to SP-B into near-term newborn rabbits induced a prominent, immediate decrease in lung compliance and anatomical changes similar to clinical RDS. A similar effect was not observed with monoclonal antibodies to SP-A (Yu et al., 1988; Robertson et al.,

1991). A recent case report of two siblings with fatal congenital alveolar proteinosis who did not have detectable SP-B mRNA or protein adds to the evidence that SP-B plays a critical role in surfactant function and metabolism (Nogee et al., 1993).

SP-C

In vitro, SP-C increases adsorption and spreading of phospholipids and lowers surface tension in response to film compression; however, the effect is less than that of native surfactant or phospholipid/SP-B mixtures. Other experiments have suggested that SP-C is involved in maintaining the lateral stability of phospholipid films. However, a discrete functional role for SP-C in vivo is not known.

SP-D

Expression of the SP-D gene of the rat is limited to pulmonary tissue and is associated with both type II cells and Clara cells of distal membranous bronchi. In the alveolar space, SP-D is localized to granular material but not to tubular myelin or lamellar bodies (Crouch et al., 1991*a,b*). Although structurally related to SP-A and designated as a surfactant-associated protein, to date there is no demonstrated role of SP-D in surfactant metabolism or function. It is proposed that one function of SP-D is related to pulmonary antimicrobial host defence based on the similarity to conglutinin and mannose binding proteins which agglutinate bacteria and activate complement. In support of this proposal, it has been found that SP-D binds *E.coli* and increases oxygen radical formation by alveolar macrophages (Kuan, Rust & Crouch, 1992; van Iwaarden, 1992).

Ontogeny

Lipids

The content of PC and saturated PC in fetal lung tissue and amniotic fluid increases during the second and third trimesters of human gestation, respectively. During most of the second trimester, the amount of saturated PC in fetal lung, expressed per mg DNA, is constant at approximately 30% of the adult value. The level begins to increase after 20 weeks gestation when type II cells containing some lamellar bodies are first detected in fetal lung tissue reaching ~35% of the adult level by 24 weeks (Fig. 2.3). There are little data for phospholipid levels in human lung

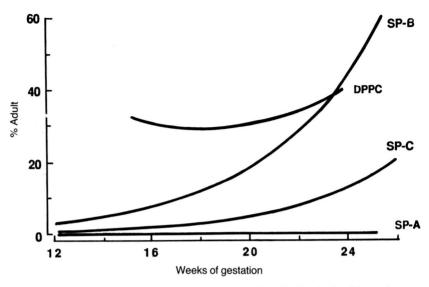

Fig. 2.3. Developmental pattern for DPPC and SP mRNAs in fetal lung tissue during the second trimesters. Best fit lines for data from 22 specimens are shown. (Reproduced with permission from Ballard, 1989.)

during the third trimester; however, in animals the content of saturated PC increases several-fold during the last quarter of gestation (Ballard, 1986). The developmental increase in saturated PC levels is likely to be due to increased rate of synthesis rather than a decrease in rate of degradation. Synthesis of saturated PC is regulated by fatty acid synthetase, a multifunctional enzyme that catalyses all of the reactions in synthesis of fatty acids, and by cholinephosphate cytidylyltransferase which is a rate limiting enzyme for the final step of PC synthesis. In animals, fatty acid synthetase activity increases late in fetal life in parallel with increasing PC content (Rooney, 1989; Batenburg, 1992). Synthetase activity is regulated by both glucocorticoids and agents that increase cAMP and both of these hormones have a similar stimulatory effect on PC synthesis and content (Ballard, 1989). These and other correlations indicate that fatty acid synthetase is probably a key regulated enzyme for production of surfactant lipids during fetal development.

There are also parallel increases in cholinephosphate cytidylyltransferase activity and the rate of PC synthesis during development and with hormonal treatment, indicating that this enzyme is also involved in developmental regulation of surfactant production. The increase in

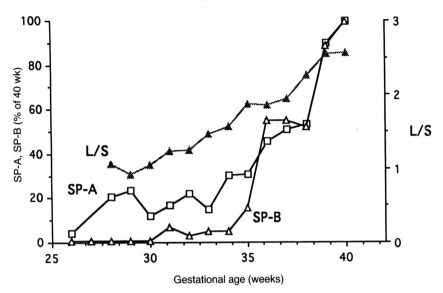

Fig. 2.4. Ontogeny of surfactant components in human amniotic fluid. Levels of SP-A and SP-B were determined by ELISA and are expressed as percent of the mean value at 40 weeks gestation. L/S = lecithin: sphingomyelin ratio. (Adapted from data of Pryhuber et al., 1991.)

cytidylyltransferase is due at least in part to increased content of lipid cofactor secondary to increased activity of fatty acid synthetase (Rooney et al., 1986). Lyso-PC: acyl CoA acyltransferase, which catalyses the remodelling of PC to the disaturated form, is under both developmental and glucocorticoid regulation in fetal animals and is likely to have a physiological role in human lung development where the percent saturation of PC increases with development.

In amniotic fluid, levels of PC (L/S ratio, saturated PC content) increase during the third trimester (Fig. 2.4) and levels are predictive of lung maturity. The increase in amniotic fluid occurs several weeks after the appearance and accumulation of lamellar bodies and saturated PC in fetal lung tissue. This temporal pattern suggests that there is also a developmental increase in the basal rate of surfactant secretion from type II cells into lung fluid. However, this has not been directly examined.

Surfactant proteins

The developmental patterns for surfactant protein mRNAs in human fetal lung are illustrated in Fig. 2.3. SP-A mRNA is undetectable or at very low concentrations compared to adult values in fetal tissue of 13–25 weeks (Ballard et al., 1986). By contrast, mRNAs for both SP-B and SP-C are detected as early as 13 weeks gestation and their content increases during the second trimester to ~50% and 15% of the adult level, respectively, at 24 weeks gestation (Liley et al., 1989). Thus expression of the SP-A gene is temporally correlated with development of differentiated type II cells whereas the genes for SP-B and SP-C are expressed prior to differentiation of pulmonary epithelial cells. There is little correlation between the content of these two mRNAs in individual lung specimens, suggesting that the two genes are independently regulated during in vivo development (Liley et al., 1989). Levels of surfactant protein mRNAs are increased by premature birth (baboon) and on exposure of newborn animals to hyperoxia (Minoo et al., 1991). The oxygen induced increase in SP-A and SP-B gene expression occurs only in Clara cells, suggesting that regulation of these two genes differs between type II and Clara cells (Wikenheiser et al., 1992).

Levels of the surfactant proteins during development appear to parallel the patterns for mRNAs. SP-A protein content by immunoassay is low or undetectable during the second trimester, and SP-A is not detected by immunofluorescence at 20–22 weeks (Ballard et al., 1986). The distribution of immunoreactive SP-B has been examined in specimens of human lung during gestation (Stahlman, Gray & Whitsett, 1992). Immunostaining was not detected in lung of <19 weeks, was present in ~50% of terminal airway cells at 19–24 weeks, and occurred in all type II cells and in some bronchioalveolar portal cells at >26 weeks. Recent immunofluorescence data indicate that SP-C protein in lung cells also parallels the developmental pattern for the mRNA (Ballard, Gonzales, Beers & Shuman, unpublished data). These observations suggest that all three surfactant proteins are primarily regulated at the transcriptional level during development, consistent with the recent finding that the major effect of glucocorticoids on SP-B and SP-C of human lung is increased rate of gene transcription (Venkatesh et al., 1993).

The developmental pattern for SP-D, which may have a role in surfactant function, is not known for the human. In fetal rats, both mRNA and protein content increase during late gestation in a pattern similar to that of surfactant lipids (Crouch et al., 1991*b*), and there are preliminary reports of precocious expression of the SP-D gene after glucocorticoid treatment.

Both SP-A and SP-B are detected in amniotic fluid as early as 30 weeks gestation and levels increase during the third trimester. The temporal pattern for SP-A is similar to that for surfactant phospholipid, whereas the major increase in SP-B appeared to occur somewhat later in this study (Fig. 2.4). At present, there are no data available for the developmental pattern of SP-C and SP-D in amniotic fluid. The delayed appearance of SP-B is unexpected since both SP-B and SP-C are felt to be packaged and secreted with lamellar bodies. By contrast, SP-A appears to be primarily secreted by a constitutive pathway independent of lamellar release. For this protein, therefore, the temporal pattern in amniotic fluid presumably directly reflects the rate of gene expression in type II cells.

Role of endogenous hormones

There is a variety of evidence that the rate of lung maturation in the developing fetus is modulated by endogenous hormones (for review see Ballard, 1986). Endogenous glucocorticoids appear to be the major modulator of lung development based on both animal studies and observations in the human. For example, hypophysectomy or adrenalectomy of fetal sheep delays the production of surfactant and replacement therapy with cortisol or ACTH stimulates production (Liggins et al., 1981). In both animals and the human there is a close temporal association between increasing levels of fetal corticoids and indices of lung maturation, and stressful interventions such as surgical procedures increase both plasma corticoids and the rate of surfactant lipid synthesis. In fetal lambs a close correlation is observed between plasma cortisol and both lung volume and saturated PC content, whereas there is less correlation between these parameters and gestational age (Kitterman et al., 1981).

The rate of lung development in animals is also influenced by thyroid hormones. Thyroidectomy of the fetal sheep delays the developmental increase in the L/S ratio in amniotic fluid and administration of T_3 in combination with cortisol stimulates lung maturation. It is likely that endogenous catecholamines and prostaglandins, acting through cAMP, also influence the rate of surfactant synthesis and release during fetal life. Administration of either of these hormones to culture systems stimulates the surfactant system, and clinically there have been numerous observations relating increased catecholamine concentrations (e.g. labour) with improved outcome for premature infants (Ballard, 1986). The data from animal studies support the concept that the rate of lung maturation is regulated by the interaction of endogenous glucocorticoids, thyroid hormones and catecholamines. In fetal sheep, the combination of these three hormones accelerated lung development more than each of the hormones administered alone (Warburton et al., 1988; Liggins et al., 1988). In cultured human tissue, as discussed below, additive or synergistic responses are observed with glucocorticoids plus either thyroid hormone or cAMP. It is important to note, however, that the lung continues to develop and achieves adequate levels of surfactant by term in the absence of the fetal pituitary (e.g. anencephaly). These observations indicate that developmental expression of key regulatory genes in lung development and production of surfactant occur even with very low levels of circulating hormones. This basal rate of development is modulated by at least three classes of hormones interacting to ensure appropriate lung maturity prior to delivery.

Functional and clinical correlations

Adequate levels of both surfactant phospholipids and proteins are essential for normal surfactant function both in vitro and in vivo. Since the surfactant components appear to be regulated independently during development, it is likely that surfactant of individual premature infants differs in composition and functional activity. Most infants born very early in the third trimester (e.g. 26 weeks gestation) are deficient in all components of surfactant and have immature peripheral lung structure. Later during gestation infants are more likely to have inadequate amounts of selected components of surfactant. There is increasing evidence of the physiological importance of SP-B for surfactant function and it is possible that a deficiency of DPPC and SP-B is most often responsible for RDS in premature infants. On the other hand, the observations of DeMello et al. (1987) suggest that a deficiency of SP-A occurs in most cases of RDS. Based on the developmental pattern for mRNA content, a developmental deficiency of SP-C is also likely with premature birth, however the physiological role of this protein is less certain. Since glucocorticoids affect all aspects of lung development, any increase in fetal corticoids before birth, for whatever reason, should be beneficial whether an infant was deficient in any one, or all components of surfactant.

Regulators of physiological importance

There is a growing list of hormones, growth factors, cytokines and other agents that have been shown to influence lung morphology, content of surfactant components or surfactant secretion (Table 2.2). Both stimulatory and inhibitory responses occur, and there are additive or synergistic interactions between agents. These findings from treatment protocols support the observations from ablation studies that lung maturation in vivo is under multi-hormonal regulation. This section discusses effects and mechanisms of those regulators that are likely to be of physiological or therapeutic relevance.

Glucocorticoids

The observations of Liggins (1969) first indicated that glucocorticoid administered to the fetus induced precocious functional lung maturation. It is now established that glucocorticoid treatment accelerates lung structural development and increases the synthesis and secretion of all major components of surfactant. The specificity and breadth of glucocorticoid responses is responsible for the clinical usefulness of prenatal glucocorticoid therapy for prevention of RDS in premature infants. All known effects of glucocorticoids in pulmonary development are mediated by glucocorticoid receptors which are present in fetal lung from early in gestation (Ballard, 1986). For example, induction of surfactant components and lipogenic enzymes occurs at nanomolar concentrations of dexamethasone and there is a close correlation between response and receptor occupancy. Only steroids with glucocorticoid activity are effective, and potency correlates with affinity for receptor. Administration of 12 mg betamethasone to women maximally increases glucocorticoid activity approximately 3-fold in fetal serum with a calculated increase in glucocorticoid occupancy from 25% to 75% (Ballard, 1986). Thus the prenatal treatment regimen for preventing RDS mimics a physiological stress response of corticosteroids, consistent with receptor mediation of in vivo responses.

Synthesis of phospholipids, in particular DPPC, in fetal lung is increased in vitro and in vivo by glucocorticoids as assessed both by the rate of precursor incorporation and content. Of the various enzymes involved in lipid synthesis, four rate-limiting enzymes are responsive to glucocorticoids. Fatty acid synthetase enzyme (FAS) activity in fetal lung explants is stimulated by dexamethasone and a similar effect is seen with in vivo treatment (fetal rat) (Gonzales et al., 1990; Rooney, 1989). Immunoprecipitation studies indicate that this effect is due to increased amounts of FAS protein and recent studies have demonstrated that FAS mRNA levels are also increased suggesting a pretranslational mechanism (Gonzales & Ballard, unpublished data).

Cholinephosphate cytidylyltransferase activity is stimulated by glucocorticoids in fetal lung of rat and other species. Stimulation in animals appears to result primarily from a glucocorticoid-induced increase in levels of lipid cofactors for enzyme activity (Rooney et al., 1986). This secondary response to glucocorticoid treatment may serve to amplify the induction of surfactant phospholipids by glucocorticoids.

Recent studies with human tissue suggest that the glucocorticoid effect on cholinephosphate cytidylyltransferase may also involve an increase in enzyme protein (Sharma, Gonzales & Ballard unpublished data). The recent availability of a cDNA probe for this enzyme should help clarify the mechanisms involved.

Two other rate limiting enzymes of the lipid synthesis pathway, lysoPC:acylCoA acyltransferase, which remodels unsaturated PC to DPPC, and phosphatidic acid phosphatase, have been shown to be responsive to glucocorticoids in fetal lung (Ballard, 1986). However, the details of the glucocorticoid effect and in vivo relevance are not yet defined.

The initial reports of glucocorticoid effects on SP-A synthesis in human fetal lung explant cultures were conflicting. It is now established that the effect of glucocorticoids on SP-A mRNA in vitro is either stimulatory or inhibitory depending on the dose and duration of exposure (Ballard, 1989). Stimulation is the initial response with dexamethasone concentrations of <10 nM but with continued exposure the degree of stimulation decreases and eventually inhibition occurs. Fig. 2.5 illustrates the biphasic nature of the response in cultured lung. At higher hormone concentrations the major response is inhibition of SP-A gene expression. The stimulatory and inhibitory responses occur simultaneously and both are receptor mediated involving pretranslational mechanisms. Two different SP-A genes have been cloned which appear to be differentially regulated by glucocorticoids.

The physiological relevance of the in vitro findings regarding SP-A regulation is uncertain. In rats, in vivo glucocorticoid treatment causes a modest stimulation of SP-A mRNA and protein at most fetal and postnatal ages, but under certain treatment conditions there was no response (Schellhase & Shannon, 1991; Phelps & Floros, 1991). Thus, the timing, dose and duration of glucocorticoid exposure may be critical factors in the response to glucocorticoids in vivo.

Glucocorticoid treatment both in vitro and in vivo increases the content of mRNAs for the two hydrophobic surfactant proteins. The stimulation, time course, dose response and requirement for ongoing protein synthesis differ for induction of the two genes in cultured human lung (Liley et al., 1989; Fig. 2.5), indicating separate and non-

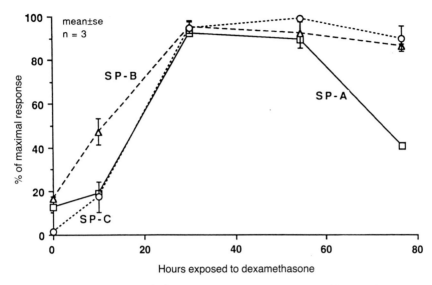

Fig. 2.5. Time course for induction of SP mRNAs in cultured human fetal lung. Explants were exposed to 10 nM dexamethasone for the times shown prior to collecting tissue for assay at 76 hours. (Data from Liley et al., 1989 and Ballard et al., 1986.)

co-ordinated mechanisms of glucocorticoid action. Glucocorticoids increase the rate of gene transcription for both SP-B and SP-C, and in addition increase the stability of SP-B mRNA (Venkatesh et al., 1993). In vivo, dexamethasone stimulates SP-B mRNA in rat and rabbit lung at all ages, however SP-C mRNA is stimulated in fetal rat lung and inhibited in the rabbit (Schellhase & Shannon, 1991; Connelly et al., 1991).

Thyroid hormones

Synthesis of surfactant phospholipids by fetal lung is stimulated by T_3, T_4 and TRH both in vitro and in vivo (Ballard, 1986). In fetal sheep, most studies find that thyroid hormone treatment increases content of DPPC in lung tissue and alveolar wash and improves lung volume and compliance. Thyroidectomy delays lung structural maturation and the developmental increase in amniotic fluid L/S value; these effects occur with normal levels of circulating cortisol suggesting that thyroid hormones act both independently and in concert with glucocorticoid. Indeed, when premature sheep fetuses are treated with a combination of corticosteroid and thyroid hormone, responses are greater than with either hormone alone (Liggins et al., 1988; Warburton et al., 1988; Ikegami et al., 1991). In one study combined treatment also increased SP-A content in lavage fluid whereas neither hormone alone was stimulatory (Ikegami et al., 1991).

Treatment of cultured lung with thyroid hormone increases synthesis (precursor incorporation) and content of phospholipids; however, saturation of PC is not affected suggesting that surfactant phospholipid synthesis is not preferentially stimulated as occurs with glucocorticoid. When glucocorticoids and thyroid hormone are added together, additive or synergistic effects on choline incorporation into PC are observed. The effects of thyroid hormones on lipids are mediated by nuclear receptors and involve increased activity of cholinephosphate cytidylyltransferase (Sharma, Gonzales & Ballard unpublished data). Other possible target enzymes of lipid synthesis have not been identified, and thyroid hormones do not induce surfactant proteins A, B, or C.

The observations of additive or synergistic responses to combined glucocorticoid and thyroid hormone treatment both in vitro and in vivo suggested potential clinical benefit. Although antenatal corticosteroid therapy reduces the incidence and severity of RDS, treatment is not effective in every infant. Recent clinical trials have examined the effect of prenatal treatment with betamethasone plus TRH compared to betamethasone alone. Combined treatment decreased the incidence and severity of RDS in premature infants and markedly reduced the occurrence of chronic lung disease (bronchopulmonary dysplasia) in premature infants (Morales et al., 1989; Ballard et al., 1992). Maternally administered TRH transiently increases fetal serum TSH, T_3 and T_4 to levels approximating those achieved on delivery, indicating placental transfer of TRH and responsiveness of the fetal pituitary–thyroid axis. The reduction in RDS and chronic lung disease with combined therapy presumably results from enhanced surfactant production and structural maturation, and possibly improved fluid clearance (see Chapter 3), but details of the mechanism are not yet known.

Cyclic AMP

Treatment with cAMP analogues or agents that increase endogenous cAMP stimulates production of most surfactant components. In one study infusion of ritodrine, a beta-mimetic, into fetal sheep increased DPPC and lung volumes, and supra-additive responses occurred in combination with cortisol and TRH (Warburton et al., 1988). In human lung explants there is a generalized response of the surfactant system to cAMP analogs and agents such as prostaglandins, terbutaline and forskolin that stimulate endogenous cAMP production. Effects include increased synthesis and content of DPPC, increased activity of fatty acid synthetase and cholinephosphate cytidylyltransferase, increased content of SP-A and SP-B mRNAs, and increased luminal space probably resulting from enhanced fluid secretion (Odom et al., 1988; Gonzales et al., 1990). Some of these responses are additive in the presence of glucocorticoids. Similar effects are found in rat and rabbit tissue plus reported stimulation of SP-C mRNA. Increasing levels of endogenous cAMP in explant tissue is in part responsible for the increased production of surfactant components that occurs during culture in the absence of serum or added hormones (Acarregui et al., 1990; Ballard et al., 1991). This observation suggests a possible role for cAMP and endogenous stimulators (e.g. prostaglandins, catecholamines) as a modulator of lung development in vivo. It is likely that cAMP acts at the level of transcription to stimulate target genes in fetal lung similar to effects characterized in other tissues.

Insulin

It has been known for a number of years that maternal diabetes is associated with respiratory distress in newborn infants. Elevated maternal serum glucose of uncontrolled diabetes crosses the placenta, producing both fetal hyperglycaemia and secondary hyperinsulinaemia. In studies with fetal sheep, Warburton (1983) found that infusion of either glucose or insulin delayed appearance and accumulation of surfactant phospholipid in tracheal fluid. Clinically, maternal diabetes is associated with delayed appearance of amniotic fluid phosphatidylglycerol which is a reliable marker of lung maturity. These effects on phospholipid production may be related to altered metabolism of glycogen which provides glucose and other metabolites for synthesis of surfactant phospholipid. It is possible that insulin/glucose acts indirectly on type II cells, since in human fetal lung explants there appears to be no effect of insulin on synthesis of phosphatidylcholine or phosphatidylglycerol content of lamellar bodies (Mendelson et al., 1981).

Recent investigations have focused on insulin regulation of SP-A. Two reports have noted decreased levels of SP-A protein in amniotic fluid from diabetic pregnancies compared to non-diabetic women (Snyder et al., 1988; Katyal et al., 1984). In cultured human lung tissue, insulin inhibits accumulation of SP-A and its mRNA during culture (Snyder & Mendelson, 1987; Dekowski & Snyder, 1992). Similarly, appearance and accumulation of SP-A mRNA was delayed in lungs of fetal and newborn pups of streptozotocin-induced diabetes in rats (Guttentag et al., 1992).

These findings indicate that fetal hyperglycemia (with normal to low insulin levels) inhibits the developmental increase in at least one surfactant protein. The mechanism of this effect is not known and could be due to decreased fetal levels of corticosterone, increased levels of β-hydroxybutyrate or direct action of excess glucose in lung cells.

Summary

Pulmonary surfactant is a complex mixture of lipids and specific proteins which when dynamically compressed at an air-liquid interface resists compression resulting in a very low surface tension. Most of the components are synthesized and packaged in type II alveolar cells, but it is becoming increasingly apparent that the metabolism of the various components is controlled independently by different hormones or hormone combinations. Glucocorticoids are the most important hormones and regulate synthesis of all components of surfactant.

References

Acarregui, M. J., Snyder, J. N., Mitchell, M. D. & Mendelson, C. R. (1990). Prostaglandins regulate surfactant protein A (SP-A) gene expression in human fetal lung in vitro. *Endocrinology*, **127(3)**, 1105–13.

Avery, M. E. & Mead, J. (1959). Surface properties in relation to atelectasis and hyaline membrane disease. *American Journal of Diseases of Children*, **97**, 517–23.

Ballard, P. L. (1989). Hormonal regulation of pulmonary surfactant. *Endocrine Review*, **10**, 165–81.

Ballard, P. L., Liley, H. G., Gonzales, L. W. et al. (1989). Interferon-gamma and synthesis of surfactant components by cultured human fetal lung. *American Journal of Respiratory Cell Molecular Biology*, **12**, 12–13.

Ballard, P. L., Hawgood, S., Liley, H. et al. (1986). Regulation of pulmonary surfactant apoprotein SP 28–36 gene in fetal human lung. *Proceedings of the National Academy of Sciences, USA*, **83**, 9527–31.

Ballard, P. L., Gonzales, L. W., Williams, M. C., Roberts, J. M. & Jacobs, M. M. (1991). Differentiation of type II cells during explant culture of human fetal lung is accelerated by endogenous prostanoids and cyclic AMP. *Endocrinology*, **128**, 2916–24.

Ballard, R. A. (1986). Antenatal glucocorticoid therapy: clinical effects. In *Hormones and Lung Maturation, Monographs on Endocrinology*, ed. P. L. Ballard. Vol. 28, Springer-Verlag, Heidelberg.

Ballard, R. A., Ballard, P. L., Creasy, R. K. et al. (1992). Respiratory disease in very low-birthweight infants after prenatal thyrotropin-releasing hormone and glucocorticoid. *Lancet*, **339**, 510–15.

Batenburg, J. J. (1992). Surfactant phospholipids: Synthesis and storage. *American Journal of Physiology*, **262**, L367–85.

Clements, J. A. (1956). Dependence of pressure–volume characteristics of lungs on intrinsic surface active material. *Journal of Physiology*, **187**, 592.

Connelly, I. H., Hammond, G. L., Harding, P. G. R. & Possmayer, F. (1991). Levels of surfactant-associated protein messenger ribonucleic acids in rabbit lung during perinatal development and after hormonal treatment. *Endocrinology*, **129**, 2583–91.

Crouch, E. C., Persson, A., Chang, D. & Parghi, D. (1991*a*). Surfactant protein D: increased accumulation in silica-induced pulmonary lipoproteinosis. *American Journal of Pathology*, **139**, 765–76.

Crouch, E. C., Rust, K., Marienchek, W., Parghi, D., Chang, D. & Persson, A. (1991*b*). Developmental expression of pulmonary surfactant protein D (SP-D). *American Journal of Respiratory Cell and Molecular Biology*, **5**, 13–18.

Dekowski, S. A. & Snyder, J. M. (1992). Insulin regulation of messenger ribonucleic acid for the surfactant-associated protein in human fetal lung in vitro. *Endocrinology*, **131**, 669–76.

DeMello, D. E., Chi, E. Y., Doo, E. & Lagunoff, D. (1987). Absence of tubular myelin in lungs of infants dying with hyaline membrane disease. *American Journal of Pathology*, **127**, 131.

Gonzales, L. W., Ertsey, R., Ballard, P. L., Froh, D., Goerke, J. & Gonzales, J. (1990). Glucocorticoid stimulation of fatty acid synthesis in explants of human fetal lung. *Biochimica et Biophysica Acta*, **1042**, 1–12.

Gruenwald, P. (1947). Surface tension as a factor in the resistance of neonatal lungs to aeration. *American Journal of Obstetrics and Gynecology*, **53**, 996–1007.

Guttentag, S. H., Phelps, D. S., Stenzel, W., Warshaw, J. B. & Floros, J. (1992). Surfactant protein A expression is delayed in fetuses of streptozotocin-treated rats. *American Journal of Physiology*, **262**, (*Lung Cellular & Molecular Physiology*, **6**), L489–94.

Hawgood, S. & Benson, B. J. (1989). The molecular biology of surfactant proteins. In *Lung Cell Biology*, ed. D. Massaro. pp 701–734. Marcel Dekker, New York.

Ikegami, M., Polk, D., Tabor, B., Lewis, J., Yamada, T. & Jobe, A. (1991). Corticosteroid and thyrotropin-releasing hormone effects on preterm sheep lung function. *American Journal of Physiology*, **70**, 2268–78.

Katyal, S. L., Amenta, J. S., Singh, G. & Silverman, J,A. (1984). Deficient lung surfactant apoproteins in amniotic fluid with mature phospholipid profile from diabetic pregnancies. *American Journal of Obstetrics and Gynecology*, **148**, 48.

Kitterman, J. A., Liggins, G. C., Campos, G. A. et al. (1981). Prepartum maturation of the lung in fetal sheep. Relation to cortisol. *Journal of Applied Physiology*, **51**, 384–90.

Kuan, S. F., Rust, K. & Crouch, E. C. (1992). Interactions of surfactant protein D with bacterial lipopolysaccharides. Surfactant protein D is an *Escherichia coli*-binding protein in bronchoalveolar lavage. *Journal of Clinical Investigation*, **90**, 97–106.

Liggins, G. C. (1969). Premature delivery of foetal lambs infused with glucocorticoids. *Journal of Endocrinology*, **45**, 515–23.

Liggins, G. C., Kitterman, J. A., Campos, G. A. et al. (1981). Pulmonary maturation in the hypophysectomized ovine fetus. Differential responses

Liggins, G. C., Schellenberg, J. C., Manzai, M., Kitterman, J. A. & Lee, C-C. (1988). Synergistic effects of cortisol and thyrotropin releasing hormone on lung maturation on fetal sheep. *Journal of Applied Physiology*, **65**, 1880–4.

to adrenocorticotropin and cortisol. *Journal of Developmental Physiology*, **3**, 1–14.

Liley, H. G., White, R. T., Warr, R. G., Benson, B. J., Hawgood, S. & Ballard, P. L. (1989). Regulation of messenger RNAs for the hydrophobic surfactant proteins in human lung. *Journal of Clinical Investigation*, **83**, 1191–7.

Liu, M., Wang, L., Li, E. & Enhorning, G. (1991). Pulmonary surfactant will secure free airflow through a narrow tube. *Journal of Applied Physiology*, **71**, 742–8.

Mendelson, C. R., Johnston, J. M., MacDonald, P. C. & Snyder, J. M. (1981). Multihormonal regulation of surfactant synthesis by human fetal lung in vitro. *Journal of Clinical Endocrinology and Metabolism*, **53**, 307–17.

Minoo, P., Segura, L., Coalson, J. J., King, R. J. & DeLemos, R. A. (1991). Alterations in surfactant protein gene expression associated with premature birth and exposure to hyperoxia. *American Journal of Physiology*, **261**, L386–92.

Morales, W. J., O'Brien, W. F., Angel, J. L., Knuppel, R. A. & Sawai, S. (1989). Fetal lung maturation: The combined use of corticosteroids and thyrotropin-releasing hormone. *Obstetrics and Gynecology*, **73**, 111–16.

Nogee, L. M., DeMello, D. E., Dehner, L. P. & Colten, H. R. (1993). Brief Report: Deficiency of pulmonary surfactant protein B in congenital alveolar proteinosis. *New England Journal of Medicine* **328**, 406–10.

Odom, M. J., Snyder, J. M., Boggaram, V. & Mendelson, C. R. (1988). Glucocorticoid regulation of the major surfactant associated protein (SP-A) and its messenger ribonucleic acid and of morphological development on human fetal lung in vitro. *Endocrinology*, **123**, 1712–19.

Pattle, R. E. (1955). Properties, function and origin of the alveolar lining layer. *Nature,* **175**, 1125–6.

Phelps, D. S. & Floros, J. (1991) Dexamethasone in vivo raises surfactant protein B mRNA in alveolar and bronchiolar epithelium. *American Journal of Physiology*, **4**, L146–52.

Pryhuber, G. S., Hull, W. M., Fink, I., McMahan, M. J. & Whitsett, J. A. (1991). Ontogeny of surfactant proteins A and B in human amniotic fluid as indices of fetal lung maturity. *Pediatric Research*, **30**, 597–605.

Robertson, B. T., Kobayashi, M., Gansuka, G., Grossman, W. Z., Li, Y. & Suzuki. (1991). Experimental neonatal respiratory failure induced by a monoclonal antibody to the hydrophobic surfactant associated protein SP-B. *Pediatric Research*, **30**, 239–43.

Robertson, B., van Golde, L. M. G. & Batenburg, J. J. (1992). (Editors). *Pulmonary Surfactant: From Molecular Biology to Clinical Practice.* Elsevier, Amsterdam.

Rooney, S. A., Dynia, D. W., Smart, D. A. et al. (1986). Glucocorticoid stimulation of choline-phosphate cytidylyltransferase activity in fetal rat lung: Receptor–response relationships. *Biochemical and Biophysical Acta*, **888**, 208–16.

Rooney, S. A. (1989). Fatty acid biosynthesis in developing fetal lung. *American Journal of Physiology*, **2257**, L195–201.

Schellhase, D. E. & Shannon, J. M. (1991). Effects of maternal dexamethasone on expression of SP-A, SP-B, and SP-C in the fetal rat lung. *American Journal of Respiratory Cell and Molecular Biology*, **4**, 304–12.

Snyder, J. M. & Mendelson, C. R. (1987). Insulin inhibits the accumulation of the major lung surfactant apoprotein in human fetal lung explants maintained in vitro. *Endocrinology*, **120**, 1250–7.

Snyder, J. M., Kwun, J. E., O'Brien, J. A., Rosenfeld, C. R. & Odom, M. J. (1988). The concentration of the 35-kDa surfactant apoprotein in amniotic fluid from normal and diabetic pregnancies. *Pediatric Research*, **24**, 728.

Stahlman, M. T., Gray, M. E. & Whitsett, J. A. (1992). The ontogeny and distribution of surfactant protein B in human fetuses and newborns. *Journal of Histochemistry and Cytochemistry*, **40**, 1471–80.

van Iwaarden, J. F. (1992). Surfactant and the pulmonary defense system. In *Pulmonary Surfactant: From Molecular Biology to Clinical Practice*, ed. B. Robertson, L. M. G. van Golde & J. J. Batenburg. pp. 215–227. Elsevier Science Publishers, Amsterdam.

Venkatesh, V. C., Ballard, P. L., Ertsey, R., Iannuzzi & D. M. (1993). Differential glucocorticoid regulation of the pulmonary hydrophobic surfactant proteins SP-B and SP-C. *American Journal of Respiratory Cell and Molecular Biology*, **8**, 222–8.

von Neergaard, K. (1929). Neue Auffassungen über einen Grundbegriff der Atemmechanik. Die Retraktionskraft der Lunge, abhängig von der Oberflächenspannung in den Alveolen. *Zeitschrift Gesamte Experimentelle Medizin.*, **66**, 373–94.

Warburton, D. (1983). Chronic hyperglycemia reduces surface active material flux in tracheal fluid of fetal lambs. *Journal of Clinical Investigation*, **71**, 550.

Warburton, D., Parton, L., Buckley, S., Cosico, L., Enns, G. & Saluna, T. (1988). Combined effects of corticosteroid, thyroid hormones, and β-agonist on surfactant, pulmonary mechanics and β-receptor binding in fetal lamb lung. *Pediatric Research*, **24**, 166–70.

Weaver, T. E. & Whitsett, J. A. (1991). Function and regulation of expression of pulmonary surfactant-associated proteins. *Biochemical Journal* **273**, 249–264.

Whitsett, J. A. & Baatz, J. E. (1992). Hydrophobic surfactant proteins SP-B and SP-C: Molecular biology structure and function. In *Pulmonary Surfactant: from Molecular Biology to Clinical Practice.* ed. B. Robertson L. M. G. van Golde & J. J. Batenburg. pp. 55–76. Elsevier Science Publishers, Amsterdam.

Wikenheiser, K. A., Wert, S. E., Wispe, J. R. *et al.* (1992). Distinct effects of oxygen on surfactant protein B expression in bronchiolar and alveolar epithelium. *American Journal of Physiology*, **262**, L32–9.

Williams, M. C., Hawgood, S. & Hamilton, R. L. (1991). Changes in lipid structure produced by surfactant proteins SP-A, SP-B, and SP-C. *American Journal of Respiratory Cell and Molecular Biology*, **5**, 41–50.

Wright, J. R. & Hawgood, S. (1989). Pulmonary Surfactant Metabolism. *Clinics in Chest Medicine*, **10**, 83–93.

Yu, S-H., Wallace, D., Bhavnani, B., Enhorning, G., Harding, G. R. & Possmayer, F. (1988). Effect of reconstituted pulmonary surfactant containing the 6000-Dalton hydrophobic protein on lung compliance of prematurely delivered rabbit fetuses. *Pediatric Research* **23**, 23–30.

3

Fetal lung liquid: secretion and absorption

DAFYDD V. WALTERS

Introduction

At birth, three important conditions must be fulfilled within the lung for adaptation to normal gas exchange to occur.

1. Pulmonary blood flow must increase tenfold.
2. Sufficient good quality surfactant must be present.
3. Secretion of lung liquid must cease and liquid present in the lumen must be removed.

It is the third process which is the subject of this chapter.

The pulmonary epithelium, or more precisely the alveolar epithelium, is unique because, at different stages of development, it has to perform two completely opposite functions. Before birth it secretes liquid to ensure that the lung is slightly distended so that a stimulus is provided for normal morphological and functional development, whereas after birth the epithelium constantly absorbs liquid, keeping the lumen of the lung relatively free of liquid in order to allow gas exchange to occur. This chapter will discuss the physiology of secretion and absorption of lung liquid and the way in which the rapid transition between the two states takes place at birth.

Fetal lung liquid secretion

Until the middle of this century, it was generally believed that any liquid in the lumen of the lung was derived from the amniotic cavity and, indeed, inhalation of amniotic fluid was claimed to have been observed directly by Preyer (1885). It was believed also, that the distal spaces of the lungs in utero were relatively empty, ready to 'spring' open with the first breath. However, Addison and How (1913) described that, on the

Table 3.1. *Selected solute composition of fetal lung liquid, fetal plasma and amniotic fluid in the sheep*

	Na^+	K^+	Cl^-	HCO_3^-	Protein
Plasma	150	4.8	107	24	4.09
Alveolar liquid	150	6.3	157	2.8	0.03
Amniotic liquid	113	7.6	87	19	0.10

Units are mM kg^{-1} water except for protein which is in g dl^{-1}.
Data from Adamson et al. (1969).

contrary, the potential air spaces were not collapsed but were filled with liquid.

The experiments of Nature described by Potter & Bolhender (1941) gave the first inkling that the presence of liquid in the fetal lung required an alternative explanation. They reported that, in the condition of congenital complete bronchial stenosis, the lung distal to the obstruction, rather than being collapsed was immensely distended with fluid. They correctly concluded that the liquid must have had a local (i.e. pulmonary) origin since there was no connection to the amniotic cavity. However, these were pathological lungs and it remained until the incidental, but none the less important, observations of the fetal endocrinologists, Jost & Policard in 1948 before the truth began to be uncovered. They tied off the necks of rabbit fetuses in utero in order to observe body growth in the absence of pituitary influence. The tracheas were obviously occluded by this intervention and, in their meticulous observations, the authors reported that the fetal lungs were distended and, furthermore, that the liquid they contained was under considerable pressure. Sham operated fetuses did not have distended lungs. A more formal series of experiments in which fetal tracheas were occluded without decapitation reported the same findings (Carmel, Friedman & Adams, 1965). From these simple observations it could be concluded that liquid is not only produced within the lung but is capable of being secreted against a hydrostatic pressure. Attention was brought to the unique composition of fetal lung liquid for the first time in 1963 by Adams, Moss & Fagan, and definitively analysed by Adamson et al. (1969). (Table 3.1).

Mechanism of secretion

It was not for another decade that the force underlying lung liquid secretion was discovered. Olver & Strang (1974) measured unidirectional isotopic ion fluxes across the fetal pulmonary epithelium of sheep and compared the observed flux ratios obtained in their experiments with the flux ratios predicted for particular ions by the Ussing flux ratio equation (Koefoed-Johnsen & Ussing, 1953). The latter equation predicts the behaviour of an ion (specifically, the ratio of its fluxes each way across the epithelium – the unidirectional fluxes) from measurement of the forces acting on the ion. The forces are chemical activity (concentration) gradient, electrical potential gradient (the electrical p.d. across the epithelium) and solvent drag (a term which makes allowance for entrainment of solute by bulk liquid movement). Agreement between observed and predicted flux ratios indicates that the ion is distributed passively as a

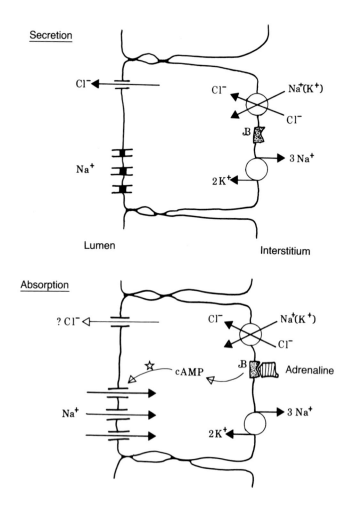

result of the forces already in existence across the epithelium. Disagreement between observed and predicted values suggests non-passive distribution, i.e. active movement of the ion. If the observed ratio is opposite to the one predicted, it is strong evidence in support of active transport of the ion. For example, if it is predicted that more chloride ions should move out of the lung lumen than into it yet the measurements show the opposite – more move into the lumen than move out – then it is likely that active movement of chloride ions into the lung lumen is present. Applying the same analysis to several ionic species led to the conclusion that there is active movement of all the halide ions (Cl^-, I^- & Br^-), and of the cations potassium and calcium into the lumen. The chloride ion is the only ion secreted in sufficient quantities by the fetal pulmonary epithelium to provide the necessary osmotic movement of water which results in fetal lung liquid secretion. Sodium was found to distribute itself passively and therefore it followed chloride, probably via a paracellular route.

There is evidence from fetal sheep and fetal guinea pig lungs that secretion of liquid is inhibited by loop diuretics (e.g. furosemide) applied to the basolateral surface (interstitial side) of the epithelium (Cassin, Gausse & Perks, 1986; Thom & Perks, 1990). This indicates the presence

---

Fig. 3.1. A diagram representing some of the secretory and absorptive mechanisms acting across the epithelium of the lung. *Secretion* which is the predominant process in the fetus. Chloride ions enter the epithelial cell on the basolateral surface by Na^+/K^+-$2Cl^-$ cotransport which can be inhibited by bumetanide and furosemide. The driving force for entry is the Na^+ gradient generated by Na^+-K^+ ATPase located on the basolateral surface of the cell. The Cl^- then passes through Cl^- channels in the apical membrane of the cell down a large electrical gradient. *Absorption* which predominates in the postnatal lung. At birth adrenaline stimulates a beta-adrenergic receptor which generates intracellular cycliccAMP which, in turn, activates or inserts Na^+ channels in the apical membrane. Na^+ ions enter the cell down a steep electrochemical gradient and are rapidly extruded by Na^+-K^+ ATPase into the interstitium. Amiloride inhibits the entry of Na^+ through the Na^+ channels in a dose dependent manner. Continued beta-adrenergic stimulation does not appear to be necessary to keep the Na^+ channels open in later life although it can increase basal liquid absorption. Whether the chloride secretory process is merely overwhelmed by Na^+ influx or whether it permanently disappears after birth is not certain, but in neonatal sheep it persists for some weeks because its presence may be unmasked by amiloride. *Indicates the probable site of the synergistic action of T3 and hydrocortisone. Other ion exchange mechanisms and transport processes (e.g. sodium linked glucose movement) have been described in the pulmonary epithelium but are not shown here because their importance to liquid movement has not been determined fully.

of a Na^+/Cl^- cotransport process on that surface and allows us to complete a theory of secondary active chloride ion transport into the lung lumen which underlies fetal lung liquid secretion. It is represented in Fig 3.1.

The presence of chloride transport in the fetal lung explains the characteristic chemical composition of fetal lung liquid whose chloride concentration is 50% greater than that of plasma (Adamson et al., 1969; See Table 3.1). Essentially, fetal lung liquid is physiological saline containing a small amount of potassium, bicarbonate, calcium and protein. The latter is present at only 1% of its concentration in plasma. The low bicarbonate concentration is the result of transport either of hydrogen ion into or of bicarbonate ion out of the lung lumen. There is some evidence for the former mechanism in the fetus (Shaw et al., 1990) and the adult lung (Nord, Brown & Crandall, 1987).

The essential prerequisite of a secretory epithelium, that it must be relatively tight (impermeable to small molecules), was established for the fetal pulmonary epithelium in 1971 by the same laboratory which reported chloride secretion by the fetal lung. The epithelium is so impermeable to small solutes that it effectively excludes all non-electrolyte water soluble molecules larger than sucrose (effective molecular radius 0.52 nm), (Normand et al., 1971). The epithelium, described in terms of pore theory, has pores or trans-membrane water filled holes of radius 0.6 nm (for comparison, mannitol has an effective radius of 0.42 nm, inulin 1.39 nm, albumin 3.5 nm & fibrinogen 11.0 nm).

These characteristics of the fetal pulmonary epithelium, namely, low permeability and an ability to secrete chloride ions appear early in gestation; certainly in the sheep by 70 days gestation (term 145 days) at which time the lung luminal volume is only a fraction of a millilitre and appears to be completely enclosed within the primitive trachea (Olver, Schneeberger & Walters, 1981).

Lung liquid volume and secretion rate

The volume of liquid contained in the mature fetal lung is about 30 ml kg^{-1} for all species studied, which includes sheep, goats, rabbits and guinea pigs. The liquid is secreted at a rate of about 4–6 ml h^{-1} (kg body wt)$^{-1}$ (Mescher et al., 1975; Olver et al., 1981, 1986; Perks & Cassin, 1989; Thom & Perks, 1990) which means that a sheep fetus, and by extrapolation a human fetus, near term secretes liquid at a rate approaching 500 ml day^{-1}. Thus it makes a considerable contribution to amniotic fluid volume and to the liquid turnover of the fetus, approaching the volume of daily fetal urine production (Tomoda, Brace & Longo, 1987). What proportion is swallowed as it passes up the trachea and how much mixes with amniotic fluid at any one time is likely to be determined by the state of arousal of the fetus. Some at least mixes into the amniotic cavity as shown by the increasing presence of pulmonary surfactant in amniotic liquor as gestation advances (see Chapter 2).

Lung liquid volume, secretion, and lung growth

The secretion of fetal lung liquid and the recoil of the fetal lung, in combination generate a small pressure difference (trachea positive) which can be measured between the fetal tracheal lumen and the amniotic cavity during periods when there are no fetal breathing movements. There seems little doubt that this pressure of a few mm H_2O, small though it is, is very important for normal lung growth. Experimental interventions which bypass the upper airway resistance produce small volume lungs containing more type II cells while those procedures which increase the resistance and thus the pressure and liquid volume, produce large lungs with relatively less type II cells (Moessinger et al., 1990). The pressure is produced by the resistance to liquid flow somewhere in the upper airway (Fewell et al., 1983) and most likely at the larynx (Fisk et al., 1992). An extended discussion of this topic and the effect of fetal breathing on fetal lung liquid volume is found in Chapter 4. How the upper airway resistance and thus the value of the pressure difference is controlled within such very precise and small limits so that the lung may develop normally, is unknown.

Absorption of lung liquid

Changes in epithelial permeability at birth

In the early 1970s, efforts were made to establish whether there were any changes in the permeability of the pulmonary epithelium at the onset of breathing and whether they could account for clearance of luminal liquid. Indeed, epithelial permeability was measured in mature sheep fetuses which were exteriorized and induced to breathe. In terms of pore theory, permeability increased from the fetal value of 0.6 nm radius pores to about 4 nm after breathing (Egan, Olver & Strang, 1975). Surprisingly, permeability was found to have returned to near fetal values in newborn lambs aged 12–60 hours (pore sizes ranging from 0.7 to 1.4 nm). It was suggested that the temporary increase in epithelial permeability was the result of stretching of the epithelium by a larger than usual luminal volume because the lung contained both liquid and gas at the start of breathing. These exteriorized fetuses had not undergone labour and were probably similar to babies delivered by elective Caesarean section. An increase in permeability of the degree described above would allow enhanced movement of liquid down a protein osmotic gradient. How much it would restrict the main solutes (Na^+ & Cl^-) in lung liquid is uncertain but it would continue to restrict protein and thus prevent entry of interstitial proteins into the lung lumen. The importance of increased epithelial permeability to clearance of lung liquid at birth under physiological conditions is not known. If it occurs at all, then its effect is probably overshadowed by the mechanism described in the subsequent paragraphs.

Birth, adrenaline and lung liquid absorption

If secretion of fetal lung liquid is followed closely through labour and delivery in sheep, it is found that secretion may decrease at first and then absorption usually occurs at a slow rate for an hour or two until the moment of birth (Brown et al., 1983). Once the fetus starts coming out of the birth canal, rapid absorption of liquid takes place across the pulmonary epithelium at rates of about 30 ml h^{-1}. (Sheep fetuses have the advantage as an experimental preparation that, if umbilical circulation is protected and the fetus kept warm, the fetus may be exteriorized and it may remain in good clinical condition after birth without breathing. This allows measurements of lung liquid movement to continue for up to several hours post partum.)

Fetal plasma adrenaline concentrations rise markedly through labour and delivery from levels which are very low in the fetus (see Fig. 3.2 and Tables 3.2 and 3.3). To establish if there was a correlation between adrenaline concentration and lung liquid absorption, Brown et al. (1983) performed experiments on mature fetuses not undergoing labour in which they infused adrenaline, measured lung liquid secretion and absorption rate and assayed adrenaline concentrations in fetal blood. They found not only good correlations between the two but that over the last few weeks of gestation, the lung became increasingly sensitive to adrenaline such that a dose of adrenaline given 2 weeks before term slowed lung liquid secretion but the same dose administered 10 days later

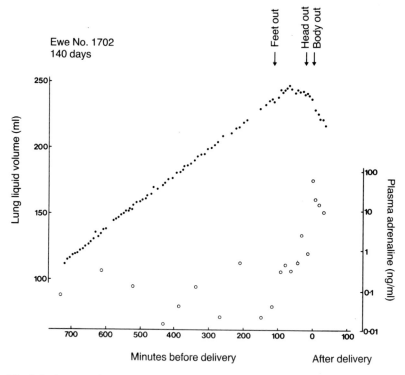

Fig. 3.2. An experiment in which cumulative lung liquid volume was measured by the impermeant tracer technique and fetal plasma adrenaline concentration was measured concomitantly during labour and delivery of a fetal sheep. Lung liquid volume is on the left-hand ordinate and time on the abscissa. An increasing lung liquid volume indicates secretion while a decreasing volume, absorption. Secretion ceases late in labour in this particular fetus and absorption starts only just before the head is delivered. The right-hand ordinate is adrenaline concentration on a log scale. Adrenaline levels rose steeply ($\times 100$) late in delivery. (Figure from Brown et al., 1993).

could produce a rapid absorption of liquid. By comparing the results of the experiments in non-labouring sheep with those undergoing labour they could explain all the observed lung liquid absorption in natural delivery by the rise in fetal adrenaline concentration, i.e. no other mechanism needed to be postulated. This does not mean that other physiological mechanisms may not be involved. Indeed, there is evidence that vasopressin can slow lung liquid secretion (Perks & Cassin, 1988; Wallace, Hooper & Harding, 1990) and vasopressin concentration rises in fetal blood during labour. However, there is as yet no unequivocal evidence that vasopressin alone can induce fetal lung liquid absorption.

Dafydd V. Walters

Table 3.2. *Pooled data from fetal sheep undergoing labour and delivery to demonstrate the timing of the onset of lung liquid absorption and the rise in fetal plasma catecholamines*

	min before delivery			min after delivery
	900–150	150–50	50–0	0–50
Jv (ml h^{-1})	7.1	−2.2	−15.2	−28.7
[Adren] ng ml^{-1}	0.09	0.52	6.86	7.17
[Norad] ng ml^{-1}	1.71	3.81	12.14	9.10

Jv is secretion or absorption rate, the latter indicated by a negative sign. Time zero is time of delivery. Data adapted from Brown et al. (1983).

Table 3.3. *Catecholamine concentration in human fetal blood during and after birth*

	Adrenaline (ng ml^{-1})	Noradrenaline (ng ml^{-1})
Cervix dilatation		
3–5 cm	0.37	1.21
6–8 cm	0.49	1.76
9–10 cm	1.03	2.91
Cord (arterial)	1.60	10.56
Breech cord (arterial)	2.57	24.00
12 h postpartum (arterial)	0.41	0.79

Note that in the sheep fetus, the concentration of adrenaline needed to stop lung liquid secretion is 0.029 ng ml^{-1}. Data are adapted from Lagercrantz et al. (1983).

The sensitivity of the mature fetal sheep lung to adrenaline is so great that very small concentrations (0.029 ng/ml) are sufficient to stop secretion. Ten times this concentration of adrenaline is achieved in human fetal blood at 2–3 cm cervical dilation in normal labour (Lagercrantz, Bistoletti & Nylund, 1983; See Table 3.3). If the human fetal lung has a similar sensitivity to adrenaline as the sheep lung, lung liquid absorption would occur much earlier in human than in sheep labour. The difference in timing may be the result of the differing modes of delivery in these species: sheep deliver feet first, then snout, then shoulders, the latter being the widest part to pass through the birth canal; in humans the head, the widest portion of the fetal body, is usually the presenting part and thus the 'stress' of delivery is likely to occur at a much earlier stage of labour.

The beta-adrenergic nature of the adrenaline response was described by Walters & Olver in 1978. Isoprenaline had the greatest effect in producing lung liquid absorption and noradrenaline the least. Furthermore the effect could be blocked by propranolol. Noradrenaline may have a beta-adrenergic effect at high concentrations and certainly such levels are seen at birth (Tables 3.2 and 3.3).

Mode of delivery and lung liquid removal

Cord blood concentrations of catecholamines in elective Caesarean section babies are as high as, if not higher than, those of babies born vaginally (Lagercrantz et al., 1983). The important point to note is that babies born normally have been exposed to adrenaline usually for some hours while those delivered by Caesarean section experience high adrenaline levels only from the moment of birth. The difference in length of exposure probably explains the increased incidence of transient tachypnoea in infants born by elective section and the increased incidence of other respiratory illnesses which include respiratory distress syndrome (RDS) (Faxelius, Bremme, & Lagercrantz, 1982). The importance of labour rather than route of delivery (vaginal or by hysterotomy) in removing lung liquid is shown by experiments on rabbits in which drier lungs were obtained in mature newborns exposed to labour regardless of whether subsequent delivery was by the normal vaginal route or by hysterotomy (Bland et al., 1980). The exposure to labour is probably the explanation for the reduced incidence of respiratory problems in babies born by emergency Caesarean section compared to those delivered by elective hysterotomy (Faxelius et al., 1982). Bland et al. (1980) also demonstrated clearly by histological sections that once liquid had been absorbed across the epithelium it collected in perivascular spaces whence it was removed more slowly over some hours into the circulation either directly (Bland et al., 1982) or via lymphatics (Normand, Reynolds & Strang, 1970).

Maturation of the adrenaline effect

The response of the fetal lung to adrenaline is very dependent on gestational age and the increase in sensitivity is particularly sharp in the last few days before delivery, see Fig. 3.3 (Brown et al., 1983). The concentration of the most active thyroid hormone, triiodothyronine (T_3), rises in fetal blood over a period which corresponds to the maturation of

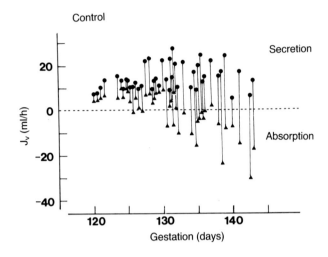

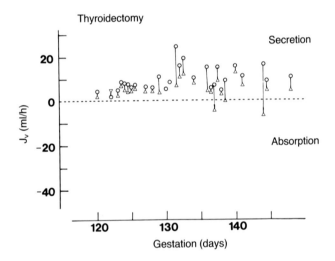

Fig. 3.3. The maturation of the lung liquid absorptive response to adrenaline in fetal sheep. Lung liquid secretion or absorption rate is on the ordinate, note the position of zero. Gestational age is on the abscissa, term in sheep is about 145 days. Each pair of data points is obtained from one experiment; the upper point is the basal secretion rate of fetal lung liquid connected to the lower point which represents the secretion or absorption rate during the infusion of a standard dose of adrenaline (0.5 μg min^{-1}). As gestation advances, absorption increasingly becomes the usual reponse. (Data prepared by P. Barker.)

the lung liquid response to adrenaline (Fisher et al., 1977; Barker, Strang & Walters, 1990). Normally, the fetus appears to be protected from the action of T_3 because the latter's concentration in fetal blood is kept low for most of gestation by peripheral fetal body enzymes which deiodinate T_4 predominantly to reverse T_3, which is inactive (Chopra et al., 1978) and by placental α-monoiodinase which converts T_3 into T_2 (Roti et al., 1982). The action of these enzymes appears, in turn, to be decreased by cortisol which also rises in fetal blood as term approaches. The net effect is that the metabolic clearance of T_3 in the fetal circulation is markedly decreased at the very end of gestation (Fraser & Liggins, 1989). Earlier in gestation the half-life of T_3 in fetal blood is only about 30 min (Fraser & Liggins, 1988) whereas in human adults it approaches 48 hours (Martindale, 1982). It was found that fetal thyroidectomy prevented the usual maturation of the adrenaline response and that infusion of T_3 was able to restore normal development (Barker, Strang & Walters, 1990). However, premature exposure to T_3 could not accelerate normal development, in other words there was yet another factor which determined the action of T_3. This factor proved to be cortisol. The actions of T_3 and cortisol are synergistic, for if either hormone was administered alone no effect on adrenaline sensitivity was observed but when they were given together in the same dosage maturation could be achieved within a few days even at a period of gestation when such a response to adrenaline would not be expected (Barker et al., 1991). Further investigation of the timing of this effect, demonstrated that as little as two hours' exposure to the two hormones was sufficient to mimic a developmental process which normally took many weeks. Furthermore, the synergistic effect was reversible, 24 hours being enough to allow reversion to the immature fetal state after discontinuation of the infusion of hormones. Together, the two hormones induce new protein(s) which must be important to the appearance of the adrenaline response because their action can be blocked by the presence of cyclohexamide, a protein synthesis inhibitor (Barker et al., 1991).

Mechanism of lung liquid absorption

The cellular mechanism by which lung liquid is absorbed from the lung, was demonstrated by the action of amiloride (a compound which inhibits sodium flux through epithelial sodium channels) when it was applied to the luminal surface of the epithelium. It blocked the absorption induced by adrenaline indicating that sodium channels are central to the absorptive process (Olver et al., 1986). Experiments, again on fetal sheep, using many different concentrations of amiloride allowed an estimate of the K_I (the concentration of amiloride which produced 50% inhibition) of the system to be established. The calculated value of 4.6×10^{-6} M is much higher than that found for amiloride's inhibitory action in kidney (about 10^{-8} M). However, work performed on sodium channels in isolated alveolar type II cells indicated that the K_I of the sodium channel in the pulmonary epithelium may indeed be high, up to $1-3 \times 10^{-5}$ M (Oh et al., 1992). In other words, the alveolar epithelium appears to express a sodium channel which has a low affinity for amiloride.

A model which explains both secretion and absorption by the same cell may be proposed where the transition from secretion to absorption at birth is accomplished by the single event of opening or activation of sodium channels on the apical (luminal) surface of the epithelium. For a detailed explanation see Fig. 3.1.

The site of action of T₃ and cortisol

It is tempting to assume that T_3 and cortisol produce their effect by increasing the numbers of beta-adrenergic receptors in lung tissue. However, this appears not to be the case and it is demonstrated by the action of dibutyryl-cyclic AMP (db-cAMP, a synthetic analogue of cAMP) on lung liquid secretion in the fetus. This compound, which mimics the effects of adrenaline on the fetal lung, stimulates the cells of the epithelium at an intracellular site which must be functionally closer to the sodium channel than the beta-receptor. During gestation, db-cAMP causes absorption at rates which increase with maturity very much like that of adrenaline (Walters, Ramsden & Olver, 1990). Thus, although T_3 and cortisol may well increase beta-receptor number in the fetal lung (Cheng et al., 1980; Giannopoulos, 1980; Warburton et al., 1988), the number of beta-receptors cannot be critical. Rather, the rate limiting step in maturation must be downstream of the generation of intracellular cAMP. This point is strengthened by the observation that fetal thyroidectomy prevents the normal increase in response to db-cAMP with maturation in exactly the same manner as it inhibits the development of the adrenaline response (Barker et al., 1988).

Postnatal lung liquid movement

Our knowledge of the way in which ions and water are handled by the postnatal pulmonary epithelium is less complete than it is for the fetus.

Primarily, this is because the postnatal lung epithelium is much more difficult to investigate because the lumen is filled with air. Nevertheless, experiments on several species in which the lung is kept alive by artificial perfusion and the lumen is filled with liquid (i.e. the postnatal lung is 'fetalized') have allowed certain conclusions to be made. Amiloride blockable sodium transport is the major mechanism of liquid absorption in adult sheep lungs (Berthiaume, Staub & Matthay, 1987), rat lung (Basset, Crone & Saumon, 1987a,b; Goodman, Kim, & Crandall, 1987) and rabbit lung (Effros et al., 1986, 1987). So far, only one group (Ramsden et al., 1992) has looked at postnatal lungs of different ages. They showed that lungs in very young lambs (less than 2 weeks old) not only stopped absorbing liquid in the presence of amiloride but started to secrete liquid, i.e. the lung reverted to the fetal state. This effect of amiloride slowly diminished with postnatal age so that, by 6 months of age, amiloride did not abolish absorption but only inhibited absorption a little. Obviously, an absorptive mechanism must appear postnatally which is either not mediated by sodium absorption or is a sodium transport system not inhibited by amiloride. Interestingly, adrenaline can increase the basal absorption rate in postnatal lungs (Berthiaume et al., 1987; Ramsden et al., 1992) but it is not the continuing stimulus causing basal absorption as is shown by the fact that propranolol, in sufficient concentration to block exogenous adrenaline, has no effect on basal absorption rates (Markiewicz & Walters, 1993).

How liquid movement across the postnatal epithelium is controlled remains a mystery. The volume of liquid lining the air filled alveolus is small, estimates varying between 1 and 6 ml 100 g lung^{-1} (Guyton et al., 1976; Gorin & Stewart, 1979) yet any change in this volume can have critical effects on lung function. It seems inherently unlikely that the volume of postnatal alveolar liquid, which appears to be so critically important, is not controlled very precisely.

Clinical relevance

The effect of T_3 and cortisol on the lung is likely to have important clinical implications. All babies demonstrate a fall in the level of their thyroid hormones during the first week of life. In premature babies the concentrations fall to even lower values (Eggermont et al., 1984; Lucas et al., 1988; Mercado et al., 1988) while, in some very immature babies (about 26 weeks), no thyroid hormones are detectable at all in blood several days after birth (personal observations). It remains to be seen how important this deficiency is and whether it can be corrected to the benefit of infants by therapeutic intervention. One might expect infants, particularly very immature ones who are deficient in thyroid hormone (with or without cortisol) to continue to secrete liquid into their lungs even in the presence of exogenously administered surfactant. This could lead to compromised respiratory function and even to long-term sequelae, such as bronchopulmonary dysplasia, in survivors because increased ventilatory support would be needed.

TRH and glucocorticoids administered to mothers in premature labour reduce the incidence of lung disease (see Chapter 2). This effect may be mediated through enhanced lung liquid absorption in addition to improved surfactant synthesis.

Surfactant and lung liquid

The surface tension at the air–liquid interface in the alveoli produces a subatmospheric pressure in the liquid which is caused by the tendency of the pockets of air to collapse because of the small radii of curvature. Laplace's equation predicts that the pressure difference across the interface of a bubble is given by $2T/r$ where T is surface tension and r the radius of curvature. (If r is in μm and T in mN m^{-1}, the pressure difference has units of kPa). The alveoli are not perfect spheres but, even so, the direction of the pressure gradient is correct – liquid phase negative with respect to the air inside the 'bubble'. The pressure is transmitted to the interstitium of the lung and is the main cause of the negative tissue pressure in this organ (Bhattacharya, Gropper, & Staub, 1984). If surface forces have any effect on liquid movement across the epithelium, they will tend to draw liquid into the lumen. In practice, the surface tension forces are normally greatly minimized by pulmonary surfactant (although T rises to over 30 mN m^{-1} on inspiration compared to values approaching zero on expiration). Furthermore, a hydrostatic pressure gradient across the pulmonary epithelium, i.e. between the interstitium and liquid in the alveolus, has not been proved to exist, in spite of efforts to measure one (Fike, Lau-Fook & Bland, 1988). Under normal circumstances, when there is sufficient surfactant present in the lung, the sodium absorptive process is likely to be more than able to overcome any liquid movement into the lung lumen from the interstitium due to surface tension forces. In the steady state which pertains in healthy air-filled lungs the constant absorption of liquid is probably balanced by the osmotic pressures generated by protein or other large molecules being concentrated in the alveolar lining liquid. (For a detailed treatment of this topic, see Walters, 1992.)

When surfactant is deficient and thus surface tension forces are much larger (values of T near those of plasma, i.e. 50 mN m^{-1}), greater hydrostatic pressure gradients will be generated within the lung. A more negative interstitial pressure will favour also a greater capillary filtration. A combination of increased pressure gradients secondary to surfactant deficiency and immature absorptive sodium transport may be the reason why liquid accumulates in both the lumen and interstitium of surfactant deficient lungs (Aherne & Dawkins, 1964; De Sa, 1969). Obviously, in severe cases of hyaline membrane disease there is breakdown of epithelial integrity (Nilsson & Robertson, 1985; Nilsson, Grossmann & Robertson, 1980) and the lung lumen is flooded with fluid containing proteins from the interstitium. Plasma proteins inhibit surfactant function (Ikegami et al., 1984; Seeger et al., 1985; Fuchimukai et al., 1987) which further compounds the pathology. Loss of epithelial integrity also means that the effect of any ion transport by the epithelium will be negated and liquid cannot be absorbed and cleared easily from the lumen.

Summary

Secretion of fetal lung liquid is important for normal development of the lung. Liquid secretion is produced by secondary active transport of chloride ions into the lung lumen by the alveolar epithelium. At birth, secretion ceases and is replaced by an absorptive process which is due to active transport of sodium ions out of the lumen into the interstitium. The acute reversal of liquid movement at birth can be accounted for totally by the rise of adrenaline concentration in fetal blood. The sensitivity of the lung to adrenaline develops in the sheep, only over the last few weeks of gestation and is controlled by the synergistic action of triiodothyronine (T_3) and hydrocortisone (HC) both of which rise in concentration in fetal blood in the last part of gestation. Relative deficiency of these two hormones (T_3 and HC) in premature babies inhibits not only normal surfactant synthesis but also may prevent the development of adequate sodium transport and thus liquid removal from the lung.

After birth at term, an ability to absorb liquid is a characteristic of postnatal lungs throughout life and is due, mostly, to active sodium transport. Nevertheless, the cellular mechanism for liquid secretion persists for a short while (weeks) after birth. Although adrenaline can increase the absorption of liquid in the postnatal lung it does not appear to be responsible for the underlying basal liquid absorption. What, if anything, controls liquid absorption from the lumen of postnatal lungs is unknown. Some of the lung disease observed in premature infants may be due not only to surfactant deficiency but to delayed clearance of lung liquid or even persisting liquid secretion by immature lungs.

References

Adams, F. H., Moss, A. J. & Fagan, L. (1963). The tracheal fluid of the foetal lamb. *Biologia Neonatorum*, **5**, 151–8.

Adamson, T. M., Boyd, R. D. H., Platt, H. S. & Strang, L. B. (1969). Composition of alveolar liquid in the fetal lamb. *Journal of Physiology*, **204**, 159–68.

Addison, W. H. F. & How, H. W. (1913). On the prenatal and neonatal lung. *American Journal of Anatomy*, **15**, 199–214.

Aherne, W. & Dawkins, M. J. R. (1964). The removal of fluid from the pulmonary airways after birth in the rabbit and the effect on this of prematurity and prenatal hypoxia. *Biologia Neonatorum*, **7**, 214–29.

Barker, P. M., Brown, M. J., Ramsden, C. A., Strang, L. B. & Walters, D. V. (1988). The effect of thyroidectomy in the fetal sheep on lung liquid reabsorption induced by adrenaline or cyclic AMP. *Journal of Physiology*, **407**, 373–83.

Barker, P. M., Strang, L. B. & Walters, D. V. (1990). The role of thyroid hormones in maturation of the adrenaline-sensitive lung liquid reabsorptive mechanism in fetal sheep. *Journal of Physiology*, **424**, 473–85.

Barker, P. M., Walters, D. V., Markiewicz, M. & Strang, L. B. (1991). Development of the lung liquid reabsorptive mechanism in fetal sheep: synergism of triiodothyronine and hydrocortisone. *Journal of Physiology*, **433**, 435–49.

Basset, G., Crone, C. & Saumon, G. (1987*a*). Significance of active ion transport in transalveolar water absorption: a study on isolated rat lung. *Journal of Physiology*, **384**, 311–24.

Basset, G., Crone, C. & Saumon, G. (1987*b*). Fluid absorption by rat lung in situ: pathways for sodium entry in the luminal membrane of alveolar epithelium. *Journal of Physiology*, **384**, 325–45.

Berthiaume, Y., Staub, N. C. & Matthay, M. A. (1987). Beta-adrenergic agonists increase lung liquid clearance in anesthetized sheep. *Journal of Clinical Investigation*, **79**, 335–43.

Bhattacharya, J., Gropper, M. A. & Staub, N. C. (1984). Interstitial fluid pressure gradient measured by micropuncture in excised dog lung. *Journal of Applied Physiology*, **56**, 271–7.

Bland, R. D., McMillan, D. D., Bressack, M. A. & Dong, L. (1980). Clearance of liquid from lungs of newborn rabbits. *Journal of Applied Physiology*, **49**, 171–7.

Bland, R. D., Hansen, T. N., Haberkern, C. N. et al. (1982). Lung fluid balance in lambs before and after birth. *Journal of Applied Physiology*, **53**, 992–1004.

Brown, M. J., Olver, R. E., Ramsden, C. A., Strang, L. B. & Walters, D. V. (1983). Effects of adrenaline and of spontaneous labour on the secretion and absorption of lung liquid in the fetal lamb. *Journal of Physiology*, **344**, 137–52.

Carmel, J. A., Friedman, F. & Adams, F. H. (1965). Foetal tracheal ligation and lung development. *American Journal of Diseases of Children*, **109**, 452–6.

Cassin, S., Gause, G. & Perks, A. M. (1986). The effects of bumetanide and furosemide on lung liquid secretion in fetal sheep. *Proceedings of the Society of Experimental Biology & Medicine*, **181**, 427–31.

Cheng, J. B., Goldfien, A., Ballard, P. L. & Roberts, J. M. (1980). Glucocorticoids increase pulmonary beta-adrenergic receptors in fetal rabbit. *Endocrinology*, **107**, 1646–8.

Chopra, I. J., Solomon, D. H., Chopra, U., Wu, S. Y., Fisher, D. A. & Nakamura, Y. (1978). Pathways of metabolism of thyroid hormones. *Recent Progress in Hormone Research*, **34**, 521–67.

De Sa, D. J. (1969). Pulmonary fluid content in infants with respiratory distress. *Journal of Pathology*, **97**, 469–80.

Effros, R. M., Mason, G. R., Silverman, P., Reid, E. & Hukkanen, J. (1986). Movement of ions and small solutes across the endothelium and epithelium of perfused rabbit lungs. *Journal of Applied Physiology*, **60**, 100–7.

Effros, R. M., Mason, G. R., Hukkanen, J. & Silverman, P. (1987). Reabsorption of solutes and water from fluid filled rabbit lungs. *American Review of Respiratory Disease*, **136**, 669–76.

Egan, E. A., Olver, R. E. & Strang, L. B. (1975). Changes in non-electrolyte permeability of alveoli and the absorption of lung liquid at the start of breathing in the lamb. *Journal of Physiology*, **244**, 161–79.

Eggermont, E., Vanderschueren-Lodeweyckx, M., De Nayer, Ph., Smeets, E. et al. (1984). The thyroid-system function in preterm infants of postmenstrual ages of 31 weeks or less: evidence for a 'transient lazy thyroid system'. *Helvetica Paediatrica Acta*, **39**, 209–22.

Faxelius, G., Bremme, K. & Largercrantz, H. (1982). An old problem revisited – hyaline membrane disease and cesarean section. *European Journal of Pediatrics*, **139**, 121–4.

Fewell, J. E., Hislop, A. A., Kitterman, J. A. & Johnson, P. (1983). Effect of tracheostomy on lung development in fetal lambs. *Journal of Applied Physiology*, **55**, 1103–8.

Fike, C. D., Lau-Fook, S. J. & Bland, R. D. (1988). Alveolar liquid pressures in newborn and adult rabbit lungs. *Journal of Applied Physiology*, **64**, 1629–35.

Fisher, D. A., Dussault, J. H., Sack, J. & Chopra, I. J. (1977). Ontogenesis of hypothalamic–pituitary thyroid function and metabolism in man, sheep and rat. *Recent Progress in Hormone Research* **33**, 59–107.

Fisk, N. M., Parkes, M. J., Moore, P. J., Hanson, M. A., Wigglesworth, J. & Rodeck, C. H. (1992). Mimicking low amniotic pressure by chronic pharyngeal drainage does not impair lung development in fetal sheep. *American Journal of Obstetrics & Gynecology*, **166**, 991–6.

Fraser, M. & Liggins, G. C. (1988). Thyroid hormone kinetics during late pregnancy in the ovine fetus. *Journal of Developmental Physiology*, **10**, 461–504.

Fraser, M. & Liggins, G. C. (1989). The effect of cortisol on thyroid hormone kinetics in the ovine fetus. *Journal of Developmental Physiology*, **11**, 207–11.

Fuchimukai, T., Fujiwara, T., Takahashi, A. & Enhorning, G. (1987). Artificial pulmonary surfactant inhibited by proteins. *Journal of Applied Physiology*, **62**, 429–37.

Giannapoulos, G. (1980). Identification and ontogeny of β-adrenergic receptors in fetal rabbit lung. *Biochemical and Biophysical Research Communications,* **95**, 388–94.

Goodman, B. E., Kim, K. J. & Crandall, E. D. (1987). Evidence for active sodium transport across alveolar epithelium of isolated rat lung. *Journal of Applied Physiology*, **62**, 2460–6.

Gorin, A. B. & Stewart, P. A. (1979) Differential permeability of endothelial and epithelial barriers to albumin flux. *Journal of Applied Physiology*, **47**, 1315–24.

Guyton, A. C., Taylor, A. E., Drake, R. E. & Parker, J. C. (1976). Dynamics of subatmospheric pressure in the pulmonary interstitial fluid. In *Lung Liquids*, ed. R. Porter & M. O'Connor. pp. 80,100. Ciba Symposium No. 38, Elsevier Press.

Ikegami, M., Jobe, A., Jacobs, H. & Lam, R. (1984). A protein from airways of premature lambs that inhibits surfactant function. *Journal of Applied Physiology*, **57**, 1134–42.

Jost, A. & Policard, A. (1948). Contribution expérimentale a l'étude du development prénatal du poumon chez le lapin. *Archives d' Anatomie Microscopique et de Morphologie Expérimentale*, **37**, 323–32.

Koefoed-Johnsen, V. & Ussing, H. H. (1953). Contribution of diffusion and flow to the passage of D_2O through living membranes. *Acta Physiologica Scandinavica* **28**, 60–76.

Lagercrantz, H., Bistoletti, P. & Nylund, L. (1983). Sympathoadrenal activity in the foetus during delivery and at birth. In *Intensive Care of the Newborn 3*, ed. L Stern. pp. 1–12. Mason Press, New York.

Lucas, A., Rennie, J., Baker, B. A. & Morley, R. (1988). Low plasma triiodothyronine concentrations and outcome in preterm infants. *Archives of Diseases of Childhood*, **63**, 1201–6.

Markiewicz, M., Barker, P. & Walters, D. V. (1990). The effect of propranolol on the postnatal absorption of luminal lung liquid in the in situ perfused sheep lung. *Journal of Physiology*, **426**, 92 P.

Martindale (1982). *The Extra Pharmacopoeia*. p. 1500, 28th edn, ed. J. E. F. Reynolds. The Pharmaceutical Press, London, UK.

Mercado, M., Yu, V. Y. H., Francis, I., Szymonowicz, W. & Gold, H. (1988). Thyroid function in very preterm infants. *Early Human Development*, **16**, 131–41.

Mescher, E. J., Platzker, A. G. C., Ballard, P. L., Kitterman, J. A., Clements, J. A. & Tooley, W. H. (1975). Ontogeny of tracheal fluid, pulmonary surfactant and plasma corticoids in the fetal lamb. *Journal of Applied Physiology*, **39**, 1017–21.

Moessinger, A. C., Harding, R. D., Adamson, T. M., Singh, M. & Kiu, G. T. (1990). Role of lung liquid volume in growth and maturation of the fetal sheep lung. *Journal of Clinical Investigation*, **86**, 1270–7.

Nilsson, R. & Robertson, B. (1985). Bronchiolar lesions in spontaneously breathing premature newborn rabbits. *Biology of the Neonate*, **48**, 357–61.

Nilsson, R., Grossmann, G. & Robertson, B. (1980). Bronchiolar epithelial lesions induced in the premature rabbit neonate by short periods of artificial ventilation. *Acta Pathologica Microbiolica Scandinavica*, **88**, 359–67.

Nord, E. P., Brown, S. E. S. & Crandall, E. D. (1987). Characterization of the sodium–proton antiport in type II alveolar cells. *American Journal of Physiology*, **252**, C490–8.

Normand, I. C. S., Olver, R. E., Reynolds, E. O. R., Strang, L. B. & Welch, K. (1971). Permeability of lung capillaries and alveoli to non electrolytes in the fetal lamb. *Journal of Physiology*, **219**, 303–30.

Normand, I. C. S., Reynolds, E. O. R. & Strang, L. B. (1970). Passage of macromolecules between alveolar and interstitial spaces in foetal and newly ventilated lungs of the lamb. *Journal of Physiology*, **210**, 151–64.

Oh, Y., Matalon, S., Kleyman, T. R. & Benos, D. J. (1992). Biochemical evidence for the presence of an amiloride binding protein in adult type II pneumocytes. *Journal of Biological Chemistry*, **267**, 18498–504.

Olver, R. E. & Strang, L. B. (1974). Ion flux across the pulmonary epithelium and the secretion of lung liquid in the fetal lamb. *Journal of Physiology*, **241**, 327–57.

Olver, R. E., Schneeberger, E. E. & Walters, D. V. (1981). Epithelial solute permeability, ion transport and tight junction morphology in the developing lung of the fetal lamb. *Journal of Physiology*, **315**, 395–412.

Olver, R. E., Ramsden, C. A., Strang, L. B. & Walters, D. V. (1986). The role of amiloride blockable sodium transport in adrenaline induced lung liquid reabsorption in the fetal lamb. *Journal of Physiology*, **376**, 321–40.

Perks, A. M. & Cassin, S. (1989). The effects of arginine vasopressin and epinephrine on lung liquid production in fetal goats. *Canadian Journal of Physiology Pharmacology*, **67**, 491–8.

Potter, E. L., & Bohlender, G. P. (1941). Intrauterine repiration in relation to development of the fetal lung. *American Journal of Obstetrics & Gynecology*, **42**, 14–22.

Preyer, W. (1885). In *Specielle Physiologie des Embryos*. Ed. L. Fernam. Th. Grieker's Verlag. Leipzig

Ramsden, C. A., Markiewicz, M., Walters, D. V. et al. (1992). Liquid flow across the epithelium of the artificially perfused lung of fetal and postnatal sheep. *Journal of Physiology*, **448**, 579–97.

Roti, E., Braverman, L. E., Fang, S. L., Alex, S. & Emerson, C. H. (1982). Ontogenesis of placental inner ring deiodinase and amniotic fluid 3,3′,5′-triiodothyronine concentration in the rat. *Endocrinology*, **111**, 959–63.

Seeger, W., Stohr, G., Wolf, H. R. D. & Neuhof, H. (1985). Alteration of surfactant function due to protein leakage: special interaction with fibrin monomer. *Journal of Applied Physiology*, **58**, 326–38.

Shaw, A. M., Ward, M. R., Steele, L. W., Butcher, P. A. & Olver, R. E. (1990). Sodium–proton exchange across the apical membrane of the alveolar type II cell of the fetal sheep. *Biochimica et Biophysica Acta*, **1028**, 9–13.

Thom, J. & Perks, A. M. (1990). The effects of furosemide and bumetanide on lung liquid production in vitro lungs from fetal guinea pigs. *Canadian Journal of Physiology & Pharmacology*, **68**, 1131–5.

Tomoda, S., Brace, R. A. & Longo, L. D. (1987). Amniotic fluid volume regulation: basal volumes and responses to fluid infusion or withdrawal in sheep. *American Journal of Physiology*, **252**, R380–7.

Wallace, J. W., Hooper, S. B. & Harding, R. D. (1990). Regulation of lung liquid secretion by arginine vasopressin in fetal sheep. *American Journal of Physiology*, **258**, R104–11.

Walters, D. V. (1992). The role of pulmonary surfactant in transepithelial movement of liquid. In *Pulmonary Surfactant: From Molecular Biology to Clinical Practice*, ed. B. Robertson, L. M. G. Van Golde & J. J. Batenburg. pp. 193–213. Elsevier Science Publishers B. V., Amsterdam.

Walters, D. V. & Olver, R. E. (1978). The role of catecholamines in lung liquid absorption at birth. *Pediatric Research*, **12**, 239–42.

Walters, D. V., Ramsden, C. A. & Olver, R. E. (1990). Dibutyryl cAMP induces a gestation-dependent absorption of fetal lung liquid. *Journal of Applied Physiology*, **68**, 2054–9.

Warburton, D., Parton, L., Buckley, S., Cosico, L., Enns, G. & Saluna, T. (1988). Combined effects of corticosteroid, thyroid hormones and beta-agonist on surfactant, pulmonary mechanics and beta-receptor binding in fetal lamb lung. *Pediatric Research*, **24**, 166–70.

4

Fetal breathing: relation to postnatal breathing and lung development

RICHARD HARDING

Introduction

The occurrence of prenatal breathing movements is now regarded as a universal phenomenon in placental (eutherian) mammals, and this probably holds for other orders that breathe air postnatally (e.g. birds, reptiles). In the context of this chapter, rhythmical activation of respiratory neurones and muscles during the prenatal period is referred to as fetal breathing movements (FBM). Most of our knowledge of FBM has been derived from two species (sheep and man), although their presence has been confirmed in other mammals, including guinea pigs, rabbits, cats and non-human primates.

Fetal breathing movements should be distinguished from other physiological events which, like FBM, intermittently lower intrathoracic pressure. The most common of these, prenatal hiccups, have been detected in several species including man. Like FBM they usually occur in episodes, but can be distinguished from FBM by the larger, briefer and more uniform changes they induce in thoracic dimensions and intrathoracic pressure. Gasping movements, which can occur in the fetus under conditions of severe hypoxia or asphyxia, are, like hiccups, considered to be physiologically distinct from FBM.

Owing to the labile nature of FBM, they can be best studied in unstressed subjects in the absence of anaesthetics or tranquillizers. These conditions are readily achieved with humans, but have proved more difficult with animals. The advent of chronic implantation techniques in animals coupled with the development of high resolution ultrasound equipment has permitted rapid advances in the understanding of FBM over the last two decades.

Ontogeny of fetal breathing

With the refinement of recording techniques has come a progressive reduction in the fetal age at which FBM-like events can be first detected in both animals and humans. However, in the very young fetus it has proved difficult to distinguish respiratory movements of the thorax or abdomen from other forms of body movement. In the human, FBM are first detected at about 10 weeks (de Vries, Visser & Prechtl, 1986), a little later than the appearance of other body movements. In sheep, which have a gestation of 145–150 days, FBM can first be detected at about 50 days (Cooke & Berger, 1990).

When first detectable, human FBM are present for approximately 2% of recording time, followed by a progressive increase in incidence to 6% at 19 weeks (de Vries et al., 1986), 11–13% at 22–24 weeks (de Vries et al., 1987), 12–14% at 24–29 weeks (Natale, Nasello-Paterson & Connors, 1988) and 31% at 30 weeks (Fox, Inglis & Steinbrecher, 1979; Patrick et al., 1980). Between 30 weeks and term, incidences of FBM between 17 and 65% have been reported, the mean value being about 30% (Fox et al., 1979; Patrick et al., 1980). Typically, studies of FBM in humans are of short duration (1–2 hours) leading to substantial variations in the measured incidence of FBM. More prolonged observations of the human fetus, such as those made by Patrick et al. (1980), as well as studies of other species, have demonstrated a high hourly variation in the incidence of FBM. Some of this variation might be attributed to fluctuations in maternal plasma glucose concentrations; for example Patrick et al. (1980) showed increased FBM after meals when maternal plasma glucose rose.

Relationship between FBM and behavioural states

As the fetal CNS matures, FBM become closely associated with other aspects of fetal behaviour, in particular the sleep/wake or rest/activity rhythm. In fetal sheep, two distinct states of electrocortical (ECoG) activity can be recognized after 120–125 days of gestation (Fig. 4.1); one in which high-voltage waves are frequent and rapid eye movements (REM) are infrequent, and one in which low voltage ECoG activity and REM predominate (Dawes et al., 1972). Breathing movements become closely associated with the latter state owing to the development of descending inhibition of the respiratory pattern generator in association with the high-voltage electrocortical state. The precise location of these inhibitory inputs is unknown, but they probably lie above the pons because transection of the brainstem at the level of the upper pons dissociates respiratory activity and behavioural states (Dawes et al., 1983).

In the human, fetal breathing movements also become associated with behavioural states as they develop during gestation. Human fetal behavioural states have been assessed by ultrasonic observations of fetal heart rate, eye movements and other body movements, the details of which are beyond the scope of this chapter. In essence, variations in fetal heart rate and other body movements have revealed the presence of alternating periods of low and high activity (or variability) during the last third of gestation (Nijhuis et al., 1982; Arduini et al., 1986). In the last 10 weeks, the relationship between periods of high heart rate variability and fetal activities such as breathing movements, eye movements and micturition becomes increasingly marked (Arduini et al., 1986) (Fig. 4.2).

Brief periods of fetal arousal have been detected in both sheep and humans. In the ovine fetus, these can be recognized by the presence of high levels of postural muscle activity (e.g. in nuchal muscles) in association with a low-voltage electrocorticogram and eye movements (Harding, 1980). It is common for FBM, fetal swallowing episodes (e.g. Fig. 4.5) and fetal micturition episodes to occur during this state (Harding et al., 1984a; Wlodek, Thorburn & Harding, 1989).

Relation between fetal breathing and postnatal breathing

Fetal breathing movements are undoubtedly a consequence of rhythmical activation of neurones in the respiratory regions of the brainstem. Micro-electrode recordings from the medulla oblongata have shown that bursts of neuronal activity coincide with activity in the phrenic and intercostal nerves (Bystrzycka, Nail & Purves, 1975). What provides the drive to these brainstem neurones is the subject of other chapters.

Information on the muscles involved in fetal breathing has been obtained principally from chronically monitored fetal sheep, in which electromyographic electrodes have been implanted. It has been found that, during late ovine gestation, the range of muscles that can be activated during fetal breathing is similar to that during postnatal breathing, provided that the effects of behavioural state are taken into account (Harding, Johnson & McClelland, 1980), so fetal breathing in the sheep during late pregnancy should only be compared with postnatal breathing that occurs during REM sleep.

The principal muscle activated at all gestational ages is the diaphragm. Not all diaphragmatic activity is related to fetal breathing, however, and

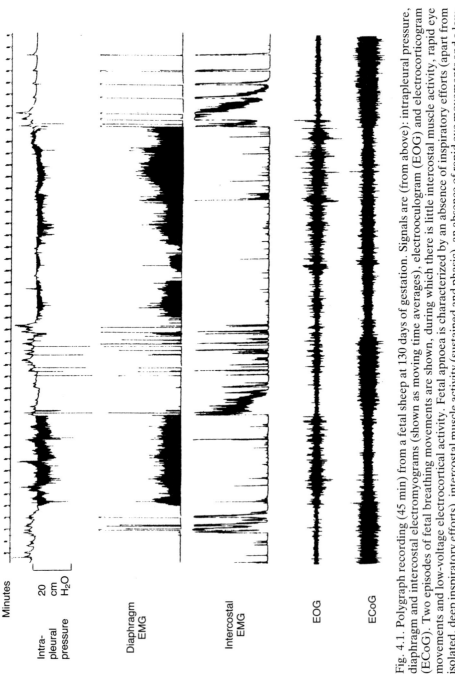

Fig. 4.1. Polygraph recording (45 min) from a fetal sheep at 130 days of gestation. Signals are (from above): intrapleural pressure, diaphragm and intercostal electromyograms (shown as moving time averages), electrooculogram (EOG) and electrocorticogram (ECoG). Two episodes of fetal breathing movements are shown, during which there is little intercostal muscle activity. Fetal apnoea is characterized by an absence of inspiratory efforts (apart from isolated, deep inspiratory efforts), intercostal muscle activity (sustained and phasic), an absence of rapid eye movements and a low-voltage electrocorticogram. (Reproduced, with permission, from Harding, 1980.)

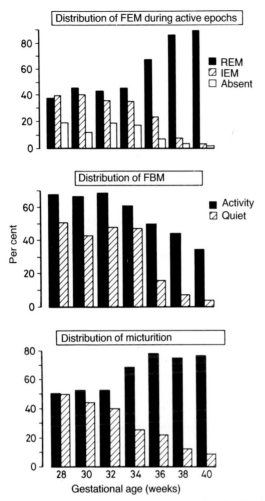

Fig. 4.2. *Upper panel*: changes with gestational age in the distribution of types of human fetal eye movements (FEM) during epochs of fetal activity, based on heart rate variability (REM, rapid eye movements; IEM intermittent eye movements). *Middle and lower panels*: distribution of fetal breathing movements (FBM) and micturition episodes in the human fetus during quiet and active phases of behaviour determined from variability of fetal heart rate. (Diagram modified from Arduini et al., 1986.)

many episodes of EMG activity appear to be related to postural adjustments. The diaphragm receives its innervation principally from the phrenic nerve which arises in the mid-cervical spinal cord. The descending motor traffic from brainstem centres is subject to modification at this

spinal level. Thus the phrenic neurogram and the diaphragmatic electromyogram may not provide a reliable expression of the output of the
central respiratory pattern generator (Bahoric & Chernick, 1975).

Data on the role of intercostal muscles in fetal breathing have been
obtained almost exclusively from fetal sheep during late gestation. Prior
to 100–110 days of gestation, bursts of EMG activity occur in the
intercostal muscles approximately in synchrony with the inspiratory
phase of the respiratory cycle (Clewlow et al., 1983). Later in gestation
(after 120 days), when electrocortical states become more clearly defined, inspiratory intercostal muscle activity becomes attenuated, and is
difficult to detect during non-stimulated fetal breathing (Harding et al.,
1980; Clewlow et al., 1983). The inhibition of intercostal muscle activation in association with breathing activity in late fetal life is probably
due to descending inhibitory neural influences arising from more rostral
brain centres, as is believed to occur postnatally. During non-breathing
periods, high levels of sustained activity are frequently seen in the
intercostal muscles, presumably in association with postural changes
involving the trunk (Harding, 1980; Clewlow et al., 1983). For technical
reasons, it has not been possible to discriminate between the activity of
internal and external intercostal muscles during fetal breathing. However, it seems likely that inspiratory-related activity is derived from the
external layer, while tonic activity, associated with fetal movements and
the high-voltage electrocortical state, is derived from the internal intercostal muscles.

Electromyographic recordings from chronically prepared fetal sheep
and ultrasonic observations of human fetuses have provided evidence
that the muscles of the upper respiratory tract are activated in association
with fetal breathing movements. In particular, data have been obtained
on the roles of muscles of the larynx, tongue and nostrils. The involvement of these muscles in different types of inspiratory effort is summarized in Table 4.1.

The principal dilator muscle of the larynx (posterior crico-arytenoid,
PCA) is activated during the inspiratory phase of each breathing movement in the fetus, as it is after birth (Harding, 1980; Harding et al., 1980).
As it is innervated from the brainstem directly by a branch of the vagus
nerve (recurrent laryngeal nerve), the PCA muscle of the fetus may
provide a more reliable expression of the phasic output from a 'central
pattern generator' than the diaphragm. The PCA muscle is increasingly
active in gestation during each period of diaphragmatic activation,
although its background level of activation may vary. An exception to this

Table 4.1. *Summary of the involvement of inspiratory muscles during fetal breathing movements, fetal hiccups (in non-ruminants) or deep inspiratory efforts (in ruminants), and fetal asphyxial gasping*

	Fetal breathing	Hiccups or deep inspiratory efforts	Asphyxial gasping
Diaphragm	+	+ +	+ +
Intercostals	−	+ ?	+
Laryngeal dilators	+	−	+ +
Pharyngeal dilators	−	−	+ +
Nasal dilators	±	?	?

+ signifies muscle activity, − signifies lack of activity.

firm relationship occurs during isolated, deep inspiratory efforts which are large reductions in intrathoracic pressure caused by diaphragmatic contraction and which are probably analogous to postnatal regurgitative efforts (Fig. 4.3) (Harding et al., 1980). Rhythmical dilation of the glottis of the human fetus has been observed by ultrasound (Cooper et al., 1985; Isaacson & Birnholz, 1991) indicating that the laryngeal dilator muscles are active in this species. Dilation of the larynx during each fetal breathing movement can cause a reduction in pressure within the upper trachea (Fig. 4.4).

In fetal sheep, recordings have been obtained from the major muscle of the tongue (genioglossus). These have shown that phasic activation of the genioglossus muscle rarely occurs in synchrony with breathing movements during unstimulated fetal breathing (Johnston, Gunn & Gluckman, 1986). The phasic bursts of EMG activity that occur in association with episodes of fetal breathing (but not in synchrony with individual FBM) are apparently related to repetitive chewing or mouthing movements, rather than to fetal breathing. Recordings from the masseter muscles show similar bouts of phasic activity (R.Harding, unpublished observations). A similar situation exists in the postnatal lamb and adult sheep, in which the genioglossus muscle, unlike that in many other species (for review see Harding, 1986), is not normally activated in association with unstimulated breathing. However, if respiratory drive is increased in lambs and ewes in response to airway obstruction the genioglossus muscle becomes active during inspiration (Harding et al., 1987). A similar respiratory activation can occur in fetal sheep in

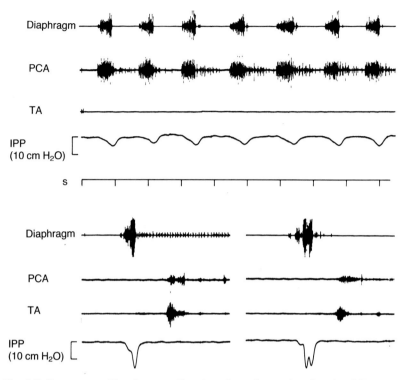

Fig. 4.3. Two types of inspiratory effort in a sheep fetus, showing the differential involvement of laryngeal muscles. Upper panel shows rapid irregular breathing movements during the low-voltage electrocortical state; lower panel shows two deep inspiratory efforts during the high-voltage electrocortical state. Tracings, from above, are: electromyograms recorded from the diaphragm, posterior crico-arytenoid (PCA, laryngeal abductor) and thyro-arytenoid (TA, laryngeal adductor) muscles, and intrapleural pressure (IPP). Fetal breathing movements are accompanied by rhythmical laryngeal dilation, whereas deep inspiratory efforts are not. (Reproduced with permission from Harding, 1980.)

response to hypercapnia (Johnston et al., 1986) and cutaneous cooling (Johnston, Gunn & Gluckman, 1988).

The nasal dilator muscles (alae nasi) may also be active in association with the inspiratory phase of fetal breathing (Jansen, Ioffe & Chernick, 1983; Johnston et al., 1986). As in sleeping preterm infants (Carlo et al., 1983), these muscles are not active with all breaths. The relationship between the inspiratory activation of the diaphragm and that of alae nasi muscles can be strengthened in fetal sheep as a result of increasing respiratory drive by the induction of hypercapnia (Johnston et al., 1986) or cutaneous cooling (Johnston et al., 1988).

Laryngeal adductor muscles are inactive in fetal sheep during periods of FBM, but they become tonically active during pauses between breathing episodes (Harding, 1980; Harding et al., 1980). During periods of fetal apnoea, these adductor muscles (principally the thyro-arytenoid muscle) are largely responsible for the increase in upper airway resistance that retards the efflux of liquid from the lungs (Fig. 4.4, Fig. 4.5). In newborn sheep, a similar relationship exists between the activation of the laryngeal constrictor muscles and behavioural state as that seen in the fetus. That is, these muscles show no respiratory-related activity during REM sleep, but during non-REM (quiet) sleep, they are active during expiration, leading to the retardation of expiratory airflow (Harding et al., 1980).

Mechanics of fetal breathing

The rhythmical activation of the respiratory muscles during FBM has a range of physical effects on the fetus. Pressure fluctuations within the thorax caused by FBM influence liquid movement within the 'airways' and may also affect cardiovascular performance. Contraction of the respiratory muscles also causes alterations in the shape of the thorax and lungs.

Thoracic pressure fluctuations

The activation of inspiratory muscles generates much larger reductions in pressure in the liquid-filled lungs of the fetus than in those of the air-breathing neonate or adult. Under basal conditions in the healthy ovine fetus, tracheal pressure (relative to amniotic sac pressure) is reduced by an average of 3.5–4.0 mmHg (Clewlow et al., 1983). During fetal hypercapnia, these may reach 12 mmHg (Rigatto et al., 1988). In the fetal pig near term, the mean amplitude of FBM was 7.6 mmHg (Harding, Fowden & Silver, 1991), considerably greater than in the ovine fetus.

The pressure fluctuations are generated as a consequence of inspiratory muscles contracting, tending to enlarge the thorax against a resistance caused by the upper respiratory tract and by the viscosity of the liquid within it. In the fetus, the diaphragm is the most important muscle contributing to this effect. However, activity of upper airway muscles may also generate reductions in tracheal pressure, independent of the diaphragm. Pressure recordings in hydraulically disconnected upper and lower sections of the trachea reveal that reductions in pressure in the

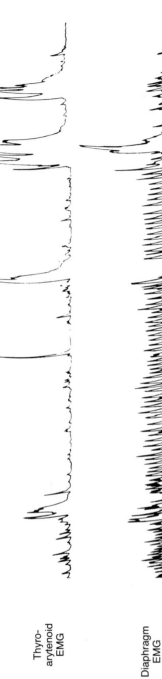
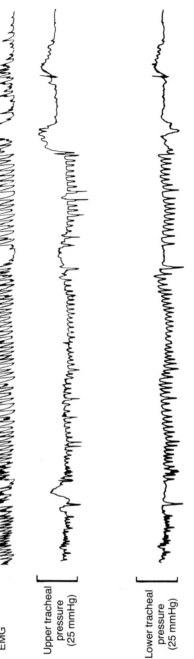

Thyro-
arytenoid
EMG

Diaphragm
EMG

Upper tracheal
pressure
(25 mmHg)

Lower tracheal
pressure
(25 mmHg)

1 min

Fig. 4.4. Polygraph recording from a fetal sheep, in which the cervical trachea was cannulated in each direction, during an episode of breathing movments. Tracings (from above) are: electromyographic activity of the thyroarytenoid (laryngeal adductor) and diaphragm muscles, recorded as moving time averages, and pressures in the upper and lower tracheal cannulae which were not connected to each other. Pressure recordings show that fetal breathing activity (diaphragm EMG) is associated with independently generated pressure fluctuations in the lower and upper trachea. Those in the upper trachea are probably due to the rhythmical dilation of the glottis by laryngeal abductor muscles. Thyroarytenoid muscle activity is coincident with increased pressure in the upper trachea, and becomes tonic after the cessation of FBM. (Reproduced, with permission, from Harding et al., 1989.)

upper trachea may approach in magnitude those developed in the lower airways by the diaphragm (Harding, Dickson & Hooper, 1989) (Fig. 4.4). The generation of sub-amniotic pressure by the larynx can be attributed to inspiratory enlargement of the larynx and confirms the presence of an effective resistance to the influx of fluid into the upper respiratory tract from the amniotic sac (Harding, Bocking & Sigger, 1986b).

As is the case with the amplitude of fetal inspiratory efforts, the frequency of FBM is highly variable. In the ovine fetus during the last third of gestation, typical mean values for the frequency of FBM within an episode are 22–32/min; the mean frequency tends to decline with age (Clewlow et al., 1983). In the fetal pig near term, the frequency of FBM was 34/min within episodes (Harding et al., 1991). Hourly averages for the human fetus range from 43–44/min at 24–25 weeks (Natale et al., 1988), 44/min at 34–35 weeks (Patrick et al., 1978), to 47/min at 38–39 weeks (Patrick et al., 1980).

Changes in thoracic dimensions

Human FBM can be detected as changes in the position of the diaphragm, abdominal wall or thoracic wall. At 34–35 weeks, each inspiratory effort causes the anterior chest wall to move inwards by 2–5 mm and the anterior abdominal wall to move outwards by 3–8 mm (Patrick et al., 1978). The retraction of the chest wall is most evident caudally, and the outward movement of the abdominal wall is usually greatest at the level of the umbilicus (Gennser & Marsal, 1979). The paradoxical movement of the thoracic and abdominal walls is compatible with the belief that FBM are essentially isovolumetric. Increased flexion of the thoracic spine also occurs during FBM (Gennser & Marsal, 1979).

Changes in thoracic dimensions induced by ovine FBM have been studied using pairs of chronically implanted ultrasound transducers in fetal sheep during the last third of gestation. Transducer pairs implanted in an anterio-posterior orientation detected inward movements of the thoracic walls of 1.7 mm during basal conditions, increasing to 3.8 mm under hypercapnic conditions (Poore & Walker, 1980). Assuming a mean anterio-posterior chest diameter of 93 mm (Harding & Poore, 1984), fetal breathing under normal conditions alters this dimension of the chest by less than 2%. In the transverse orientation, the chest also became narrower with each inspiratory effort; the size of these changes (mean 2.7 mm) was greater than those in the anterio-posterior plane, indicative of the greater compliance of the thoracic wall of the ovine fetus in this plane. Assuming a mean chest diameter in the transverse plane of 65 mm

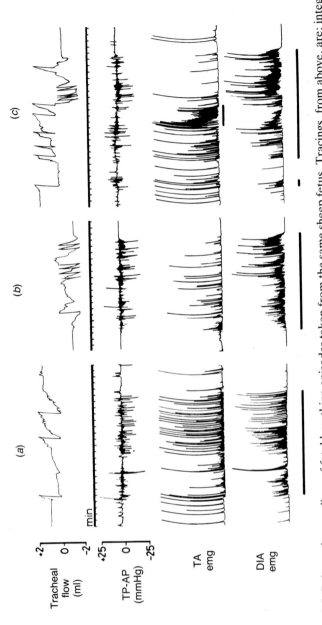

Fig. 4.5. Polygraph recordings of fetal breathing episodes taken from the same sheep fetus. Tracings, from above, are: integrated tracheal fluid flow, tracheal pressure after subtraction of amniotic sac pressure (TP-AP), and moving time averages of electromyographic activity in the thyro-arytenoid (TA) and diaphragm (DIA) muscles. Episodes of fetal breathing are indicated by bars beneath DIA EMG tracing, and an episode of fetal swallowing is indicated by a bar beneath TA emg tracing. Recording *a* shows bars beneath DIA EMG tracing, and an episode of fetal swallowing is indicated by a bar beneath TA emg tracing. Recording *a* shows the most common pattern, a net efflux of tracheal fluid during the fetal breathing episode. Recording *b* shows a net influx of fluid, and recording *c* shows both efflux and influx. Little flow of tracheal fluid occurs in the absence of FBM. (Reproduced, with permission from Harding et al., 1989.)

(Harding & Poore, 1984), this diameter varies by approximately 4% during fetal breathing. In summary, FBM cause minor fluctuations (<2–4%) in the dimensions of the thorax, and by inference, in the dimensions of the fetal lungs.

Tracheal fluid movement during FBM

Early recordings of tracheal fluid movement using electromagnetic flow-meters in fetal sheep indicated that small oscillatory fluid fluxes occurred in association with individual inspiratory efforts. Peak tracheal flow rates of up to 6 ml/s were recorded but the net change in tracheal volume during each 'breath' was normally less than 0.5 ml (i.e. less than one tenth of tracheal volume (Dawes et al., 1972; Maloney et al., 1975). Oscillatory flow of tracheal fluid has also been detected in the human fetus (26–29 weeks) using pulsed Doppler ultrasound. The mean flow velocity during each breath was 15–25 cm/s and the calculated maximum tidal volume was about 6 ml, much less than that in the newborn (Utsu et al., 1983).

Episodes of FBM are usually associated with an increased rate of tracheal fluid flow from the lungs (i.e. greater than the rate of pulmonary fluid production) (Harding et al., 1984*b*; Dickson, Maloney & Berger, 1987) (Fig. 4.5). In contrast, periods of fetal apnoea are associated with a rate of efflux considerably less than the rate of fluid production. These differences are due to changes in the behaviour of muscles which affect the resistance of the upper respiratory tract. During episodes of FBM, upper airway resistance is reduced by active glottic dilation, due to rhythmical PCA muscle activation, allowing fluid to leave the lungs as a result of their elastic recoil (Harding, Bocking & Sigger, 1986*a*,*b*). When breathing movements cease, the absence of rhythmic active dilation of the glottis, coupled with a sustained low level of activity in the laryngeal constrictor muscles, increases the resistance of the upper airway, thereby retarding the efflux of liquid from the lungs (Harding et al., 1986*a*,*b*). The net effect, in a late gestation ovine fetus, is a small (<2 ml, 1–2% of total liquid volume) reduction in lung liquid volume during episodes of FBM and the re-establishment of the original volume during the intervening periods of apnoea (Dickson et al., 1987; Harding & Bocking, 1990).

Other forms of inspiratory effort in the fetus

In addition to rhythmical breathing movements, which can be regarded as being analogous to postnatal breathing, a second type of inspiratory effort has been identified in healthy fetuses of several species. These have been given different names in different species, but probably all represent the same phenomenon.

Trains of deep inspiratory efforts (initially termed 'gasps') were first described by Dawes et al. (1972) in healthy fetal sheep. They cause large reductions in intrathoracic pressure (10–20 mmHg) at intervals of 20–60 s, and typically occur in episodes which occupy about 3 minutes per hour. These inspiratory efforts are unique in that the diaphragm is activated in the absence of increased activation of the laryngeal dilator muscles (Fig. 4.3) (Harding, 1980; Harding et al., 1980). In this respect, and in their timing and association with the high-voltage electrocortical state (Harding et al., 1980) they resemble the deep inspiratory efforts against a closed glottis that immediately precede each regurgitive effort in the mature sheep, and other ruminants. In the fetus, however, there is no evidence that gastric contents are moved orally along the oesophagus during these inspiratory efforts.

Sudden, deep inspiratory efforts resembling hiccups have been detected during fetal life in several non-ruminant species, including humans (Norman, 1942; de Vries et al., 1986), baboons (R. Stark, personal communication) and pigs (Harding et al., 1991). Similar events have been described in fetal guinea pigs (Kendall, 1977) and rabbits (J.S. Robinson, personal communication). It seems likely that hiccups, which are powerful inspiratory efforts in association with glottic closure (Newsom Davis, 1970) are a universal phenomenon amongst non-ruminant mammalian fetuses. In the human fetus, they are particularly common during early gestation, and occur largely in association with the 'active' behavioural state. Their incidence falls from about 10% of recording time at 14–18 weeks to 2–4% close to term (Pillai & James, 1990). It is of interest that the incidence of hiccups in preterm infants 3–80 days after birth was, on average, 2.5% of recording time (Brouillette et al., 1980), similar to that in the near-term fetus. The functional significance of hiccupping is unknown, but it is more likely to be related to digestion than to respiration.

Asphyxial gasping

Hypoxia normally inhibits FBM, but if it becomes severe, gasping movements may become initiated. These are much more powerful than rhythmic FBM and involve strong activation of the upper airway dilator muscles (Harding, 1986) (Table 4.1).

Fetal breathing movements and lung development

The rediscovery of FBM in the 1960s and 1970s prompted a search for their functional role. Many years earlier, Ballantyne (1902) had likened FBM to thoracic gymnastics in preparation for the great extrauterine function of atmospheric respiration. The notion that FBM benefit respiratory muscle development has not, apparently, been the subject of experimentation. However, considerable interest has been directed at the possibility that FBM are necessary for normal lung development in the fetus. This section deals with the influence of FBM on fetal lung development and the underlying mechanisms. In general, data on FBM and lung development have been obtained from human infants in whom FBM were absent due to congenital abnormalities or from fetal animals (mainly sheep) in which FBM have been experimentally abolished or impaired.

As fetal breathing movements during late gestation are principally diaphragmatic, they can be most readily abolished experimentally by section of the phrenic nerves. This has been done in three studies using fetal sheep (Alcorn et al., 1980; Fewell, Lee & Kitterman, 1981; Nagai et al., 1988). Each of these reported that prolonged phrenic nerve section during late gestation led to significant lung hypoplasia, as assessed by reduced pulmonary DNA content, tissue weight and lung volume. This procedure also causes atrophy of the diaphragm muscle (Fewell et al., 1981; Kitterman, 1984) and a profound reduction in lung liquid volume at postmortem (Alcorn et al., 1980; Fewell et al., 1981). It is likely that a prolonged reduction in lung volume as a consequence of phrenic nerve section was the cause of the reduction in lung growth as a direct relationship between fetal lung expansion (i.e. lung liquid volume) and growth of the lung has been well documented (Alcorn et al., 1977; Moessinger et al., 1990; Hooper, Han & Harding, 1993). The hypoplastic effect of phrenic nerve section on the fetal lungs is similar to, but less dramatic than, that of chronically reducing lung volume by the continuous drainage of lung liquid.

The congenital absence of phrenic nerves in a human fetus has also been shown to result in lung hypoplasia and upward displacement of the diaphragm (Goldstein & Reid, 1980). Similarly, lung hypoplasia has been observed in anencephalic infants with intact diaphragms in whom fetal breathing movements were absent (Dornan, Ritchie & Meban, 1984).

Another method of experimentally abolishing fetal breathing movements is by transection of the spinal cord above the level of the phrenic motoneurones which lie in the mid-cervical cord. This technique avoids denervation-atrophy of the diaphragm muscle; however, the effects on fetal lung development are similar to those of phrenic nerve section. That is, in both fetal rabbits (Wigglesworth & Desai, 1979) and fetal sheep (Liggins et al., 1981a) subjected to transection of the upper cervical spinal cord, the lungs became hypoplastic. However, lung liquid volumes were not measured. Recently, we have measured lung liquid volume in fetal sheep following high cervical spinal section and have found it to be reduced, on average, by 34% between 121 and 134 days of gestation (Harding, Hooper & Han, 1993). This effect cannot be attributed to a reduction in lung liquid secretion as it was found to be increased compared to control fetuses. A further study, in which FBM were abolished for 48 h by blocking the phrenic nerves with tetrodotoxin, confirmed the role of FBM in maintaining lung expansion (Miller, Hooper & Harding, 1993).

The reason for the reduced lung expansion following the abolition of FBM by phrenic nerve blockade or spinal cord transection is not immediately obvious. It is unlikely to be due to atrophy of the diaphragm muscle (this would not necessarily lead to lengthening of the muscle), nor to the possible abolition of a tonic excitation of the muscle, as no such activity has been detected in the fetus. It cannot be attributed to a reduction in lung liquid secretion, as it was found to be unaltered or increased (Fewell et al., 1981; Harding & Hooper, 1992). The reduced expansion cannot be due to an absence of phasic lung expansion by FBM, as it is known that individual FBM have little effect on lung volume, and that episodes of FBM are more commonly associated with a reduction, rather than an increase, in lung liquid volume (Harding et al., 1984b; Dickson et al., 1987).

It is likely that prolonged abolition of the diaphragmatic contractions leads to upward displacement of the diaphragm, due to the elastic properties of the lung. In the intact fetus the pulmonary recoil pressure is partially opposed by diaphragmatic contractions during episodes of FBM, and in the absence of FBM episodes it is opposed by the constrictor action of the larynx (Fig. 4.6). Several lines of evidence support the existence in the fetus of a small, sustained transpulmonary recoil pressure which tends to collapse the lungs. (Of course, surface tension forces are not present in the liquid-filled lungs of the fetus.)

1. When FBM cease in a normal fetus, the pulmonary luminal pressure (measured in the trachea) rapidly becomes 1–3 mm Hg greater than amniotic sac pressure (Vilos & Liggins, 1982; Harding, Hooper &

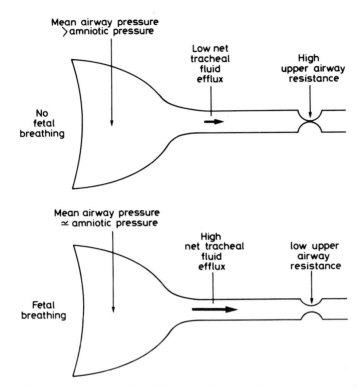

Fig. 4.6. Diagram summarizing differences in intra-pulmonary pressure (relative to amniotic sac pressure), tracheal fluid flow and upper airway resistance during episodes of breathing movements and apnoea in fetal sheep. During apnoea, lung liquid accumulates in lungs owing to a high resistance in the upper airway. During episodes of FBM, increased efflux of lung liquid occurs because the recoil pressure of the lungs is no longer opposed by a high resistance in the upper airway.

Dickson, 1990). This effect is dependent on the presence of a resistance in the upper respiratory tract, principally in the larynx and is abolished by tracheo-amniotic shunt (Fewell & Johnson, 1983).

2. At postmortem, when the fetal thorax is opened, the liquid-filled fetal lungs collapse down to a smaller size than in the intact thorax.

3. If the resistive effects of the upper airway are abolished by the creation of a tracheo-amniotic shunt, lung liquid rapidly flows out of the trachea, leading to a large reduction in the volume of the lungs (Harding et al., 1986a).

4. During episodes of FBM, when the resistance of the upper airway (larynx) is reduced, lung liquid tends to leave the lungs at an increased rate than during periods of apnoea (Harding et al., 1984b).

Owing to the elastic recoil of the fetal lungs, the prolonged absence of episodes of the diaphragmatic component of FBM (e.g. following spinal cord section or phrenic nerve section or blockade) in the presence of a normally functioning upper airway is likely to result in gradual pulmonary collapse in spite of the continued secretion of lung liquid. In the intact fetus diaphragmatic contractions during FBM act to limit reductions in thoracic volume and lung expansion by their tendency to oppose the elastic recoil of the lungs at times (i.e. during FBM episodes) when upper airway resistance is low. Although the rate of fluid efflux is normally greater during FBM episodes than during apnoea, the rate of efflux would be even greater in the absence of the thoracic component of FBM. That is, in the absence of the diaphragmatic component of FBM, but in the presence of continued FBM-related activation of the laryngeal muscles, lung liquid will be lost from the lungs at a greater rate than if the diaphragm were rhythmically active. It is likely, therefore, that the inhibitory effects of abolishing the thoracic component of FBM by spinal section of phrenic nerve section on fetal lung growth are principally due to a prolonged reduction in lung expansion.

Another experimental approach to determine the effects of the thoracic component of FBM on fetal lung development was to diminish the fluctuations in intrathoracic pressure caused by them. This was achieved by surgically replacing, bilaterally, parts of the thoracic walls of fetal sheep with silicone rubber membranes, thereby increasing the compliance of the thoracic wall (Liggins et al., 1981b). This had the effect, after 32 days, of reducing the dry weight, DNA content and distensibility of the lungs. These effects may have been due to a reduction in fetal lung liquid volume, although it was not measured. The tendency for the lungs to collapse would be less effectively opposed in the presence of the membrane, resulting in a reduced degree of lung expansion.

The effects of totally abolishing fetal breathing activity (thoracic and upper airway components) on lung development remain to be determined, and will probably depend on the ability of the upper airway to retard the efflux of lung liquid.

Future directions

It is apparent that the dominant physical factor mediating fetal lung growth is the basal degree of distension by liquid, although phasic distortion of the lungs may also play a role. Therefore, an analysis of the molecular and cellular responses to tonic stretch of the developing lungs is clearly warranted. Previous experiments have focused on the effects of abolishing fetal breathing movements on lung development. In future, it may be possible to determine whether lung growth and maturation can be enhanced by their augmenation in the absence of other factors likely to affect lung development. It may also be possible to perform in vivo experiments aimed at confirming the in vitro experiments of Skinner (1989) which have demonstrated the stimulation of pulmonary cell division in response to rhythmical stretching. The relationship between lung expansion, fetal breathing and the synthesis and release of surfactant phospholipids (Higuchi et al., 1991) also deserves investigation in an animal model.

References

Alcorn, D., Adamson, T. M., Lambert, T. F., Maloney, J. E., Ritchie, B. C. & Robinson, P. M. (1977). Morphological effects of chronic tracheal ligation and drainage in the fetal lamb lung. *Journal of Anatomy*, **123**, 649–60.

Alcorn, D., Adamson, T. M., Maloney, J. E. & Robinson, P. M. (1980). Morphological effects of chronic bilateral phrenectomy or vagotomy in the fetal lamb lung. *Journal of Anatomy*, **130**, 683–95.

Arduini, D., Rizzo, G., Giorlandino, C., Valensise, H., Dell'aqua, S. & Romanini, C. (1986). The development of fetal behavioural states: a longitudinal study. *Prenatal Diagnosis*, **6**, 117–24.

Bahoric, A. & Chernick, V. (1975). Electrical activity of phrenic nerve and diaphragm in utero. *Journal of Applied Physiology*, **39**, 513–18.

Ballantyne, J. W. (1902). *Manual of Antenatal Pathology and Hygiene*. Green, Edinburgh.

Brouillette, R. T., Thach, B. T., Abu-Osba, Y. K. & Wilson, S. L. (1980). Hiccups in infants: characteristics and effects on ventilation. *Journal of Pediatrics*, **96**, 219–25.

Bystrzycka, E., Nail, B. & Purves, M. J. (1975). Central and peripheral neural respiratory activity in the mature sheep foetus and newborn lamb. *Respiration Physiology*, **25**, 199–215.

Carlo, W. A., Martin, R. J., Abboud, E. R., Bruce, E. N. & Strohl, K. P. (1983). Effect of sleep state and hypercapnia on alae nasi and diaphragm. *Journal of Applied Physiology*, **54**, 1590–6.

Clewlow, F., Dawes, G. S., Johnston, B. M. & Walker, D. W. (1983). Changes in breathing, electrocortical and muscle activity in unanaesthetized fetal lambs with age. *Journal of Physiology*, **341**, 463–76.

Cooke, I. R. C. & Berger, P. J. (1990). Precursor of respiratory pattern in the early gestation mammalian fetus. *Brain Research*, **522**, 333–6.

Cooper, C., Mahoney, B. S., Bowie, J. D., Albright, T. O. & Callen, P. W. (1985). Ultrasound evaluation of the normal fetal upper airway and esophagus. *Journal of Ultrasound in Medicine*, **4**, 343–6.

Dawes, G. S., Fox, H. E., Leduc, B. M., Liggins, G. C. & Richards, R. T. (1972). Respiratory movements and rapid eye movement sleep in the fetal lamb. *Journal of Physiology*, **220**, 119–43.

Dawes, G. S., Gardner, W. N., Johnston, B. M. & Walker, D. W. (1983). Breathing in fetal lambs: the effect of brain stem section. *Journal of Physiology*, **335**, 535–53.

de Vries, J. I. P., Visser, G. H. A. & Prechtl, H. F. R. (1986). Fetal behaviour in early pregnancy. *European Journal of Obstetrics and Gynecology and Reproductive Biology*, **21**, 271–6.

de Vries, J. I. P., Visser, G. H. A., Mulder, E. J. H. & Prechtl, H. F. R. (1987). Diurnal and other variations in fetal movement and heart rate patterns at 20–22 weeks. *Early Human Development*, **15**, 333–48.

Dickson, K. A., Maloney, J. E. & Berger, P. J. (1987). State-related changes in lung liquid secretion and tracheal flow rate in fetal lambs. *Journal of Applied Physiology*, **62**, 34–8.

Dornan, J. C., Ritchie, J. W. K. & Meban, C. (1984). Fetal breathing movements and lung maturation in the congenitally abnormal human fetus. *Journal of Developmental Physiology*, **6**, 367–75.

Fewell, J. E. & Johnson, P. (1983). Upper airway dynamics during breathing and during apnoea in fetal lambs. *Journal of Physiology*, **339**, 495–504.

Fewell, J. E., Lee, C. C. & Kitterman, J. A. (1981). Effects of phrenic nerve section on the respiratory system of fetal lambs. *Journal of Applied Physiology*, **51**, 293–7.

Fox, H. E., Inglis, J. & Steinbrecher, M. (1979). Fetal breathing movements in uncomplicated pregnancies. 1. Relationship to gestational age. *American Journal of Obstetrics and Gynecology*, **134**, 544–6.

Gennser, G. & Marsal, K. (1979). Fetal breathing movements monitored by real-time B-mode ultrasound: basal appearance and response to challenges. *Contributions to Obstetrics and Gynecology*, **6**, 66–79.

Goldstein, J. D. & Reid, L. M. (1980). Pulmonary hypoplasia resulting from phrenic nerve agenesis and diaphragmatic amyoplasia. *Journal of Pediatrics*, **97**, 282–7.

Harding, R. (1980). State-related and developmental changes in laryngeal function. *Sleep*, **3**, 307–22.

Harding, R. (1986). The upper respiratory tract in perinatal life. In *Respiratory Control and Lung Development in the Fetus and Newborn*, ed. B. M. Johnston & P. D. Gluckman. pp. 331–76. Perinatology Press, Ithaca, New York.

Harding, R. & Bocking, A. D. (1990). Fetal lung growth. In *Handbook of Human Growth and Developmental Biology*, vol. III, Part B, ed. E. Meisami & P. S. Timiras. pp. 131–148. CRC Press, Boca Raton.

Harding, R., Bocking, A. D. & Sigger, J. N. (1986*a*). Influence of upper respiratory tract on liquid flow to and from fetal lungs. *Journal of Applied Physiology*, **61**, 68–74.

Harding, R., Bocking, A. D. & Sigger, J. N. (1986*b*). Upper airway resistances in fetal sheep: the influence of breathing activity. *Journal of Applied Physiology*, **60**, 160–5.

Harding, R., Buttress, J. A., Caddy, D. J. & Wood, G. A. (1987). Respiratory and upper airway responses to nasal obstruction in awake lambs and ewes. *Respiration Physiology*, **68**, 177–88.

Harding, R., Dickson, K. A. & Hooper, S. B. (1989). Fetal breathing, tracheal fluid movement and lung growth. In *Advances in Fetal Physiology*, ed. P. D. Gluckman, B. M. Johnston & P. W. Nathanielsz. pp. 153–75. Perinatology Press, Ithaca, New York.

Harding, R., Fowden, A. L. & Silver, M. (1991). Respiratory and non-respiratory thoracic movements in the fetal pig. *Journal of Developmental Physiology*, **15**, 263–9.

Harding, R., Hooper, S. B. & Han, V. K. M. (1993). Abolition of fetal breathing movements by spinal cord transection leads to reductions in fetal lung liquid volume, lung growth, and IGF-II gene expression. *Pediatric Research*, **34**, 148–53.

Harding, R., Hooper, S. B. & Dickson, K. A. (1990). A mechanism leading to reduced lung expansion and lung hypoplasia in fetal sheep during oligohydramnios. *American Journal of Obstetrics and Gynecology*, **163**, 1904–13.

Harding, R., Johnson, P. & McClelland, M. E. (1980). Respiratory function of the larynx in developing sheep and the influence of sleep state. *Respiration Physiology*, **40**, 165–79.

Harding, R. & Poore, E. R. (1984). The effects of myometrial activity on fetal thoracic dimensions and uterine blood flow during late gestation in the sheep. *Biology of the Neonate*, **45**, 244–51.

Harding, R., Sigger, J. N., Poore, E. R. & Johnson, P. (1984*a*) Ingestion in fetal sheep and its relation to sleep states and breathing movements. *Quarterly Journal of Experimental Physiology*, **69**, 477–86.

Harding, R., Sigger, J. N., Wickham, P. J. D. & Bocking, A. D. (1984*b*). The regulation of flow of pulmonary fluid in fetal sheep. *Respiration Physiology*, **57**, 47–59.

Higuchi, M., Hirano, H., Gotoh, K., Takahashi, H & Maki,M. (1991). Relationship of fetal breathing movement pattern to surfactant phospholipid levels in amniotic fluid and postnatal respiratory complications. *Gynecological and Obstetrical Investigation*, **31**, 217–21.

Hooper, S. B., Han, V. K. M. & Harding, R. (1993). Changes in lung expansion alter pulmonary DNA synthesis and IGF–II gene expression in fetal sheep. *American Journal of Physiology*, **265**, L403–9.

Isaacson, G. & Birnholz, J. C. (1991). Human fetal upper respiratory tract function as revealed by ultrasonography. *Annals of Otology, Rhinology and Laryngology*, **100**, 743–7.

Jansen, A. H., Ioffe, S. & Chernick, V. (1983). Drug-induced changes in fetal breathing activity and sleep state. *Canadian Journal of Physiology and Pharmacology*, **61**, 315–24.

Johnston, B. M., Gunn, T. R. & Gluckman, P. D. (1986). Genioglossus and alae nasi activity in fetal sheep. *Journal of Developmental Physiology*, **8**, 323–31.

Johnston, B. M., Gunn, T. R. & Gluckman, P. D. (1988). Surface cooling rapidly induces coordinated activity in the upper and lower airway muscles of the fetal lamb in utero. *Pediatric Research*, **23**, 257–61.

Kendall, J. Z. (1977). Respiratory movements in the fetal guinea pig in utero. *Journal of Applied Physiology*, **42**, 661–3.

Kitterman, J. A. (1984). Fetal lung development. *Journal of Developmental Physiology*, **6**, 67–82.

Liggins, G. C., Vilos, G. A., Campos, G. A., Kitterman, J. A. & Lee, C. H. (1981*a*). The effect of spinal cord transection on lung development in fetal sheep. *Journal of Developmental Physiology*, **3**, 267–74.

Liggins, G. C., Vilos, G. A., Campos, G. A., Kitterman, J. A. & Lee, C. H. (1981*b*). The effect of bilateral thoracoplasty on lung development in fetal sheep. *Journal of Developmental Physiology*, **3**, 275–82.

Maloney, J. E., Adamson, T. M., Brodecky, V., Cranage, S., Lambert, T. F. & Ritchie. (1975). Diphragmatic activity and lung liquid flow in the unanesthetized fetal sheep. *Journal of Applied Physiology*, **39**, 423–8.

Millar, A. A., Hooper, S. B. & Harding, R. (1993). Role of fetal breathing movements in control of fetal lung distension. *Journal of Applied Physiology*, **75**, 2711–17.

Moessinger, A. C., Harding, R., Adamson, T. M., Singh, M. & Kiu, G. T. (1990). Role of lung fluid volume in the growth and maturation of the fetal sheep lung. *Journal of Clinical Investigation*, **86**, 1270–7.

Nagai, A., Thurlbeck, W. M., Jansen, A. H., Ioffe, S. & Chernick, V. (1988). The effect of chronic biphrenectomy on lung growth and maturation in fetal lambs. *American Review of Respiratory Diseases*, **137**, 167–72.

Natale, R., Nasello-Paterson, C., & Connors, G. (1988). Patterns of fetal breathing activity in the human fetus at 24 to 28 weeks of gestation. *American Journal of Obstetrics and Gynecology*, **158**, 317–21.

Newsom Davis, J. (1970). An experimental study of hiccup. *Brain*, **93**, 851–72.

Nijhuis, J. G., Prechtl, H. F. R., Martin, C. B. & Bots, R. S. G. M. (1982). Are there behavioural states in the human fetus? *Early Human Development*, **6**, 177–95.

Norman, H. N. (1942). Fetal hiccups. *Journal of Comparative Psychology*, **34**, 65–73.

Patrick, J., Fetherston, W., Vick, H. & Voegelin, R. (1978). Human fetal breathing movements and gross fetal movements at weeks 34 to 35 of gestation. *American Journal of Obstetrics and Gynecology*, **130**, 693–9.

Patrick, J., Campbell, K., Carmichael, L., Natale, R. & Richardson, B. (1980). Patterns of human fetal breathing during the last 10 weeks of pregnancy. *Obstetrics and Gynecology*, **56**, 24–30.

Pillai, M. & James, D. (1990). Hiccups and breathing in human fetuses. *Archives of Disease in Childhood*, **65**, 1072–5.

Poore, E. R. & Walker, D. W. (1980). Chest wall movements during fetal breathing in the sheep. *Journal of Physiology*, **301**, 307–15.

Rigatto, H., Lee, D., Davi, M., Moore, M., Rigatto, E. & Cates, D. (1988). Effect of increased arterial CO_2 on fetal breathing and behavior in sheep. *Journal of Applied Physiology*, **64**, 982–7.

Skinner, S. J. M. (1989). Fetal breathing movements: a mechanical stimulus for fetal lung cell growth and differentiation. In *Advances in Fetal Physiology*, ed. P. D. Gluckman, B. M. Johnston & P. W. Nathanielsz. pp. 133–51. Perinatology Press: Ithaca, New York.

Utsu, M., Sakakibara, S., Ishida, T., Chiba, Y. & Hasegawa, T. (1983). Dynamics of tracheal fluid flow in the human fetus, studied with pulsed doppler ultrasound. *Acta Obstetrica Gynaecologica Japan*, **35**, 2017–18.

Vilos, G. A. & Liggins, G. C. (1982). Intrathoracic pressures in the fetal sheep. *Journal of Developmental Physiology*, **4**, 247–56.

Wigglesworth, J. S. & Desai, R. (1979). Effects of cervical cord section in the rabbit fetus. *Early Human Development*, **3**, 51–65.

Wlodek, M. E., Thornburn, G. D. & Harding, R. (1989) Bladder contractions and micturition in fetal sheep: their relation to behavioral states. *American Journal of Physiology*, **257**, R1526–32.

5

Peripheral control of breathing

CARLOS E. BLANCO

Introduction

The mechanisms responsible for rhythmic breathing are not completely understood. It is suggested that groups of neurones in the brain stem are primarily responsible for generation of the rhythmic pattern of respiration (Karczewski, 1974; Mitchell & Berger, 1975; Wyman, 1977). Several possibilities have been proposed for the central respiratory controller including inherent rhythmic pacemaker cells, a bi-stable oscillator system and an inhibitory phasing network of cells (Mitchell & Berger, 1975). Afferent respiratory stimuli are thought to play a role modulating influences on the basic respiratory rhythm. It is reported that when unanaesthetized adult animals are in NREM sleep, withdrawal of their vagal and chemoreceptor afferent input significantly reduces respiratory activity (Philipson, 1978; Sullivan et al., 1978). The fetus experiences no changes in temperature, little cutaneous sensations and no light. The airway is full of lung fluid, pulmonary circulation is minimal and blood gases show little variation due to a constant gas exchange through the placenta. In this situation most, if not all, of the classical stimuli which regulate and control breathing activity are absent, or if present their stimulatory effects seem to be below threshold.

Nevertheless breathing activity is present in utero from early gestation despite an environment almost free of stimuli, although it seems to be under very little reflex control (Barcroft & Barron, 1937; Dawes et al., 1972). The presence of fetal breathing movements (FBM) is almost continuous and very irregular in frequency and amplitude in early gestation, and it should reflect spontaneous activity of central structures in the brain stem. These movements represent brain stem output since they are associated with phrenic and diaphragmatic activity and they produce small tidal movements of tracheal fluid (Bahoric & Chernick, 1975; Maloney et al., 1975a). Until late in pregnancy there is no evidence of any central or peripheral mechanisms regulating this activity. The first evidence of some type of regulation becomes evident with the differentiation of the electroencephalographic activity (ECoG) and behavioural states (Dawes et al., 1972; Patrick et al., 1980; Trudinger & Knight, 1980).

Breathing movements appear to be a spontaneous and random activity, provided that the fetus is in the behavioural state when breathing is allowed. This is to be expected since breathing activity does not seem to be regulated by peripheral mechanisms and is not expected to respond to demands of gas exchange. The lack of peripheral control is suggested by several experiments; vagotomy (Dawes et al., 1972; Boddy et al., 1974; Condorelli & Scarpelli, 1976) or chemoreceptor denervation (Jansen et al., 1981; Rigatto et al., 1988; Koos & Sameshima, 1988; Moore et al., 1989) does not modify the incidence of breathing activity. However, Murai et al. (1985) suggested participation of the carotid chemoreceptors in the regulation of spontaneous fetal breathing activity because they described an initial reduction of FBM in recordings made soon after surgery; however the incidence of FBM tended to increase later on. Therefore, peripheral chemoreceptors do not seem to be involved in the regulation of spontaneous FBM. This is interesting since it is known that, in fetal sheep in utero, carotid chemoreceptors show spontaneous activity and are responsive to hypoxia (Blanco et al., 1984a) although their increased activity in hypoxia fails to stimulate FBM (Boddy et al., 1974). These observations suggest that either the evoked activity of the chemoreceptors is not strong enough to elicit a respiratory response or that predominately inhibitory mechanisms exist within the brain stem which make the respiratory centres insensitive to this afferent input. Evidence for the latter could be found in experiments in fetal lambs where the carotid and aortic chemoreceptors were denervated and either the brainstem was transected (Moore et al., 1989; Koos, Chao & Doany, 1992) or lesions were made the lateral pons (Gluckman & Johnston, 1987; Johnston & Gluckman, 1989; Johnston, 1991). In those experiments, brain stem transection or lesions in the lateral pons 'permitted' a respiratory response during fetal hypoxia. However, after carotid chemoreceptor denervation, this response disappeared and the incidence of FBM during normoxia decreased. This indicates again that peripheral chemoreceptors can exert a tonic stimulatory respiratory drive but in the intact fetus this activity remains below threshold in the brain stem.

Other peripheral afferent inputs such as cutaneous cooling can also influence breathing activity in utero (Gluckman, Gunn & Johnston, 1983). This will be discussed in more detail below.

Breathing after birth is continuous throughout all behavioural states and is regulated to meet the gas exchange requirements of the neonate. Birth brings the fetus into contact with many potentially relevant stimuli: tactile stimuli, light, lower environmental temperature, mild asphyxia, the removal of the umbilical circulation, arousal, lung expansion with gas, a larynx free of fluid, contact of the airway with O_2 and CO_2, increase in oxygen consumption, full right ventricular output increasing pulmonary blood flow which exposes pulmonary receptors to changing CO_2 (Fitzgerald & Lahiri, 1986), higher arterial PO_2, blood gas oscillations perfusing the peripheral chemoreceptors and vagal afferent input from mechanoreceptors. We will examine the role of these peripheral stimuli below.

Chemoreceptors

Hypoxaemia is a potent respiratory stimulant producing an increase in ventilation ($\dot{V}_E$) and arousal from sleep in adult man and animals. This response is mediated almost totally by the peripheral chemoreceptors. During the early neonatal period, a decrease in inspired PO_2 always causes an increase in $\dot{V}_E$ in all species studied, even though this is only transient (Brady & Ceruti, 1966; Schweiler, 1968; Brady & Dunn, 1970; Rigatto, 1977; Sankaran et al., 1979; Grunstein, Hazinski & Schleuter, 1981; LaFramboise et al., 1981; Woodrum et al., 1981; Blanco et al., 1984*b*). It may be expected that, at birth, when the fetus is hypoxaemic and needs to establish breathing, hypoxia would play an important role. Yet acute reduction of fetal PaO_2 in utero causes reduction and eventual cessation of FBM in animals (Boddy et al., 1974; Maloney et al., 1975*b*; Martin, Murata & Ikenoue, 1975) and man (Ritchie, 1980). There is also a reduction in the incidence of limb movements (Natale, Clewlow & Dawes, 1981) and hindlimb polysynaptic reflexes (Blanco, Dawes & Walker, 1983*a*) and absence of fetal arousal. The fetal response to hypoxia is the reverse of that expected after birth and it could be regarded as appropriate for conservation of oxygen (Parer, 1980). Blanco et al., (1987*a*) showed that moderate hypoxia delayed the establishment of breathing when the fetus was delivered and the umbilical cord clamped (see Fig. 5.1). However, these inhibitory effects of hypoxia at birth were overridden by hypercapnia, cold and an increase in general afferent input.

The inhibitory effects of hypoxia before and at birth suggest that the peripheral chemoreceptors play little or no role in the establishment of

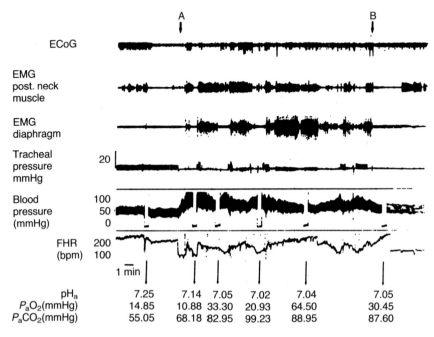

Fig. 5.1. Recording from a sheep fetus of 133 days GA in utero 4 days after operation. Traces from the top are: electrocortical activity (ECoG); posterior neck muscle EMG; diaphragm EMG; tracheal pressure; arterial pressure; fetal heart rate. At A the cord was occluded and mechanical ventilation was stopped. At B the cord occlusion was released. Blood gases and pH values are indicated at the points when samples were taken. Note the failure to achieve continuous breathing for prolonged periods after cord occlusion in the presence of hypoxia.

breathing. However, at birth after cord clamping cardiovascular changes occur (bradycardia & hypertension) showing an active chemoreflex. Direct recordings from afferent fibres showed that the carotid chemoreceptors are functionally active and responsive to hypoxia in the last third of gestation in the fetal lamb (Blanco et al., 1984a). Therefore, fetal carotid chemoreceptor activity is sufficient to produce cardiovascular changes, which will assure perfusion of fetal organs, but it is not adequate to produce a ventilatory stimulation or arousal. That this chemoreceptor activity is not followed by stimulation of breathing and arousal suggests suprapontine inhibitory mechanisms overriding respiratory responses (Dawes et al., 1983). Furthermore, chemodenervation before birth does not impair the establishment of breathing at birth (Harned et al., 1967; Herrington et al., 1971; Jansen et al., 1981).

After birth, afferent activity of the carotid chemoreceptors plays a key role in reversing central inhibition triggered by hypoxaemia as shown in carotid denervated newborn lambs (Blanco, Dawes & Walker, 1983*b*) and in carotid denervated adult man (Honda & Hashizume, 1991).

Resetting of chemoreceptor sensitivity

Chemoreceptor sensitivity to hypoxia does not change rapidly after birth from fetal to the adult range. Direct evidence for this was provided by recording the afferent neural activity of the carotid sinus nerve in fetal and newborn lambs and by measuring the steady-state ventilatory response to isocapnic hypoxia in newborn lambs (Blanco et al., 1982; Blanco et al., 1984*a*; Blanco et al., 1987*b*; Blanco, Hanson & McCooke, 1988*a*, see Fig. 5.2). The conclusion from this work was that arterial chemoreceptors are active and responsive in the fetus and almost silenced by the rise in PaO_2 after birth (Blanco et al., 1982; Blanco et al., 1984*a*). The range of their sensitivity to changes in PaO_2 appears to be reset to its adult position over the first few days postnatally (Blanco et al., 1988*a*) and it seems to be dependent on gestational age (Blanco et al., 1987*b*). Indirect evidence which supports this comes from the diminished ventilatory response to hypoxia during the first 24–48 hours after birth (Miller & Behrle, 1954; Miller & Smull, 1955; Belenky, Standaert & Woodrum, 1979; Bureau & Begin, 1982; Blanco et al., 1982; Blanco et al., 1984*a*). Also, an intravenous bolus of dopamine (which suppresses chemoreceptor activity, Nishino & Lahiri, 1981) produced a greater reduction of $\dot{V}_E$ in older new-born lambs than during the first day of life (Maycock et al., 1983). A similar response was obtained in newborn infants when they were given 100% O_2 to breathe for 30 seconds (Hertzberg & Lagercrantz, 1987). These observations confirm the idea that chemoreceptor activity is decreased during the first few days after birth. It would not therefore be expected to play a large role in defending the body against hypoxia at this time: in this respect it is interesting that lambs that were carotid body denervated, at 2 days of life, died unexpectedly only after the third week of life and not in the newborn period (Bureau et al., 1985).

The role of CO_2 sensitivity of the peripheral chemoreceptors and its contribution to the ventilatory response to CO_2 inhalation is less clear. It is reported that the ventilatory response (breathing frequency) to inhaled CO_2 increases with postnatal age in premature infants. However, this work did not differentiate peripheral from central components (Rigatto, Brady & de la TorreVerduzco, 1975). It has been stated already that the fetal peripheral chemoreceptors are responsive to changes in PaO_2 and in

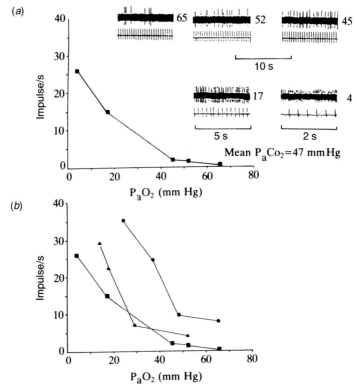

Fig. 5.2. Examples of hypoxic response curves of carotid chemoreceptors of lambs after ventilation in utero. (*a*) A carotid chemoreceptor hypoxic response curve of a fetus ventilated with O_2 for 6 h. Inset are sections of the chemoreceptor recording (upper trace) and the electrocardiogram (lower trace) at each P_aO_2 studied (indicated on the right of each trace). Discharge increases as P_aO_2 falls. (*b*) Sample individual curves from the three group of fetuses. (●) Fetus ventilated with O_2/CO_2 for 30 h; (■) fetus ventilated with O_2/CO_2 for 6 h; (▲) fetus ventilated with N_2/CO_2 for 31 h.

$PaCO_2$ and that the range for hypoxic sensitivity changes to the adult range within 24–48 hours after birth. As the responses to CO_2 and hypoxia interact positively at the carotid body, this change would be expected to produce an increase in the steady state response of CO_2. It is not known whether the sensitivity to changes in CO_2 resets after birth. There are reasons for not expecting this: first, the changes in $PaCO_2$ after birth are not so dramatic as for PaO_2; secondly, CO_2 has a very important contribution in the control of breathing and its establishment at birth. Recent data indicate that peripheral chemoreceptors are responsive to CO_2 challenges from the second day of life in piglets and kittens and that this response does not change with postnatal age (Wolsink et al., 1991; Watanabe, Kumar & Hanson, 1993*a*). Since both reports included newborn animals from the second day of life, it is not known whether CO_2 sensitivity was reset earlier as is the case for PaO_2. Even though CO_2 sensitivity of the peripheral chemoreceptors does not change with postnatal age, increases in environmental temperature seem to reduce its gain (Watanabe, Kumar & Hanson, 1993*b*). This may predispose neonates to respiratory failure at warmer environmental temperature.

Responses to changes in blood gases

Oscillations

Peripheral chemoreceptors are not only responsive to changes in the mean level of blood gas tensions under steady state conditions but it is known that their discharge oscillates with respiration (Goodman, Nail & Torrance, 1974; Cross et al., 1986). Carotid chemoreceptors can detect small changes in PaO_2 and $PaCO_2$ at least at a frequency of 15 breaths per minute in the adult cat (Kumar & Nye, 1985; Kumar, Nye & Torrance, 1988). These changes in blood gas are directly related to tidal volume and indirectly to respiratory frequency (Lamb, Anthonisen & Tenney, 1965; Purves, 1966). It is also postulated that the transducing capability of the carotid chemoreceptors decreases at frequencies above 70/minute (Fitzgerald, Leitner & Liaubet, 1969).

These oscillations in chemoreceptor discharge lead to measurable changes in respiratory variables. In adult man and cat breath-by-breath variations in alveolar PO_2 induced changes in several respiratory variables (e.g. tidal volume, frequency, inspiratory and expiratory times, etc.) (Ward et al., 1979; Kumar, Nye & Torrance, 1983).

In the newborn period, respiratory variables are also influenced by induced oscillations in the chemoreceptor discharge. Alternations in F_iO_2 produce alternations in several respiratory variables in newborn kittens (Hanson, Kumar & Williams, 1987, 1989), newborn lambs (Williams & Hanson, 1990) and in newborn infants (Blanco et al., 1988*b*; Williams et al., 1991). Bilateral carotid chemoreceptor denervation in newborn lambs abolished the effect of F_iO_2 alternation on respiratory variables (Williams & Hanson, 1990, see Fig. 5.3).

The response to F_iO_2 alternations in the newborn infant is dependent on postnatal age: although it is present within 24 hours after birth it is significantly weaker than thereafter (Williams et al., 1991, see Fig. 5.4).

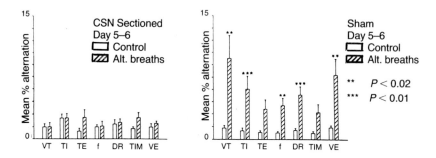

Fig. 5.3. The mean percentage breath-by-breath alternation for five carotid sinus nerve (CSN) sectioned and five sham-operated lambs on postnatal day 5–6. Mean responses ± SEM are shown during control (open bars) and test runs (hatched bars) for tidal volume (VT), inspiratory time (TI), expiratory time (TE), frequency (f), inspiratory drive (DR), timing (TIM) and instantaneous ventilation (VE). **,*** show significant difference between control and test runs $P <$ 0.02 and $P < 0.01$ respectively by Student's paired t-test. (Reproduced with permission from Williams & Hanson, 1990.)

This supports the results of previous observations in fetal and newborn lambs which showed a resetting period for the sensitivity of chemoreceptors shortly after birth (Blanco et al., 1984a, 1988a; Kumar & Hanson, 1989). The respiratory response of newborn infants to exaggeration of blood gas oscillations induced by breath-to-breath alternation in F_iO_2 is an indication of chemoreceptors resetting/functioning. This method could be clinically valuable in detecting deviations of chemoreceptor sensitivity during the first months of life.

Pulmonary afferents

In utero the lungs are expanded with about 30 ml/kg body weight of fluid at term and are not exposed to phasic changes in alveolar volume since FBM move only around 1 ml of tracheal fluid (Dawes et al., 1972; Maloney et al., 1975a; see also Chapter 4). Moreover, vagotomy does not affect FBM (Dawes et al., 1972; Condorelli & Scarpelli, 1976). This suggests that, at resting lung volume, there is neither an overall excitatory nor an inhibitory vagal input to the central respiratory pattern generator. Even though pulmonary afferents seem not to be actively involved in the regulation of breathing activity in utero, their effects can be elicited when the fetal lung is inflated or deflated (Maloney et al., 1975b; Blanco et al., 1987c, see Fig. 5.5). After birth, in the newborn and preterm infant, mechanoreceptor activity in the lung is important in the maintenance of lung volume and in promoting inflation (Olinsky, Bryan & Bryan, 1974;

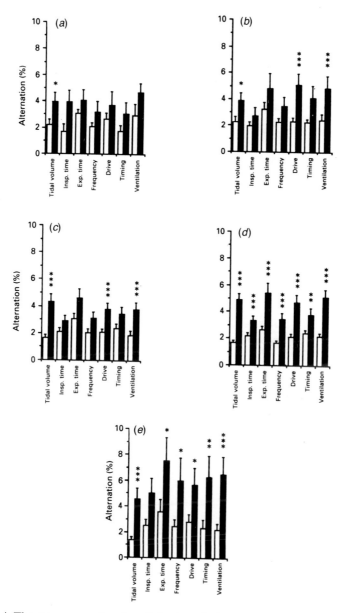

Fig. 5.4. The mean percentage breath-by-breath alternation for infants at postnatal ages of 3–10 h (*a*: *n* = 12 runs from 6 infants), 12–24 h (*b*: *n* = 24 runs from 12 infants), 24–48 h (*c*: *n* = 36 runs from 18 infants), 3–4 days (*d*: *n* = 42 runs from 21 infants) and 5–8 days (*e*: *n* = 14 runs from 7 infants). Mean responses (±SEM) are shown during control (open bars) and test runs (filled bars) for tidal volume, inspiratory time, expiratory time, breath frequency, inspiratory drive, timing and instantaneous ventilation. Asterisks show significant differences between control and test runs; *$P < 0.05$, **$P < 0.02$, ***$P < 0.01$ by Student's paired t-test. (Reproduced with permission from Williams et al., 1991.)

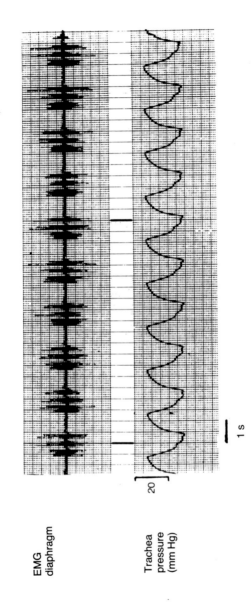

EMG
diaphragm

Trachea
pressure
(mm Hg)

20

1 s

Fig. 5.5. Chronically instrumented fetal lamb at 132 days GA ventilated with 95% O_2 and 5% CO_2. Note inhibition of spontaneous phasic diaphragm EMG activity during inflation of the lung by the ventilator. (Reproduced with permission from Blanco et al., 1987c.)

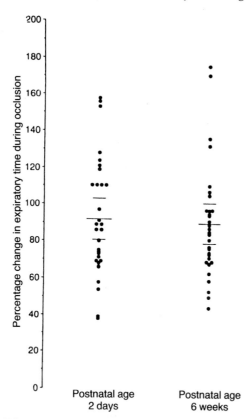

Fig. 5.6. Effects of end-inspiratory occlusion on expiratory time during week 1 and week 6 measurements. Each point represents mean value from five occlusions in each infant. Mean and 95% confidence intervals of groups are also shown. Occlusion resulted in a lengthening of expiratory time by >38% in all infants. (Reproduced with permission from Rabbette et al., 1991.)

Henderson-Smart & Read, 1979). The lung inflation reflex (Hering–Breuer) is an important vagally mediated mechanism for regulating the rate and depth of respiration in newborn mammals during the first week of life since loss of end-expired pressure or vagotomy modified the breathing pattern in newborn animals (Fedorko, Kelly & England, 1988; Grunstein, Younes & Milic-Emili, 1973). It can be demonstrated by end-expiratory occlusions (Cross et al., 1960; Kirkpatrick et al., 1976; Gerhardt & Bancalari, 1981; Witte & Carlo, 1987) or end inspiratory occlusion (Rabbette, Costeloe & Stocks, 1991) that it is present also in newborn and premature healthy infants and that it persists during the first 2 months of life in infants (Rabbette et al., 1991, see Fig. 5.6) and in lambs (Andrews, Symonds & Johnson, 1991) (see also Chapter 7). In the adult, the Hering–Breuer reflex is weak or active only at large changes in lung volume (Guz et al., 1964; Clark & Von Euler, 1972; Green & Kaufman, 1990).

Irritant receptors

Irritant receptors are located throughout the epithelium of the upper and lower airway; they are sensitive to mechanical irritation. In utero these receptors are exposed to lung fluid at a constant temperature. There is no evidence for any function of these receptors during fetal life. It is known that cough could not be elicited in unanaesthetized fetal lambs in utero either by noxious stimulation of the laryngeal region, by electrical stimulation of the laryngeal nerve (Johnson, Salisbury & Storey, 1975) or by air ventilation in utero (Blanco et al., 1987c). After birth irritant receptor activity can elicit typical adult responses after 35 weeks of gestational age (Fleming, Bryan & Bryan, 1978).

Phrenic afferents and respiratory control

It is known that nociceptive afferents are present in the phrenic nerve. It is estimated that 10–25% of the myelinated axons of the phrenic nerve are afferents (Hinsey, Hare & Phillips, 1939; Duron, Jung-Caillol & Marlot, 1978). There is only a small quantity of smaller diameter myelinated afferents corresponding to gamma fibres (Gasser & Grundfest, 1939; Duron & Condamin, 1970) which may correspond to the small proportion of muscle spindles found in the diaphragm. This could explain the absence of diaphragmatic load compensation. There is no evidence that phrenic afferents have an influence on muscle activation during eupnoeic breathing. However, experiments on the isolated diaphragm of adult dogs showed that the stimulation of diaphragmatic thin-fibre afferents had an excitatory effect on inspiratory motor drive (Hussain et al., 1990). The role of these afferent inputs in the regulation of breathing activity before birth and in the neonatal period is not known. For further reading see reviews by Road (1990), Frazier & Revelette (1991).

Somatic afferent input

In utero there are no changes in temperature or other conditions which could increase the peripheral input to the CNS although sound can be transmitted to the fetal ear. This environment most probably determines the absence (or limited presence) of wakefulness within the fetal behavioural repertoire (Ruckebusch, 1972; Natale et al., 1981; Rigatto, Blanco & Walker, 1982; Rigatto, 1984). For the same reason it would not be expected that peripheral input would have any role in the regulation of spontaneous FBM. However, FBM can be influenced by experimental changes of the intrauterine environment. Peripheral cooling results in a shift of the CO_2 response curve to the left, (Moss, Mautone & Scarpelli, 1983) and alters the fetal behaviour to an aroused state resulting in increased breathing (Gluckman et al., 1983). The same effect can be produced by application of ice-cold water to the snout region of the fetus still in utero (Dawes, 1968; Merlet et al., 1967). Since this effect is rapid, cutaneous receptors seem to mediate the response. Later, there may be a fall in central temperature, which will affect the central thermoreceptors and increase activity of brainstem reticular neurones. However, electrical stimulation of the peroneal or sciatic nerves does not affect FBM, ECoG or nuchal activity in fetal sheep (Blanco et al., 1983a). In utero changes in peripheral input do not play a defined role but at birth they are important in the initiation and maintenance of breathing (Blanco et al., 1987a).

During the first half-hour after birth, rectal temperature falls rapidly in normal infants and animals (Engstrom et al., 1966). Several experiments indicate that cold stimulation of the body in general, or of the facial region in particular, may initiate breathing (Barcroft, 1947; Dawes & Mott, 1959a; Cross, Dawes & Mott, 1959; Ceruti, 1966; Dawes, 1968; Harned & Ferreiro, 1973). Conversely, if babies (Oliver, 1963) or newborn lambs (Harned, Herrington & Ferreiro, 1970) are placed in warm water, respiration is greatly reduced. It has also been shown that cold stimuli at birth can override the negative effects of hypocapnia or moderate hypoxia in newborn lambs (Blanco et al., 1987a). At birth, prompt arousal is manifest by increasing muscle tone, opening of the eyes, increasing body activity, the appearance of purposeful movements and crying (Desmond et al., 1963). The fetus seems to emerge from an inhibitory state as described by Barcroft (1947). The mechanisms for this 'release' from inhibition are not known, but may involve the increase in plasma catecholamines (Lagercrantz, Bistoletti & Nylund, 1981). This might be an important mechanism for the establishment of breathing because of the close relationship between respiratory activity and arousal (Wallace, Benson & Wilson, 1971). Moreover, it is probable that, at the moment of birth, respiration is maintained in part by non-specific external and internal stimuli. These provide important afferent 'noise'

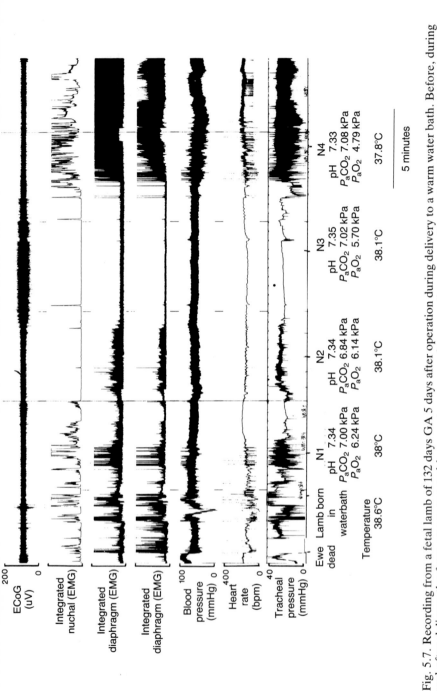

Fig. 5.7. Recording from a fetal lamb of 132 days GA 5 days after operation during delivery to a warm water bath. Before, during and after delivery the fetus was supported by an extra-corporeal oxygenation system. Traces from the top are: electrocortical activity (ECoG); integrated activity of the nuchal muscle EMG; integrated diaphragm EMG, 2 pairs of electrodes; arterial blood pressure; fetal heart rate and tracheal pressure. The cord occluder was inflated, the ewe was sacrificed with overdose of pentobarbital and the fetus delivered by Caesarian section. Note that breathing activity did not start after birth and remained associated with low voltage electrocortical activity. N1–N4 denote points at which blood samples were taken. (Kuipers & Blanco, personal observation.)

which in some way maintains a rhythmic discharge of respiratory neurones (Burns, 1963; Sullivan et al., 1978) and enhances the ventilatory response to hypoxia and hypercapnia (Bowes & Phillipson, 1984).

The use of an extra-corporeal oxygenation system (ECMO) in chronically instrumented fetal lambs allowed delivery of fetuses while maintaining fetal blood gases constant. In Fig. 5.7 it can be seen that breathing activity remained periodic and associated with low voltage electrocortical activity after cord clamping when the fetus was delivered into a warm water bath (Kuipers & Blanco, unpublished observations).

In conclusion, the increase in non-specific afferent input reaching the brainstem reticular formation and the associated increase in CO_2 production play a very effective role in the establishment and maintenance of breathing. These effects are not dependent on peripheral chemoreceptors or vagal receptors. Cold seems to play an important role in producing arousal and overriding inhibition caused by moderate hypoxia at birth.

Mixed venous, intrapulmonary and vagal chemoreceptors

At birth, after cord clamping, there is a rearrangement of the circulation, whereby for the first time the whole right ventricular output flows through the lungs and CO_2 excretion has to be handled by the neonatal lungs. There are three points here that are new to the fetus and are worth consideration: first, metabolic CO_2 production increases significantly at birth (Dawes & Mott, 1959b; Lister et al., 1979; Andrews et al., 1991); secondly, CO_2 may come in contact with possible chemosensitive areas in the lungs and pulmonary vessels; thirdly, oscillations in arterial PCO_2 occur, due to cyclic alveolar ventilation, which will affect chemoreceptor activity (Kumar & Nye, 1985).

There are data, albeit conflicting (Comroe, 1939; Coleridge, Coleridge & Howe, 1967; Cropp & Comroe, 1961; Dawes & Comroe, 1954), supporting the existence of pulmonary artery or mixed venous chemoreceptors which stimulate ventilation (Riley, 1963; Armstrong et al., 1961; Sheldon & Green, 1982). Kollmeyer & Kleinman (1975) reported evidence of venous chemoreceptors sensitive to both PO_2 and PCO_2 in puppies but not in adult dogs. They used an extracorporeal venous–venous circuit to change venous blood gases, and showed a resulting alteration of ventilation.

There are conflicting observations on the role of the increase in CO_2 production and hence the rise in CO_2 flow to the lungs on ventilatory stimulation during exercise (Wasserman et al., 1977; Cross et al., 1987). Nevertheless, there seems to be agreement that inhalation of CO_2 modifies breathing frequency and this effect is vagally mediated. Since vagotomy does not affect fetal breathing activity, the function of these receptors seems to be of no importance in utero. There are no data of their function during the neonatal period.

Abdominal chemoreceptor afferents in the vagus have been identified in the adult rat. These receptors are believed to be concerned with cardiovascular control rather than with respiration (Howe, Pack & Wise, 1981). Whether these mechanisms have any role in the establishment of continuous breathing at birth has not been well studied. However, if they do, it does not seem critical because breathing at birth can be established in vagotomized and chemodenervated animals.

Summary

In summary, peripheral information to the respiratory centres in the brainstem is an important modulator of breathing activity. This afferent input does not seem to be necessary for the presence of spontaneous respiratory activity in utero, even though changes in input can elicit changes in FBM. After birth, some of the peripheral receptors are exposed to adequate stimuli for the first time and the new environment begins to exert its influence on respiratory control. Chemoreception seems to need a period of days before it reaches its adult sensitivity level. Abnormalities in this adaptation could predispose the newborn to a vulnerable period in control of breathing.

References

Andrews, D. C., Symonds, M. E. & Johnson, P. (1991). Thermoregulation and the control of breathing during non-REM sleep in the developing lamb. *Journal of Developmental Physiology*, **16**, 27–36.

Armstrong, B. W., Hurt, H. H., Blide, R. W. & Worckman, J. M. (1961). The humoral regulation of breathing. *Science*, **133**, 1897–906.

Bahoric, A. & Chernick, V. (1975). Electrical activity of phrenic nerve and diaphragm in utero. *Journal of Applied Physiology* **39**, 513–18.

Barcroft, J. (1947). *Researches on Prenatal Life*, pp. 260–264. Charles C. Thomas, Springfield, Illinois.

Barcroft, J. & Barron, D. H. (1937). The genesis of respiratory movements in the fetus of the sheep. *Journal of Physiology*, **88**, 56–61.

Belenky, D. A., Standaert, T. A. & Woodrum, D. E. (1979). Maturation of hypoxic ventilatory response of the newborn lamb. *Journal of Applied Physiology*, **47**, 927–30.

Blanco, C. E., Dawes, G. S., Hanson, M. A. & McCooke, H. B. (1982). The arterial chemoreceptors in fetal sheep and newborn lamb. *Journal of Physiology*, **330**, 38P.

Blanco, C. E., Dawes, G. S. & Walker, D. W. (1983*a*). Effects of hypoxia on polysynaptic hindlimb reflexes of unanaesthetized fetal and newborn lambs. *Journal of Physiology*, **339**, 453–66.

Blanco, C. E., Dawes, G. S. & Walker, D. W. (1983*b*). Effects of hypoxia on polysynaptic hind-limb reflexes before and after carotid denervation. *Journal of Physiology*, **339**, 467–74.

Blanco, C. E., Dawes, G. S., Hanson, M. A. & McCooke, H. B. (1984*a*). The response to hypoxia of arterial chemoreceptors in fetal sheep and newborn lamb. *Journal of Physiology*, **351**, 25–37.

Blanco, C. E., Hanson, M. A., Johnson, P. & Rigatto, H. (1984*b*). Breathing pattern of kittens during hypoxia. *Journal of Applied Physiology*, **56**, 12–17.

Blanco, C. E., Martin, C. B., Jr, Hanson, M. A. & McCooke, H. B. (1987*a*). Determinants of the onset of continuous air breathing at birth. *European Journal of Obstetrics, Gynecology and Reproductive Biology*, **26**, 183–92.

Blanco, C. E., Hanson, M. A., McCooke, H. B. & Williams, B. A. (1987*b*). The effect of premature delivery on chemoreceptor sensitivity in the lamb. In *Chemoreceptors in Respiratory Control*, ed. J. A. Ribeiro. pp. 216–20. Croom Helm, Kent.

Blanco, C. E., Martin, C. B. Jr, Hanson, M. A. & McCooke, H. B. (1987*c*). Breathing activity in fetal sheep during mechanical ventilation of the lungs in utero. *European Journal of Obstetrics, Gynecology and Reproductive Biology*, **26**, 175–82.

Blanco, C. E., Hanson, M. A. & McCooke, H. B. (1988*a*). Effects of carotid chemoreceptor resetting of pulmonary ventilation in the fetal lamb in utero. *Journal of Developmental Physiology*, **10**, 167–74.

Blanco, C. E., Degraeuwe, P. L. G., Hanson, M. A., Kumar, P. & Williams, B. A. (1988*b*). Chemoreflex responses to alternations of F_iO_2 in the newborn infant. *Journal of Physiology*, **403**, 102P.

Boddy, K., Dawes, G. S., Fisher, R., Pinter, S. & Robinson, J. S. (1974). Foetal respiratory movements, electrocortical and cardiovascular responses to hypoxemia and hypercapnia in sheep. *Journal of Physiology*, **243**, 599–618.

Bowes, G. & Phillipson, E. A. (1984). Arousal responses to respiratory stimuli during sleep. In *Sleep and Breathing*. (Lung Biol. Health Dis. Ser.). pp. 137–161. Dekker, New York.

Brady, J. P. & Ceruti, E. (1966). Chemoreceptor reflexes in the new-born infant: Effects of varying degrees of hypoxia on heart rate and ventilation in a warm environment. *Journal of Physiology*, **184**, 631–45.

Brady, J. P. & Dunn, P. M. (1970). Chemoreceptor reflexes in the newborn infant: effects of CO_2 on the ventilatory response to hypoxia. *Pediatrics*, **45**, 206–215.

Bureau, M. A. & Begin, R. (1982). Postnatal maturation of the respiratory response to O_2 in awake newborn lamb. *Journal of Applied Physiology*, **52**, 428–33.

Bureau, M. A., Lamarche, J., Foulon, P. & Dalle, D. (1985). Postnatal maturation of respiration in intact and carotid body denervated lambs. *Journal of Applied Physiology*, **59**, 869–74.

Burns, B. D. (1963). Central control of respiratory movements. *British Medical Bulletin*, **19**, 7–9.

Ceruti, E. (1966). Chemoreceptor reflexes in the newborn infant: effects of cooling on the response to hypoxia. *Pediatrics*, **37**, 556–64.

Clark, F. J. & Von Euler, C. (1972). On the regulation of depth and rate of breathing. *Journal of Physiology*, **222**, 267–95.

Coleridge, H. M., Coleridge, J. C. G. & Howe, A. (1967). Search for pulmonary arterial chemoreceptors in the cat, with a comparison of the blood supply of the aortic bodies in the newborn and adult animal. *Journal of Physiology*, **191**, 353–74.

Comroe, J. H. Jr (1939). The location and function of the chemoreceptors of the aorta. *American Journal of Physiology*, **127**, 176–91.

Condorelli, S. & Scarpelli, E. M. (1976). Fetal breathing: Induction in utero and effects of vagotomy and barbiturates. *Journal of Pediatrics*, **88**, 94–101.

Cropp, G. J. A. & Comroe, J. H. Jr (1961). Role of mixed venous blood PCO_2 in respiratory control. *Journal of Applied Physiology*, **16**, 1029–33.

Cross, K. W., Dawes, G. S. & Mott, J. C. (1959). Anoxia, oxygen consumption and cardiac output in new-born lambs and adult sheep. *Journal of Physiology*, **146**, 316–43.

Cross, K. W., Klaus, M., Tooley, W. H. & Weisser, K. (1960). The response of the new-born baby to inflation of the lungs. *Journal of Physiology*, **151**, 551–65.

Cross, B. A., Leaver, K. D., Semple S. J. G. & Stidwill, R. P. (1986). The effects of small changes in arterial carbon dioxide tension on carotid chemoreceptor activity in the cat. *Journal of Physiology*, **380**, 415–27.

Cross, B. A., Stidwill, R. P., Leaver, K. D. & Semple, S. J. G. (1987). Derivation of CO_2 output from oscillations in arterial pH. *Journal of Applied Physiology*, **62**, 880–91.

Dawes, G. S. & Comroe, J. H. Jr (1954). Chemoreflexes from the heart and lungs. *Physiology Review*, **34**, 167–201.

Dawes, G. S. & Mott, J. C. (1959a). Reflex respiratory activity in the newborn rabbit. *Journal of Physiology*, **145**, 85–97.

Dawes, G. S. & Mott, J. C. (1959b). The increase in oxygen consumption of the lamb after birth. *Journal of Physiology*, **146**, 295–315.

Dawes, G. S. (1968). *Foetal and Neonatal Physiology*, pp. 131–3. Year Book Medical Publishers, Chicago, Illinois.

Dawes, G. S., Fox, H. E., Leduc, B. M., Liggins, G. C. & Richards, R. T. (1972). Respiratory movements and rapid eye movements sleep in the foetal lamb. *Journal of Physiology*, **220**, 119–43.

Dawes, G. S., Gardner, W. N., Johnston, B. M. & Walker, D. W. (1983). Breathing in fetal lambs: The effects of brain stem section. *Journal of Physiology*, **335**, 535–53.

Desmond, M. M., Franklin, R. R., Vallbona, C., Hill, R. M., Plumb, R., Arnold, H. & Watts, J. (1963). The clinical behavior of the newly born. *Journal of Pediatrics*, **62**, 307–325.

Duron, B. & Condamin, M. (1970). Etude au microscope électronique de la composition du nerf phrénique du chat. *CR Seances Soc Biol*, **164**, 577–83.

Duron, B., Jung-Caillol, M. C. & Marlot, D. (1978). Myelinated nerve fiber supply and muscle spindles in the respiratory muscles of the cat: a quantitive study. *Anatomy and Embryology*, **152**, 171–92.

Engstrom, L., Karlberg, P., Rooth, G. & Tunell, R. (1966). *The Onset of Respiration.* Association Aid Crippled Children, New York.

Fedde, M. R. (1970). Peripheral control of avian respiration. *Federal Proceedings*, **29**, 1664–73.

Fedorko, L., Kelly, E. N. & England, S. J. (1988). Importance of vagal afferents in determining ventilation in newborn rats. *Journal of Applied Physiology*, **65**, 1033–9.

Fitzgerald, R. S., Leitner, L. M. & Liaubet, M. J. (1969). Carotid chemoreceptor response to intermittent or sustained stimulation in the cat. *Respiration Physiology*, **6**, 395–402.

Fitzgerald, R. S. & Lahiri, S. (1986). Reflex responses to chemoreceptor stimulation. In *Handbook of Physiology. The Respiratory System. American Physiological Society*, sect. 3, Vol. II, pt 1, chap. 3. pp. 324–5. Bethesda, MD.

Fleming, P., Bryan, A. C. & Bryan, M. H. (1978). Functional immaturity of pulmonary irritant receptors and apnea in newborn preterm infants. *Pediatrics*, **61**, 515–8.

Frazier, D. T. & Revelette, W. R. (1991). Role of phrenic afferents in the control of breathing. *Journal of Applied Physiology*, **70**, 491–6.

Gasser, H. S. & Grundfest, H. (1939). Axon diameters in relation to spike dimensions and the conduction velocity in mammalian fibers. *American Journal of Physiology*, **127**, 393–414.

Gerhardt, T. & Bancalari, E. (1981). Maturational changes of reflexes influencing inspiratory timing in newborns. *Journal of Applied Physiology*, **50**, 1282–5.

Gluckman, P. D., Gunn, T. R. & Johnston, B. M. (1983). The effects of cooling on breathing and shivering in unanaesthetized fetal lambs in utero. *Journal of Physiology*, **343**, 495–506.

Gluckman, P. D. & Johnston, B. M. (1987). Lesions in the upper lateral pons abolish the hypoxic depression of breathing in unanaesthetized fetal lambs in utero. *Journal of Physiology*, **382**, 373–83.

Goodman, N. W., Nail, B. S. & Torrance, R. W. (1974). Oscillations in the discharge of single carotid chemoreceptor fibers of the cat. *Respiration Physiology*, **20**, 251–69.

Green, J. F. & Kaufman, M. P. (1990). Pulmonary afferent control of breathing as end-expiratory lung volume decreases. *Journal of Applied Physiology*, **68**, 2186–94.

Grunstein, M. M., Younes, M. & Milic-Emili, J. (1973). Control of tidal volume and respiratory frequency in anesthetized cats. *Journal of Applied Physiology*, **35**, 463–76.

Grunstein, M. M., Hazinski, T. A. & Schleuter, M. A. (1981). Respiratory control during hypoxia in newborn rabbits: implied action of endorphins. *Journal of Applied Physiology*, **51**, 122–30.

Guz, A., Noble, M. I. M., Trenchard, D., Cochrane, H. L. & Makey, A. R. (1964). Studies on the vagus nerves in man: their role in respiratory and circulatory control. *Clinical Science*, **27**, 293–304.

Hanson, M. A., Kumar, P. & Williams, B. A. (1987). Developmental changes in the reflex respiratory response to alternations of FiO2 in the newborn kitten. *Journal of Physiology*, **394**, 69P.

Hanson, M. A., Kumar, P. & Williams, B. A. (1989). The effects of chronic hypoxia upon the development of respiratory chemoreflexes in the newborn kitten. *Journal of Physiology*, **411**, 563–74.

Harned, H. S. Jr, Griffin, C. A. III, Berryhill, W. S. Jr, MacKinney, L. G. & Sugioka, K. (1967). Role of carotid chemoreceptors in the initiation of effective breathing of the lamb at term. *Pediatrics*, **39**, 329–36.

Harned, H. S., Herrington, R. T. & Ferreiro, J. I. (1970). The effects of immersion and temperature on respiration in newborn lambs. *Pediatrics*, **45**, 598–605.

Harned, H. S. & Ferreiro, J. (1973). Initiation of breathing by cold stimulation: effects of changes in ambient temperature on respiratory activity of the full-term lamb. *Journal of Pediatrics*, **83**, 663–9.

Henderson-Smart, D. J. & Read, D. J. C. (1979). Reduced lung volume during behavioural active sleep in the newborn. *Journal of Applied Physiology*, **46**, 1081–5.

Herrington, R. T., Harned, H. S. Jr, Ferreiro, J. I. & Griffin, C. A. (1971). III. The role of central nervous system in perinatal respiration: Studies of chemoregulatory mechanisms in the term lamb. *Pediatrics*, **47**, 857–64.

Hertzberg, T. & Lagercrantz, H. (1987). Postnatal sensitivity of the peripheral chemoreceptors in newborn infants. *Archives of Disease in Childhood*, **62**, 1238–41.

Hinsey, J. C., Hare, K. & Phillips, R. A. (1939). Sensory components of the phrenic nerve in the cat. *Proceedings of the Society for Experimental Biology and Medicine*, **41**, 411–14.

Honda, Y. & Hashizume, I. (1991). Evidence for hypoxic depression of CO_2-ventilation response in carotid body-resected humans. *Journal of Applied Physiology*, **70**, 590–3.

Howe, A., Pack, R. J. & Wise, J. C. (1981). Arterial chemoreceptor-like activity in the abdominal vagus of the rat. *Journal of Physiology*, **320**, 309–18.

Hussain, S. N. A., Magder, S., Chatillon, A. & Roussos, C. (1990). Chemical activation of thin-fiber phrenic afferents: respiratory responses. *Journal of Applied Physiology*, **69**, 1002–11.

Jansen, A. H., Ioffe, S., Russell, B. J. & Chernick, V. (1981). Effect of carotid chemoreceptor denervation on breathing in utero and after birth. *Journal of Applied Physiology*, **51**, 630–3.

Johnson, P., Salisbury, D. M. & Storey, A. T. (1975). Apnea induced by stimulation of sensory receptors in the larynx. In *Symposium on Development of Upper Respiratory Anatomy and Function.* ed. Bosma & Showacre. Chapter 11. pp. 160–183. US Govt Printing Office, Washington, DC.

Johnston, B. M. (1991). Brain stem inhibitory mechanisms in the control of fetal breathing movements. In *The Fetal and Neonatal Brain Stem: Developmental and Clinical Issues*, ed. M. A. Hanson. pp. 21–47. University Press, Cambridge.

Johnston, B. M. & Gluckman, P. D. (1989). Lateral pontine lesions affect central chemosensitivity in unanaesthetized fetal lambs. *Journal of Applied Physiology*, **67**, 1113–8.

Karczewski, W. A. (1974). Organization of the brainstem respiratory complex. In *MTP International Review of Science. Respiratory Physiology.* Physiology Series 1 vol. 2, chap 7, pp. 197–219. Butterworths, London.

Kirkpatrick, S. M., Olinsky, L. A., Bryan, M. H. & Bryan, A. C. (1976). Effect of premature delivery on the maturation of the Hering-Breuer inspiratory inhibitory reflex in human infants. *Journal of Pediatrics*, **88**, 1010–14.

Kollmeyer, K. R. & Kleinman, L. I. (1975). A respiratory venous chemoreceptor in the young puppy. *Journal of Applied Physiology*, **38**, 819–26.

Koos, B. J. & Sameshima, H. (1988). Effects of hypoxaemia and hypercapnia on breathing movements and sleep state in sinoaortic denervated fetal sheep. *Journal of Developmental Physiology*, **10**, 131–44.

Koos, B. J., Chao, A. & Doany, W. (1992). Adenosine stimulates breathing in fetal sheep with brain stem section. *Journal of Applied Physiology*, **72**, 94–9.

Kumar, P., Nye, P. C. G. & Torrance, R. W. (1983). Reflex responses to dynamic stimulation of the feline respiratory system. *Journal of Physiology*, **345**, 174P.

Kumar, P. & Nye, P. C. G. (1985). Comparison of responses of cat carotid chemoreceptor to oscillations of PCO_2, PO_2 and asphyxia. *Journal of Physiology*, **369**, 146P.

Kumar,P., Nye, P. C. G. & Torrance, R. W. (1988). Do oxygen tension variations contribute to the respiratory oscillations of chremoreceptors discharge in the cat? *Journal of Physiology*, **395**, 531–52.

Kumar, P & Hanson, MA (1989). Re-setting of the hypoxic sensitivity of aortic chemoreceptors in the new-born lamb. *Journal of Developmental Physiology*, **11**, 199–206.

LaFramboise, W. A., Standaert, T. A., Woodrum, D. E. & Guthrie, R. D. (1981). Occlusion pressures during the ventilatory response to hypoxemia in the newborn monkey. *Journal of Applied Physiology*, **51**, 1169–74.

Lagercrantz, H., Bistoletti, P. & Nylund, L. (1981). Sympatho-adrenal activity in the foetus during delivery and at birth. In *Intensive Care of the Newborn III*, ed. L. Stern. pp. 1–12. Masson, New York.

Lamb, T. W., Anthonisen, N. R. & Tenney, S. M. (1965). Controlled frequency breathing during muscular exercise. *Journal of Applied Physiology*, **20**, 244–8.

Lister, G., Walter, T. K., Versmold, H. T., Dalman, P. R. & Rudolph, A. M. (1979). Oxygen delivery in lambs: cardiovascular and hematologic development. *American Journal of Physiology*, **237**, H668–75.

Maloney, J. E., Adamson, T. M., Brodecky, V., Cranage, S., Lambert, T. F. & Ritchie, B. C. (1975a). Diaphragmatic activity and lung liquid flow in the unanaesthetized fetal sheep. *Journal of Applied Physiology*, **39**, 423–8.

Maloney, J. E., Adamson, T. M., Brodecky, V., Dowling, M. H. & Ritchie, B. C. (1975b). Modifications of respiratory center output in the unanaesthetized fetal sheep in utero. *Journal of Applied Physiology*, **39**, 552–8.

Martin, C. B., Murata, Y. & Ikenoue, T. (1975). Effects of PO_2 and PCO_2 on fetal breathing movements in rhesus monkeys. *Gynecologic Investigation*, **6**, 74.

Maycock, D. E., Standaert, R. D., Guthrie, R. D. & Woodrum, D. E. (1983). Dopamine and carotid body function in the newborn lamb. *Journal of Applied Physiology*, **54**, 814–20.

Merlet, C., Leandri, J., Rey, P. & Tchobroutsky, C. (1967). Action du refroidissement localisé dans le declenchement de la réspiration chez l'agneau à la naissance. *Journal de Physiologie* (Paris), **59**, 457–8.

Miller, H. C. & Behrle, F. C. (1954). The effects of hypoxia on the respiration of new-born infants. *Pediatrics*, **14**, 93–103.

Miller, H. C. & Smull, N. W. (1955). Further studies on the effects of hypoxia on the respiration of new-born infants. *Pediatrics*, **16**, 93–103.

Mitchell, R. A. & Berger, A. J. (1975). Neural regulation of respiration. *American Review of Respiratory Diseases*, **111**, 206–24.

Moore, P. J., Parkes, M. J., Nijhuis, J. G. & Hanson, M. A. (1989). The incidence of breathing movements of fetal sheep in normoxia and hypoxia after peripheral chemodenervation and brain-stem transection. *Journal of Developmental Physiology*, **11**, 147–51.

Moss, I. R., Mautone, A. J. & Scarpelli, E. M. (1983). Effects of temperature on regulation of breathing and sleep/wake state in the fetal lambs. *Journal of Applied Physiology*, **54**, 536–43.

Murai, D. T., Lee, C. C. H., Wallen, L. D. & Kitterman, J. A. (1985). Denervation of peripheral chemoreceptors decreases breathing movements in fetal sheep. *Journal of Applied Physiology*, **59**, 575–9.

Natale, R., Clewlow, F. & Dawes, G. S. (1981). Measurement of fetal forelimb movements in the lamb in utero. *American Journal of Obstetrics & Gynecology*, **140**, 545–51.

Nishino, T. & Lahiri, S. (1981). Effects of dopamine on chemoreflexes in breathing. *Journal of Applied Physiology*, **50**, 892–7.

Olinsky, A. M., Bryan, H. & Bryan, A. C. (1974). Influence of lung inflation on respiratory control in neonates. *Journal of Applied Physiology*, **36**, 426–9.

Oliver, T. K., Jr (1963). *Neonatal Respiratory Adaptation*. pp. 117. Public Health Service Publication 1432, US Department of health, Education and Welfare, Bethesda, Maryland.

Parer, J. T. (1980). The effects of acute maternal hypoxia on the fetal oxygenation and the umbilical circulation in the sheep. *European Journal of Obstetrics, Gynecology and Reproductive Biology*, **10**, 125–36.

Patrick, J., Campbell, K., Carmichael, L., Natale, R. & Richardson, B. (1980). A definition of human fetal apnea and the distribution of fetal apneic intervals during the last ten weeks of pregnancy. *American Journal of Obstetrics and Gynecology*, **136**, 471–7.

Philipson, E. A. (1978). Control of breathing during sleep. *American Review of Respiratory Disease*, **118**, 909–39.

Purves, M. J. (1966). Fluctuations of arterial oxygen tension which have the same period as respiration. *Respiration Physiology*, **1**, 281–96.

Rabbette, P. S., Costeloe, K. L. & Stocks, J. (1991). Persistence of the Hering–Breuer reflex beyond the neonatal period. *Journal of Applied Physiology*, **71**, 474–80.

Rigatto, H. (1977). Ventilatory response to hypoxia. *Seminars in Perinatology*, **1**, 357–62.

Rigatto, H. (1984). A new window on the chronic fetal sheep. In *Animal Models in Fetal Medicine (III)*, ed. P. W. Nathanielsz. pp. 57–67. Perinatology Press, Ithaca, New York.

Rigatto, H., Brady, J. P. & de la Torre Verduzco, R. (1975). Chemoreceptor reflexes in preterm infants:II. The effect of gestational age on the ventilatory response to inhaled carbon dioxide. *Pediatrics*, **55**, 614–20.

Rigatto, H., Blanco, C. E. & Walker, D. W. (1982). The response to stimulation of hindlimb nerves in fetal lambs in utero during the different phases of electrocortical activity. *Journal of Developmental Physiology*, **4**, 175–83.

Rigatto, H., Hasan, S. U., Jansen, A., Gibson, D. & Nowaczyk, B. (1988). The effects of total peripheral denervation on fetal breathing and on the establishment of breathing at birth in sheep. In *Fetal and Neonatal Development*, ed. C. T. Jones. pp. 613–621. Perinatology Press, Ithaca, New York.

Riley, R. L. (1963). The hyperpnea of exercise. In *The Regulation of Human Respiration*. ed. D. J. C. Cunningham & B. B. Lloyd, pp. 525–534. Blackwell: Oxford, U. K.

Ritchie, K. (1980). The fetal response to changes in the composition of maternal inspired air in human pregnancy. *Seminars in Perinatology*, **4**, 295–9.

Road, J. D. (1990). Phrenic afferents and ventilatory control. *Lung*, **168**, 137–49.

Ruckebusch, Y. (1972). Development of sleep and wakefulness in the foetal lamb. *Electroencephalography and Clinical Neurophysiology*, **32**, 119–28.

Sankaran, K., Wiebe, H., Seshia, M. M. K., Boychuk, R. B., Cates, D. & Rigatto, H. (1979). Immediate and late ventilatory response to high and low O_2 in preterm infants and adult subjects. *Pediatric Research*, **13**, 875–8.

Schweiler, G. H. (1968). Respiratory regulation during postnatal development in cats and rabbits and some of its morphological substrate. *Acta Physiologica Scandinavia Supplement*, **304**, 49–63.

Sheldon, M. I. & Green, J. F. (1982). Evidence for pulmonary CO_2 chemosensitivity: effects on ventilation. *Journal of Applied Physiology (Respiratory, Environmental & Exercise Physiology)*, **52**, 1192–7.

Sullivan, C. E., Kozar, L. F., Murphy, E. & Phillipson, E. A. (1978). Primary role of respiratory afferents in sustaining breathing rhythm. *Journal of Applied Physiology*, **45**, 11–17.

Trudinger, B. J. & Knight, P. C. (1980). Fetal age and patterns of human fetal breathing movements. *American Journal of Obstetrics and Gynecology*, **137**, 724–8.

Wallace, R. K., Benson, H. & Wilson, A. F. (1971). A wakeful hypometabolic physiologic state. *American Journal of Physiology*, **221**, 795–9.

Ward, S. A., Drysdale, D. B., Cunningham, D. J. C. & Petersen, E. S. (1979). Inspiratory-expiratory responses to alternate-breath oscillation of $PaCO_2$ and PaO_2. *Respiration Physiology*, **36**, 311–25.

Wasserman, K., Whipp, B. J., Casaburi, R. & Beaver, W. L. (1977). Carbon dioxide flow and exercise hyperpnea. *American Review of Respiratory Disease*, **115** Suppl, 225–37.

Watanabe, T., Kumar, P. & Hanson, M. A. (1993*a*). Comparison of respiratory responses to CO2 and hypoxia in neonatal kittens. *Journal of Physiology*, **459**, 141P.

Watanabe, T., Kumar, P. & Hanson, M. A. (1993*b*). Effects of warm environmental temperature on the gain of the respiratory chemoreflex in the kitten. *Journal of Physiology,* **459**, 336P.

Williams, B. A. & Hanson, M. A. (1990). Role of the carotid chemoreceptors in the respiratory response of newborn lambs to alternate 2-breaths of air and a hypoxic gas. *Journal of Developmental Physiology*, **13**, 157–64.

Carlos E. Blanco

Williams, B. A., Smyth, J., Boon, A. W., Hanson, M. A., Kumar, P. & Blanco, C. E. (1991). Development of respiratory chemoreflexes in response to alternations of fractional inspired oxygen in the newborn infant. *Journal of Physiology*, **442**, 81–90.

Witte, M. K. & Carlo, W. A. (1987). Prolongation of inspiration during lower airway occlusion in children. *Journal of Applied Physiology*, **62**, 1860–4.

Wolsink, J. G., Berkenbosch, A., DeGoede, J. & Olievier, C. N. (1991). Ventilatory sensitivities of peripheral and central chemoreceptors of young piglets to inhalation of CO_2 in air. *Pediatric Research*, **30**, 491–95.

Woodrum, D. E., Standaert, T. A., Maycock, D. E. & Guthrie, R. D. (1981). Hypoxic ventilatory response in the newborn monkey. *Pediatric Research*, **15**, 367–70.

Wyman, R. J. (1977). Neural generation of the breathing rhythm. *Annual Review of Physiology*, **39**, 417–48.

6

Control of breathing: central influences

PETER J. MOORE and MARK A. HANSON

Introduction

Breathing is often thought of simply as the mechanism by which the lungs are mechanically ventilated with air to facilitate the acquisition of oxygen, the removal of carbon dioxide and hence the control of arterial pH. However the same respiratory processes are involved in such diverse functions as speech and temperature regulation. The respiratory muscles are also used for maintaining posture.

Discussion of the control of breathing falls naturally into three parts: 1) Afferents: the chemo-, mechano- and thermoreceptor inputs from receptors located peripherally and in the CNS which determine the force of the ventilation required to maintain a constant internal environment. 2) Efferents: the muscular control and co-ordination which causes the pressure changes required to move gas into or out of the lungs. 3) Central control: the mechanism by which all of the diverse influences that impinge on breathing are integrated so that breathing rate and timing are set appropriately. 1) and 2) are dealt with in Chapters 5 and 7, respectively. This chapter concerns the question of central control, but it must be pointed out that the distinction drawn is conceptual rather than real: indeed, as we do not fully understand the processes by which the CNS controls breathing in the perinatal period (or in the adult for that matter) we are forced to discuss central *influences* on breathing. As will become apparent, some of these could be classified as afferent inputs to a 'controller', e.g. the effects of CO_2 or hypoxia on brain stem neurones; other influences could be considered as efferents from the 'controller', e.g. the projections from one group of neurones to another. It may even be that CO_2 and hypoxia act directly on the 'controller' itself. We cannot address these issues in this chapter but hope that, by discussing central *influences* in this way, we will stimulate thought about the ways in which breathing is controlled in the perinatal period.

Relation of fetal breathing to postnatal breathing

Obviously any breathing exhibited by the fetus has little to do with blood gas homeostasis, but it may still be driven by the same muscles and controlled by the same neural processes as postnatally. The question of whether postnatal breathing is a continuation of a prenatal exercise, or the display of a new pattern of behaviour, has been debated for many years. Drawing on data collected from anaesthetized sheep, Barcroft (1946) saw breathing as a new activity for a new environment. The first neonatal breath, he wrote, is 'an event so dramatic as to have stamped itself on the imagination of the idealist as the earnest of a new vital principle; to the realist, the first breath is the necessary initiation of life in a new environment'. Indeed, many at that time believed that any fetal breathing movements seen were an artefact due to the recording method (Snyder, 1949).

Since Barcroft's time it has been established that fetal breathing movements (FBM) are part of the normal behaviour of a fetus (Dawes et al., 1972). They are due to contraction of the diaphragm (Maloney et al., 1975) in response to activity of the phrenic nerves (Chernick & Bahoric, 1974; Bahoric & Chernick, 1975; Hanson, Moore & Nijhuis, 1987) and of the intercostal muscles (Bystrzycka, Nail & Purves, 1973, 1975). Recordings made under ketamine anaesthesia in exteriorized fetal sheep showed that medullary respiratory motoneurones were active, with inspiratory: expiratory discharge time ratios similar to those of the neonate (Bystrzycka et al., 1973; Chernick & Bahoric, 1974). So it is clear that FBM are indeed due to similar muscular processes as occur during postnatal breathing and, consequently, they have often been assumed to be precursors of postnatal breathing.

Recently, however, this assumption has been questioned in the light of evidence showing that, whilst the mechanical processes of FBM and postnatal breathing are in many ways similar, their control is different. First of all, rather than being stimulated, FBM are reduced or inhibited by hypoxia (Boddy et al., 1974). Secondly, in contrast to the adult, the peripheral chemoreceptors play little or no role in the control of FBM (Jansen et al., 1981; Murai et al., 1985; Koos & Sameshima, 1988; Rigatto et al., 1988; Moore et al., 1989*b*). Thirdly, the effects on FBM of several drugs are different from those on postnatal breathing, e.g. the respiratory stimulant almitrine stimulates postnatal breathing but inhibits FBM (Moore, Hanson & Parkes, 1989*a*).

So the question remains: is the breathing seen after birth a purely neonatal phenomenon, or do the same controlling influences act both pre- and postnatally? The hypothesis advanced in this chapter is that FBM and postnatal breathing *are* controlled by a collection of similar mechanisms in the CNS. The resulting output of the CNS in terms of breathing movements depends, however, on the balance of several interacting processes. Apparent changes occurring through development are not due to the sudden appearance of new control mechanisms, but to a shift in the relative importance of pre-existing ones.

In approaching this task, we will start by considering the central chemoreceptors in order to see whether current evidence is compatible with the theory that central chemoreception is a similar process in the adult, neonate and fetus. Then we will turn our attention to the effects of hypoxia on the fetal and neonatal CNS in relation to breathing. Lastly, we will note some of the other CNS influences which play an important, if poorly understood, role in the control of breathing in the perinatal period.

Central chemoreceptors

Since 1868, when Pflüger reported that hypoxia and hypercapnia were both respiratory stimulants, two questions have been prominent. 1) What do 'chemoreceptors' detect, and 2) Where are they located? We will first look at the current opinions about central chemoreception in adults, before considering the data from fetal and neonatal mammals.

The stimulus to the central chemoreceptors

It is well known that the respiratory response to CO_2 and $[H^+]$ is maintained after removal of peripheral chemoreception by section of the carotid sinus nerves and vagi in adult mammals, indicating a prominent site of chemoreception within the CNS. Miescher-Rusch (1885) showed that acids could elicit a respiratory response similar to CO_2 and, in 1888, Lehmann proposed that this was due to the change in pH caused by the presence of CO_2 (Lehmann, 1888). As this idea developed, it became known as the 'reaction theory'. However, a given reduction of pH caused by CO_2 causes greater respiratory effects than an equivalent reduction caused by fixed acids (Hooker, Wilson & Connett, 1917; Eldridge, Kiley & Millhorn, 1985). The greater effect of CO_2 is because it diffuses much more rapidly into cells than do H^+ ions, and thus produces a more rapid swing in intracellular pH. Such a rapid swing depends on the presence of carbonic anhydrase within the cell, which permits the swing in pH to outstrip the cell's mechanisms for intracellular pH stabilization. This concept is supported by the effects of acetazolamide, a carbonic anhydrase inhibitor which is able to enter cells; it slows the respiratory responses to a rapid change in PCO_2 (Hanson, Holman & McCooke, 1984). It explains the observations from an in vitro preparation (Harada, Kuno & Wang, 1985a; Harada, Wang & Kuno, 1985b) that phrenic nerve activity is enhanced transiently by hypercapnia at constant pH, but increased only slowly after lowering pH at constant PCO_2 (Fig. 6.1).

It thus appears that the intracellular pH of 'central chemoreceptor' neurones is critical in providing the adequate stimulus to them, as opposed to the CSF pH as was formerly thought (see Loeschcke, 1982). Techniques have been developed which use small H^+-sensitive electrodes to measure the pH of the CSF and of the medullary ECF independently (Ahmad & Loeschcke, 1982; Eldridge et al., 1985; Kiley, Eldridge & Millhorn, 1985). Changing the pH of the CSF by adding an acid phosphate buffer had little effect on the ECF pH and no effect on phrenic activity. However, a brief cessation of ventilation, which reduced ECF pH without affecting CSF pH, caused a marked increase in phrenic activity (Kiley et al., 1985).

The site of central chemoreception

In 1812, Le Gallois proposed a medullary site for chemoreception, but it was not until 1958 that Loeschcke showed clear evidence for central chemoreceptors. Two gross locations were subsequently identified, bilaterally on the ventral surface of the medulla: one was between the pyramidal tracts and the point where the vagus nerves enter the medulla (Mitchell et al., 1963a,b), and the other medial to the rootlets of the hypoglossal nerve (Loeschcke et al., 1979; Schlaefke et al., 1979). Loeschcke and coworkers (Dev & Loeschcke, 1979; Loeschcke & Fukuda, 1979; Loeschcke, 1982) subsequently came to the conclusion that the medullary chemoreceptors had a muscarinic synapse, from the results obtained by topically applying acetylcholine or a variety of muscarinic antagonists. However, the effects of such agents could be very widespread.

There is now a wealth of literature describing the search for the specific location and cell type of these receptors, which has so far been unsuccessful (for reviews see Schlaefke, 1981; Millhorn & Eldridge, 1986; Konig & Seller, 1991). It is, however, agreed that the ventral surface of the

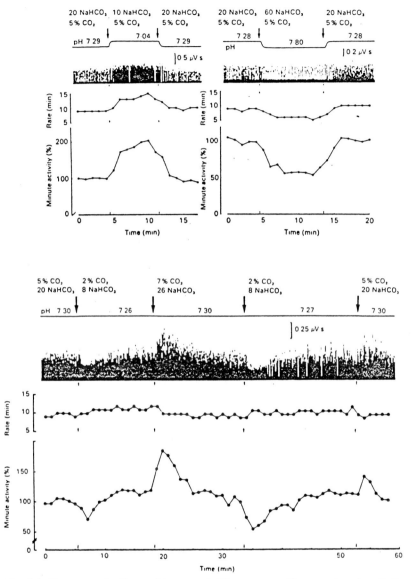

Fig. 6.1. *Upper panel*: effects of decreased pH at constant P_{CO_2} on phrenic activity of isolated brain stem and spinal cord preparation in vitro. Traces from top are: perfurate pH; integrated phrenic activity; respiratory rate; phrenic minute activity as a percentage of control. Reducing (left) or increasing (right) pH produced marked sustained change in phrenic activity even at constant PCO_2. *Lower panel*: As above, but showing the effects of changing P_{CO_2} while pH was held relatively constant. Note that changing CO_2 percentage produces only transient effect on phrenic output. (From Harada et al., 1985*b*.)

medulla is sensitive to changes in pH, especially those brought about by changes in PCO_2, and that carbonic anhydrase is necessary for producing a swing in intracellular pH at the receptors. Whilst carbonic anhydrase-containing neurones have been found in the ventral medulla, the enzyme is present in most parts of the brain (Ridderstrale & Hanson, 1985), but there are still no unequivocal reports of recordings from chemoreceptor cells in the VLM.

In fact, there is no reason to assume that changes in intracellular pH would affect neuronal function only on the surface of the medulla. In their review of central chemoreception, Millhorn & Eldridge (1986) pointed out that Mitchell et al. (1963a) and Schlaefke, See & Loeschke (1970) used large changes in pH applied to the ventral surface and produced only small changes in tidal volume. Thus the possibility exists that changes in pH were induced throughout the brain stem and thus affected neuronal function at more distant sites, producing the effect on breathing. Furthermore, peripherally chemodenervated adult cats still show a marked increase in ventilation with CO_2 inhalation after a local anaesthetic had been placed on the surface of the medulla (Cozine & Ngai, 1967).

Miles (1983) has recorded chemoreceptor activity in neurones ventro-lateral to the solitary tract. Once again it has been found that tonically active neurones excited by changes in ECF $[H^+]$ are not restricted to the ventral surface of the medulla, but are also to be found in the 'vicinity of the ventral respiratory group neurones, and in the dorsal area of the area ventral to the solitary tract' (Arita, Kogo & Ichikawa, 1988).

That neurones in the region of the nucleus tractus solitarius (NTS) are themselves 'chemosensitive', whether or not they receive an input from more remote chemoreceptors, has been shown in vitro for the adult rat using brain stem slices which include the NTS but exclude all of the VLM. In such preparations, CO_2 depolarized neurones (Dean, Lawing & Millhorn, 1989). In vivo, Seller, Konig & Czachurski (1990) showed that, whilst CO_2 excites neurones in the ventral medulla and the NTS to a greater extent than does HCl, the excitation was unaffected by block-ade of synaptic input by topical application of $CoCl_2$. Also, working with excitatory amino acids Nattie et al. (1988) showed that topical application of kainic acid to the VLM initially stimulates, and then inhibits, phrenic output. As kainic acid first stimulates, and then destroys, cell bodies, its effect on respiratory activity is consistent with a stimulation and then destruction of chemoreceptors that serve to increase ventilation.

Central chemoreception in the fetus and neonate

Owing to the inherent inaccessibility of the fetus, data on central chemical control of FBM is sparse. Hohimer et al. (1983) and Koos (1985) showed that infusing an acidic artificial CSF into the cerebral ventricles induced a gradual increase in the amplitude of FBM, the increase taking 1 hour to become maximal. Sustained and vigorous FBM are also produced by infusing NH_4Cl or HCl, again with a time lag of over an hour from the start of the infusion to the point of maximal response (Molteni et al., 1980).

NaCN injected onto the floor of the fourth ventricle of exteriorized anaesthetized fetal sheep induced a sequence of 'gasps' (Jansen & Chernick, 1974). Acids or alkali placed on the ventral medulla also produce effects on breathing in neonatal guinea pigs and rabbits (Wennergren & Wennergren, 1980) after a delay of up to a minute (Fig. 6.2). This is consistent with the concept that the 'central chemoreceptors' do not simply detect immediate changes in the composition of the CSF bathing the ventral medulla, and so fits with the data derived from adult animals. Breathing may not be affected until the chemical stimulus has diffused to a sufficiently large population of neurones.

In contrast to the slow effects of ventriculo-cisternal perfusion with acidic CSF on FBM, fetal hypercapnia leads to a rapid increase in FBM in both intact (Boddy et al., 1974; Chapman et al., 1980), and peripherally chemodenervated fetuses (Koos & Sameshima, 1988). Administration of the carbonic anhydrase inhibitor acetazolamide also stimulates FBM

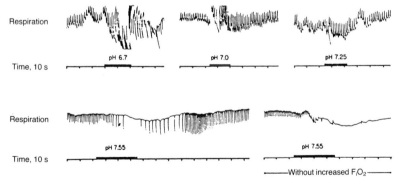

Fig. 6.2. Effect on breathing of a newborn rabbit a few hours old of superfusing the ventral medullary surface with mock CSF of various pH values. Note that low pH stimulates, and high pH inhibits breathing but the effects take some time to be manifest. In the last sequence, the animal breathes air, in the preceding ones, 40% O_2. (From Wennergren & Wennergen, 1980.)

owing to the central acidosis which develops, appearing to be similar to the effect seen postnatally (Hohimer et al., 1985*a*).

In the neonate, CO_2 inhalation stimulates breathing rapidly in both intact and peripherally chemodenervated animals (Fewell et al., 1989; Johnson, 1989; Carroll, Canet & Bureau, 1991). Wolsink et al. (1991) have now used a technique for producing step changes in end-tidal CO_2, whilst monitoring its effect on ventilation. Using the difference in the speed of response of peripheral and central chemoreceptor reflex loops and the difference in transport time of the CO_2 challenge to the site of chemoreception, the contributions made by peripheral and central chemoreceptors can be assessed individually. They did not find an increase in either the peripheral or central component over the first few days postnatally in the piglet, which strengthens the idea that CO_2 chemoreception is functional in fetal life and matures little in the neonatal period.

Further information suggesting that similar 'chemosensitive' mechanisms exist pre- and postnatally came from the work of Hanson et al. (1988). They showed that FBM could be stimulated with the muscarinic agonist pilocarpine, a process similar to the stimulation of adult breathing described by Loeschcke and coworkers above. That this stimulation is centrally mediated, and is not a product of peripheral chemoreceptor stimulation, was demonstrated as it still occurred in peripherally chemodenervated fetuses, and it could be blocked by atropine, but not by atropine methlynitrate which cannot cross the blood–brain barrier.

Hypoxia and drugs which mimic its action

One of the first observations made about FBM was that they are inhibited by fetal hypoxia induced by giving the ewe a low F_iO_2 to breathe (Boddy et al., 1974). This was proposed to be due to active inhibitory mechanisms arising from, or with pathways running through, the upper pons; fetuses in which the brain stem had been transected at the level of the colliculi (Dawes et al., 1983), or in which more discrete lesions had been placed in the ventrolateral pons (Parkes et al., 1984; Gluckman & Johnston, 1987) show an *increase* in respiratory activity in hypoxia.

The inhibition of FBM is not limited to hypoxaemia produced by lowering the arterial PO_2, but may be produced by fetal anaemia (Koos, Sameshima & Power, 1987), carboxyhaemoglobinaemia (Koos, Matsuda & Power, 1988) and methaemoglobinaemia (Koos, Matsuda & Power, 1990). This is interesting because these latter conditions reduce arterial

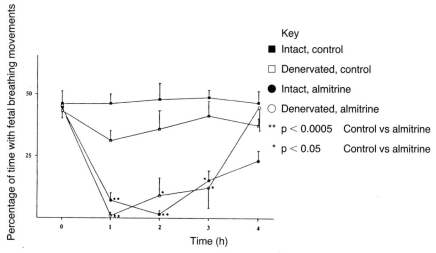

Fig. 6.3. The effect on the incidence of fetal breathing movements in intact or carotid sinus denervated fetuses of 10 mg almitrine in 2 ml 10 mM HCl or of 2 ml 10 mM HCl alone each given at time zero.

oxygen content without changing arterial PO_2. This suggests that a change in brain tissue PO_2 initiates the response. It does not reveal anything about the location in the brain involved. It is possible that, in some areas, the increase in local blood flow during hypoxia (see Jensen & Berger, 1991) limits the fall in local PO_2.

The mitochondrial ATPase inhibitor oligomycin B also inhibits FBM (Koos, Sameshima & Power, 1986). This drug causes a decrease in oxidative phosphorylation (Lardy, Tousky & Johnson, 1965) by reducing electron transfer in the respiratory chain (Tzagoloff, 1982). Thus it may be considered to mimic hypoxia and it may act via a similar mechanism. A second pharmacological agent which appears to mimic hypoxia is almitrine. This drug is a respiratory stimulant postnatally, acting by increasing peripheral chemoreceptor discharge (Laubie & Schmitt, 1980; Bisgard, 1981; Roumy & Leitner, 1981). Almitrine is again thought to act by blocking the mitochondrial electron transport chain (Mottershead, Nye & Quirk, 1988). Almitrine inhibits FBM in normoxia in both intact and peripherally chemodenervated fetuses (Fig. 6.3) (Moore et al., 1989a) so, like hypoxia, its action appears to be predominantly in the CNS. In fetuses in which lesions were placed in the brainstem at sites which result in a stimulation of FBM in hypoxia, almitrine also stimulates

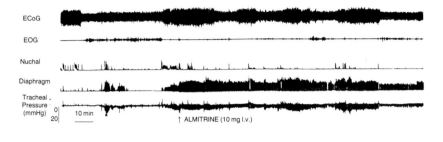

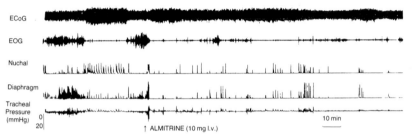

Fig. 6.4. *Upper panel*: Polygraph record from a fetus in which lesions had been placed in the upper pons such that hypoxia *stimulated* breathing. Traces show effect of 10 mg almitrine administered intravenously as a bolus injection over a 60 s period. EOG: electrooculogram. Breathing movements as shown by diaphragm activity and tracheal pressure became continuous through both LV and HV ECoG. Eye movements and nuchal activity still show their normal association with ECoG state, but the activity of both is depressed, an effect that is seen in normal fetal lambs during hypoxia. *Lower panel*: Polygraph record showing effect of almitrine in a fetus in which lesions had been placed in the pons, such that hypoxia *inhibited* breathing as normal. Breathing movements are almost totally abolished. Amplitude and incidence of eye movements and nuchal activity are reduced as in hypoxia.

FBM; in fetuses with brainstem lesions at other sites, in which hypoxia produced an inhibition of FBM, almitrine still inhibited FBM (Fig. 6.4) (Johnston et al., 1990). In the former group, it appears that the lesions unmasked the stimulatory effect of the drug on the peripheral chemoreceptors.

The purine nucleoside adenosine is a metabolite of adenosine monophosphate produced in large quantities during hypoxia (Bardenheuer & Schrader, 1986). Adenosine is known to stimulate the peripheral chemoreceptors in the adult (McQueen & Ribeiro, 1981), and it has also been implicated in respiratory depression via an action in the CNS. Thus it is interesting that its effects on FBM are very similar to those of almitrine.

Administration of adenosine intra-arterially depresses FBM (Koos & Matsuda, 1990) and in fetuses with brain stem transections in which hypoxia stimulates FBM, adenosine stimulates FBM (Koos, Chao & Doany, 1992).

Taken together, the work described above is consistent with the idea that, whilst in the fetus the peripheral chemoreceptors are stimulated by hypoxia, adenosine or almitrine, they are prevented from producing a stimulation of FBM owing to the over-riding action of some inhibitory CNS process. This would explain why appropriate placement of lesions or transections in the brainstem unmasks a stimulation of FBM by hypoxia and these drugs.

At birth, breathing becomes continuous and after a few days a sudden decrease in the inspired oxygen fraction (F_iO_2) produces an increase in minute ventilation ($\dot{V}_E$). This increase is due to stimulation of the peripheral chemoreceptors. However, 2–3 min later $\dot{V}_E$ falls to, or to below, its control value, much in the same way that FBM are depressed (Cross & Oppé, 1952; Brady & Ceruti, 1966; Schwieler, 1968; Cotton & Grunstein, 1980).

This effect occurs even though carotid sinus nerve activity is sustained throughout the hypoxic episode (Biscoe & Purves, 1967; Blanco et al., 1984). Several groups suggested that this secondary fall in $\dot{V}_E$ is due to the operation of an inhibitory mechanism in the CNS. Once again, the mechanism may originate, or have a pathway running through, the upper pons. It may even be the same inhibitory mechanism that operates in the fetus.

There are a number of strands of evidence for this hypothesis, none of which on their own would be strong enough to prove the case, but which taken collectively constitute a reasonably strong argument. Performing transections in the brainstem of neonatal rats and rabbits at a similar level to those made in fetal sheep removes the secondary fall in $\dot{V}_E$ in hypoxia (Martin-Body & Johnston, 1988; Williams & Hanson, 1989). Furthermore, electrical stimulation of the ventrolateral pons in the area adjacent to the middle cerebellar peduncle causes normoxic newborn lambs to become apnoeic (Coles, Kumar & Noble, 1989). Noble and coworkers (see Noble, 1991) have also shown that there are neurones in the same region whose discharge increases in hypoxia.

In order to pursue the idea of a pontine inhibitory mechanism further, Moore and coworkers have developed a technique that allows specific areas of the brainstem of neonatal sheep to be cooled. This effectively produces a lesion (Benita & Conde, 1972) but has the advantage that the

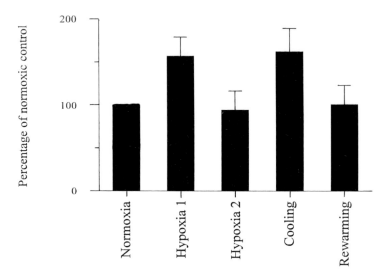

Fig. 6.5. Effect of focal cooling in the upper pons on respiratory response, shown as peak phrenic discharge/inspiratory time, produced by isocapnic hypoxia (P_aO_2 = 37 ± 2 mmHg) in anaesthetized lamb aged 4–8 days. Note that respiratory drive increased above control after 1–2 min of hypoxia (hypoxia 1) but then fell to control over next 5 min (hypoxia 2) although hypoxia was maintained. Cooling the probe tip to 30°C permitted breathing to increase to a similar value to Hypoxia 1, and rewarming reduced it to a similar value to Hypoxia 2, the P_aO_2 being held constant throughout. (From Moore et al., 1991.)

lesion can be removed by rewarming the area. Animals can be used as their own controls, thus increasing the value of the data collected in each experiment. With this technique, it has been shown that the secondary fall in ventilation that occurs in hypoxia can be abolished by unilaterally cooling an area of the rostral pons, and that it returns as soon as the area is rewarmed (Fig. 6.5) (Moore et al., 1991).

The inhibitory response described above is removed by cooling the probe from 39 to 30°C. Benita & Conde (1972) showed that synaptic transmission was reduced in the brain stem if local temperatures were reduced to 20°C, but temperatures approaching 0°C were required to block pathways. Taken together, this is the first data to suggest that the effects in the pons are not simply due to the passage of a pathway through the area, but are due to activity of cell bodies in this area.

None of the above procedures targets highly specific groups of cells in the brainstem, suggesting that, as is the case with the central chemoreceptors, the effects of hypoxia on respiratory activity are caused by a change in the balance of the activity of a diffuse population of neurones. This is seen most clearly from the work of Moore and coworkers (1991) where the cooling probe was placed unilaterally in the brainstem, but it is also true of lesion and transection experiments, which produce highly variable damage. In the case of unilateral cooling, the effects seen cannot be attributed to a bilateral blockade of specific groups of cells. Instead, they are likely to be due to an alteration in the gross balance of inputs to the neurones controlling respiratory output. Indeed, Heywood, Moosavi and Guz (1992) have recently shown that human adults with a unilateral brainstem lesion have an impaired CO_2 sensitivity. This does not contradict the results from studies using transections (Dawes et al., 1983) or electrolytic lesions (Gluckman & Johnston, 1987), as procedures used in both of these studies may have simply been disturbing the balance of inputs within the brainstem, and thus affecting FBM.

There is, of course, an alternative strategy which could be adopted to get a handle on some of the CNS processes described above: this is a pharmacological approach. Micro-injection of excitatory neurotransmitters such as glutamate into areas proposed to be involved in control has been widely used in other contexts, and may assist in mapping the brainstem areas involved, for example in the neonatal response to hypoxia. More specifically, micro-injection of kainic acid could help to establish whether the hypoxia-sensitive neurones are confined to a small region of the brainstem, for if this is the case micro-injection into adjacent areas should cause little or no effect. Application of such techniques will be necessary to examine the possible central action of agents such as the prostaglandins (see below) or progesterone (Skatrud, Dempsey & Kaiser, 1978; Kimura et al., 1984) on breathing.

Adrenergic agonists and antagonists have also been used to investigate the role of catecholamines in the central control of FBM. Murata et al. (1981), working on the fetal rhesus monkey, showed that noradrenaline inhibits FBM, while isoproterenol, a β-adrenergic agonist had a stimulatory effect on FBM. However, Bamford et al. (1986) showed that the α_2-agonist, clonidine, inceased FBM and the α_2-antagonist idazoxan inhibits it. As α_2-adrenoreceptors exert a pre-synaptic inhibition on noradrenaline release, this data suggests that noradrenaline stimulates FBM rather than inhibiting it as indicated by Murata et al. (1981).

In a subsequent study, Bamford and Hawkins (1990) showed that the α_2-adrenergic antagonist MSD L–657,743 also stimulated FBM in normoxia, and also allowed FBM to continue in hypoxia, an effect that Giussani et al. (1993) have recently reported of phentolamine (an α_1- & α_2-antagonist). Furthermore, Joseph and Walker (1990) blocked the reuptake of noradrenaline from the synaptic cleft and showed that FBM were initially increased and then decreased presumably owing to a depletion of pre-synaptic stores of noradrenaline. Fig. 6.6 shows a schematic representation of a noradrenergic synapse showing how these reports of catecholaminergic control of FBM can be integrated. The conclusion drawn is that noradrenaline stimulates FBM, but that the predominant action of drugs is on the pre-synaptic α_2-adrenergic receptor, which when stimulated inhibits endogenous release of noradrenaline. A central neuropharmacological approach may provide an indication of which areas of the brainstem merit further study.

The discussion above has focused largely on the fetus and neonate. However, the mechanisms involved are not necessarily confined to the early stages of life and hypoxia can elicit an inhibitory influence on respiratory control via apparently similar mechanisms in adult humans (Easton, Slykerman & Anthonisen, 1986), rats (Martin-Body, Robson & Sinclair, 1985) and cats (Spode & Schlaefke, 1975). It may be that understanding of fetal and neonatal control mechanisms will shed light on those operating in the adult.

Cerebral blood flow

Tissue PO_2 in the CNS not only depends on the PaO_2 but also on the perfusion of the tissue. Cerebral blood flow increases in hypoxia in the fetus (Carter & Gu, 1988) and the neonate (Massik et al., 1989; Suguihara, Bancalari & Hehre, 1990), and this increase will serve to restrict the fall in PO_2 to which neurones are exposed. This effect of hypoxaemia is most likely to be via a direct effect on cerebral blood vessels, but it is also part of the reflex redistribution of cardiac output in hypoxaemia in both fetus and neonate (Giussani et al., 1992). The rise in blood flow will also produce a fall in tissue PCO_2, particularly as metabolism may also fall. Thus it is possible that a reduction in the stimulus to breathe in hypoxia may result from a reduced stimulus to 'central chemoreceptors' (see above). The idea that an increase in blood flow may therefore account for the second phase of the biphasic response has been discussed

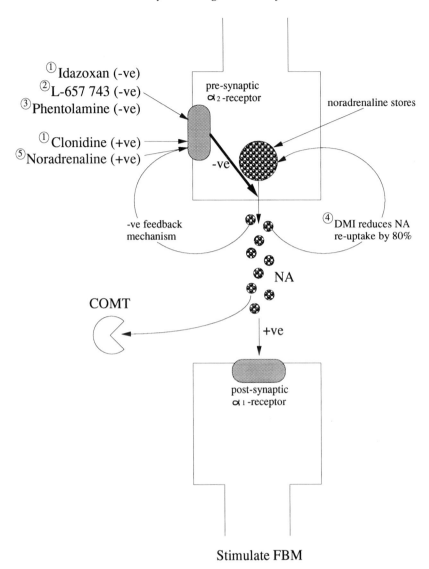

Fig. 6.6. Diagram to summarize concepts about central adrenergic agonists and antagonists on fetal breathing in terms of actions at an adrenergic synapse involved in modulating breathing activity. 1. Bamford et al., 1986; 2. Bamford & Hawkins, 1990; 3. Giussani et al., 1992; 4. Joseph & Walker, 1990; 5. Murata et al., 1981. For discussion, see text.

in the litreature for many years. Suzuki et al., (1989) found in adult humans that there was no correlation between jugular venous PCO_2 and the ventilatory response to sustained hypoxia. There have been also some tests of the hypothesis in the neonate, which to date have not confirmed it. Thus Brown & Lawson (1988) found that medullary ECF pH continued to fall during the second phase as ventilation declined, rather than increasing as would be expected if tissue PCO_2 were falling.

Other influences

To leave a discussion of central influences of the control of breathing here, would grossly oversimplify the picture. The brainstem integrates a host of information from different regions.

Sleep–wake state

Tenney & Ou (1977) pointed out that as sleep affects the rate and depth of breathing (Bulow, 1963), the ventilatory response to hypercapnia (Honda & Natsui, 1967) and to hypoxia (Robin et al., 1958), a rostral influence on breathing is implicated. They showed the presence of both facilitatory and inhibitory influences on medullary respiratory neurones that descend from the diencephalon and cerebrum, respectively. Sleep/wake state is now regarded as an important regulator of the gain of respiratory, metabolic and cardiovascular reflexes (see Chapter 8).

Hypothalamus

The defence reaction initiated in the hypothalamus also has a major influence on respiratory control (Redgate & Gellhorn, 1958). Electrical stimulation of the pre-fornical region of the hypothalamus results in tachypnoea and hyperpnoea (Ballantyne et al., 1988), and thermal stimulation of the hypothalamus results in respiratory rates >100 per min in the adult cat.

Prostaglandins

Prostaglandins exert a powerful influence on FBM and postnatal breathing. Prostaglandin E_2 (PGE_2) decreases the incidence of FBM (Kitterman et al., 1983), whilst meclofenamate and indomethacin, inhibitors of its synthesis, increase FBM (Kitterman et al., 1979; Wallen et al., 1986;

Patrick, Challis & Cross, 1987*a*). The effect of prostaglandins appears to be central, as it is independent of the peripheral chemoreceptors (Murai et al., 1987) and because central administration of meclofenamate stimulates FBM (Koos, 1982, 1985). The same effects can be produced postnatally, with PGE_2 decreasing (Guerra et al., 1988), and meclofenamate and indomethacin increasing, ventilation in lambs (Long, 1988; Guerra et al., 1989). However the change in the concentration of PGE_2 that occurs around birth cannot be solely responsible for either the decrease in FBM seen immediately before birth (Patrick et al., 1987*b*; Wallen et al., 1988), or the onset of continuous breathing postnatally (Lee et al., 1989).

It is, of course, possible that PGE_2 exerts its influence on FBM via changes in cerebral blood flow or metabolism. Indomethacin decreases blood flow to the cerebral hemispheres, subcortical regions, pons and medulla, and increases sagittal vein PCO_2 and $[H^+]$ in fetal sheep (Hohimer et al., 1985*b*), suggesting that the stimulation of FBM by indomethacin could be due to increased $[H^+]$ at the central chemoreceptors. Indomethacin also decreases cerebral blood flow velocities in human infants and cerebral perfusion in adults (Lundell, Sonesson & Sundell, 1989). Murai et al. (1984) reported that, whilst indomethacin increased blood glucose concentrations, this increase could not be held responsible for the increase in FBM seen. Furthermore, glucose infusions during PGE_2-induced inhibition of FBM did not over-ride the inhibition.

Cerebellum

The cerebellum is not commonly discussed in terms of respiratory control. Indeed, Parkes et al. (1984) found that cerebellectomy had no influence on FBM, and neuronal recordings from the brainstem are often made with the cerebellum removed. Recently, however, its role has been discussed (see Paton & Spyer, 1992) in the light of evidence that the cerebellar posterior vermis (uvula) may play a role in cardiorespiratory control, affecting the NTS and the VLM via the parabrachial nuclear complex.

Pons

The 'pnuemotaxic centres' of the pons that are situated around the nucleus parabrachialis medialis and the Kölliker–Fuse nucleus play a fundamental role in respiratory control (Lumsden, 1923; Bertrand & Hugelin, 1971; Cohen, 1971; Bertrand, Hugelin & Vibert, 1973). These areas project to the respiratory-related neurones in the rostral pons by multiple and diffuse pathways, each of which may have only one synapse (Bianchi & St John, 1982; St John, 1986). Pathways exist that allow each 'pneumotaxic centre' to influence both its ipsilateral and its contralateral medullary respiratory centre. Ipsilateral connections appear to be made by direct descending neurones, whilst in contralateral connections, neurones either decussate within the pons and then descend to the medulla, or descend to the medulla before decussating.

Metabolism and thermoregulation

Postnatally, ventilation must be linked to metabolic drive, and the increase in metabolic rate which occurs at birth is clearly an important stimulus for continuous breathing. The precise mechanisms by which ventilation is matched to metabolism have not been established, but their operation is shown by procedures such as exposing newborn lambs to cold stress, which induces thermogenesis and also increases ventilation (Andrews, Symonds & Johnson, 1991). It is interesting to note again that there are descending inhibitory influences on thermogenesis, as lesions in the lateral hypothalamus or transection through the upper pons increases brown adipose tissue (BAT) metabolism (Benzi et al., 1988). Pontine and hypothalamic influences have also been reported to operate in the effects of starvation on metabolism (Keesey et al., 1984; Corbett, Kaufman & Keesey, 1988). The way in which metabolism can affect ventilation in hypoxia is shown by two further observations: first, the secondary fall in ventilation in hypoxia is less in mice and rats which have a genetic BAT deficiency (Hanson & Williams, 1987); secondly, raising the environmental temperature appears to reduce the gain of chemoreflex responses to rapid changes in PO_2 in conscious kittens (Watanabe, Kumar & Hanson, 1992).

Upper airway

Respiratory related upper airway muscle function is important in maintaining upper airway patency (Brouillette & Thach, 1980). In preterm babies these muscles are poorly coordinated with the major muscles of breathing, i.e. diaphragm and intercostals. It has been suggested that this is due to an immaturity in the organization of brainstem neurones mediating upper airway reflexes (Watchko et al., 1989).

The recruitment of muscles that maintain patency of the upper airway (e.g. genioglossus) which occurs in hypoxia is very poor immediately after birth and increases with postnatal age. Even then it is not always sustained. Possibly it too is influenced by a similar mechanism to that which inhibits breathing in hypoxia. Recently, a study by Smith, Li & Noble (1992), involving recording both extra- and intra-cellularly from hypoglossal motoneurones, supports this view: they showed that, although large populations of motoneurones increase their activity during hypoxia, more than 50% do not sustain it, and others are inhibited.

Conclusion

This chapter has two related tenets. The first is that the CNS processes which affect respiratory control in the perinatal period are diverse, not only with respect to their locations in the CNS but also in the stimuli which act on them. The pathways which connect such locations appear to be numerous. As we do not know the anatomical correlates of these influences, we cannot say whether stimuli such as hypoxia or CO_2 act on the same neurones or whether there are specialised receptors for them. The second tenet is that similar CNS processes are involved in the control of fetal and neonatal breathing, but that the balance alters during development, the greatest change occurring at birth, giving the appearance of the involvement of different underlying processes during different periods. The next decade will see major advances in this area, as recently developed techniques for studying CNS function increase our understanding of this important area of physiology.

Acknowledgements

The authors are grateful to The Wellcome Trust for financial support.

References

Ahmad, H. R. & Loeschcke, H. H. (1982). Transcient and steady state responses of pulmonary ventilation to the medullary extracellular pH after rectangular changes in alveolar PCO_2. *Pflugers Archiv,* **395**, 285–92.

Andrews, D. C., Symonds, M. E. & Johnson, P. (1991). Thermoregulation and the control of breathing during non-REM sleep in the developing lamb. *Journal of Developmental Physiology,* **16**, 27–36.

Arita, H., Kogo, N. & Ichikawa, K. (1988). Locations of medullary neurons with non-phasic discharges excited by stimulation of central and/or peripheral chemoreceptors and by activition of nociceptors in cat. *Brain Research,* **442**, 1–10.

Bahoric, A. & Chernick, V. (1975). Electrical activity of phrenic nerve and diaphragm in utero. *Journal of Applied Physiology*, **39**, 513–18.

Ballantyne, D., Jordan, D., Spyer, K. M. & Wood, L. M. (1988). Synaptic rhythm of caudal medullary expiratory neurones during stimulation of the hypothalamic defence area of the cat. *Journal of Physiology*, **405**, 527–46.

Bamford, O. S., Dawes, G. S., Denny, R. & Ward,R. A. (1986). Effects of the α_2-adrenergic agonist clonidine and its antagonist idazoxan on the fetal lamb. *Journal of Physiology*. **381**, 29–37.

Bamford, O. S. & Hawkins, R. L. (1990). Central effects of an alpha$_2$-adrenergic antagonist on fetal lambs: a possible mechanism for hypoxic apnea. *Journal of Developmental Physiology*, **13**, 353–8.

Barcroft, J. (1946). *Researches on Pre-natal Life*. Blackwell Scientific Publications, Oxford.

Bardenheuer, H. & Schrader, J. (1986). Supply-to-demand ratio for oxygen determines formation of adenosine by the heart. *American Journal of Physiology*, **250**, H173–80.

Benita, M. & Conde, H. (1972). Effects of local cooling upon conduction and synaptic transmission. *Brain Research*, **36**, 133–51.

Benzi, R. H., Shibata, M., Seydoux, J. & Girardier, L. (1988). Prepontine knife cut-induced hyperthermia in the rat. Effect of chemical sympathectomy and surgical denervation of brown adipose tissue. *Pflugers Archiv*, **411**, 593–9.

Bertrand, F. & Hugelin, A. (1971). Respiratory synchronizing function of nucleus parabrachialis medialis; Pneumotaxic mechanisms. *Journal of Neurophysiology*, **34**, 189–207.

Bertrand, F., Hugelin, A. & Vibert, J. F. (1973). Quantitative study of anatomical distribution of respiration related neurons in the pons. *Experimental Brain Research*, **16**, 383–99.

Bianchi, A. L. & St. John, W. M. (1982). Medullary axonal projections of respiratory neurones of pontile pneumotaxic center. *Respiration Physiology*, **48**, 357–73.

Biscoe, T. J. & Purves, M. J. (1967). Carotid body chemoreceptor activity in the new-born lamb. *Journal of Physiology*, **190**, 443–54.

Bisgard, G. E. (1981). The response of few-fibre carotid chemoreceptor preparations to almitrine in the dog. *Canadian Journal of Physiology*, **59**, 396–401.

Blanco, C. E., Hanson, M. A., Johnson, P. & Rigatto, H. (1984). Breathing pattern of kittens during hypoxia. *Journal of Applied Physiology*, **56(1)**, 12–17.

Boddy, K., Dawes, G. S., Fisher, R., Pinter, S. & Robinson, J. S. (1974). Foetal respiratory movements, electrocortical and cardiovascular responses to hypoxemia and hypercapnia in sheep. *Journal of Physiology*, **243**, 599–618.

Brady, J. P. & Ceruti, E. (1966). Chemoreceptor reflexes in the newborn infant: effects of varying degrees of hypoxia on heart rate and ventilation in a warm environment. *Journal of Physiology*, **184**, 631–45.

Brouillette, R. T. & Thach, B. T. (1980). Control of genioglossus muscle inspiratory activity. *Journal of Applied Physiology*, **49**, 801–8.

Brown, D. L. & Lawson, E. E. (1988). Brain stem extracellular fluid pH and respiratory drive during hypoxia in newborn pigs. *Journal of Applied Physiology*, **64**, 1055–9.

Bulow, K. (1963). Respiration and wakefulness in man. *Acta Physiologica Scandinavica*, **209**, 1–110.

Bystrzycka, E., Nail, B. S. & Purves, M. J. (1973). Central respiratory activity in the mature sheep foetus. *Journal of Physiology*, **236**, 36–7P.

Bystrzycka, E., Nail, B. S. & Purves, M. J. (1975). Central and peripheral neural respiratory activity in the mature sheep fetus and newborn lamb. *Respiration Physiology*, **25**, 199–215.

Carroll, J. L., Canet, E. & Bureau, M. A. (1991). Dynamic ventilatory responses to CO_2 in the awake lamb: role of the carotid chemoreceptors. *Journal of Applied Physiology*, **71**, 2198–205.

Carter, A. M. & Gu, W. (1988). Cerebral blood flow in the fetal guinea pig. *Journal of Developmental Physiology*, **10(2)**, 123–9.

Chapman, R. L. K., Dawes, G. S., Rurak, D. W. & Wilds, P. L. (1980). Breathing movements in fetal lambs and the effect of hypercapnia. *Journal of Physiology*, **302**, 19–29.

Chernick, V. & Bahoric, A. (1974). Output of the fetal respiratory centre in utero. *Pediatric Research*, **8**, 465.

Cohen, M. I. (1971). Switching of the respiratory phases and evoked phrenic responses produced by rostral pontine electrical stimulation. *Journal of Physiology*, **217**, 133–58.

Coles, S. K., Kumar, P. & Noble, R. (1989). Pontine sites inhibiting breathing in anaesthetized neonatal lambs. *Journal of Physiology*, **409**, 66P.

Corbett, S. W., Kaufman, L. N. & Keesey, R. E. (1988). Thermogenesis after lateral hypothalamic lesions: Contributions of brown adipose tissue. *American Journal of Physiology*, **255**, E708–15.

Cotton, E. K. & Grunstein, M. M. (1980). Effects of hypoxia on respiratory control in neonates at high altitude. *Journal of Applied Physiology*, **48**, 587–95.

Cozine, R. A. & Ngai, S. H. (1967). Medullary surface chemoreceptors and regulation of respiration in the cat. *Journal of Applied Physiology*, **22**, 177–21.

Cross, K. W. & Oppé, T. E. (1952). The effect of inhalation of high and low oxygen concentrations on the respiration of the premature infant. *Journal of Physiology*, **117**, 38–55.

Dawes, G. S., Fox, H. E., Leduc, B. M., Liggins, G. C. & Richards, R. C. (1972). Respiratory movements and rapid eye movement sleep in the fetal lamb. *Journal of Physiology*, **220**, 119–43.

Dawes, G. S., Gardner, W. N., Johnston, B. M. & Walker, D. W. (1983). Breathing in fetal lambs: the effect of brainstem section. *Journal of Physiology*, **335**, 535–53.

Dean, J. B., Lawing, W. L. & Millhorn, D. E. (1989). CO_2 decreases membrane conductance and depolarizes neurons in the nucleus tractus solitarii. *Experimental Brain Research*, **76**, 656–61.

Dev, N. B. & Loeschcke, H. H. (1979). A cholinergic mechanism involved in the chemosensitivity of the medulla oblongata in the cat. *Pflugers Archiv*, **379**, 29–36.

Easton, P. A., Slykerman, L. J. & Anthonisen, N. R. (1986). Ventilatory response to sustained hypoxia in normal adults. *Journal of Applied Physiology*, **61(3)**, 906–11.

Eldridge, F. L., Kiley, J. P. & Millhorn, D. E. (1985). Respiratory responses to medullary hydrogen ion changes in cats: different effects of respiratory and metabolic acidoses. *Journal of Physiology*, **358**, 285–97.

Fewell, J. E., Kondo, C. S., Dascalu, V. & Filyk, S. C. (1989). Influence of carotid-denervation on the arousal and cardiopulmonary responses to alveolar hypercapnia in lambs. *Journal of Developmental Physiology*, **12(4)**, 193–9.

Giussani, D. A., Moore, P. J., Bennet, L., Spencer, J. A. D. & Hanson, M. A. (1992). Phentolamine increases the incidence of fetal breathing movements both in normoxia and in hypoxia in term fetal sheep. *Journal of Physiology*, **452**, 320P.

Giussani, D. A., Spencer, J. A. D., Moore, P. J., Bennet, L. & Hanson, M. A. (1993). Afferent and efferent components of the cardiovascular reflex responses to acute hypoxia in term fetal sheep. *Journal of Physiology*, **461**, 431–49.

Gluckman, P. D. & Johnston, B. M. (1987). Lesions in the upper lateral pons abolish the hypoxic depression of breathing in unanaesthetized fetal lambs in utero. *Journal of Physiology*, **382**, 373–83.

Guerra, F. A., Savich, R. A., Clyman, R. I. & Kitterman, J. A. (1989). Meclofenamate increases ventilation in lambs. *Journal of Developmental Physiology*, **11**, 1–6.

Guerra, F. A., Savich, R. D., Wallen, L. D. et al. (1988). Prostaglandin E2 causes hypoventilation and apnea in newborn lambs. *Journal of Applied Physiology*, **64**, 2160–6.

Hanson, M. A. & Williams, B. A. (1987). A role for brown adipose tissue in the biphasic ventilatory response of the newborn rat to hypoxia. *Journal of Physiology*, **386**, 70P.

Hanson, M. A., Holman, R. B. & McCooke, H. B. (1984). Further studies of carbonic anhydrase at the medullary chemoreceptors of the cat. In *The Peripheral Arterial Chemoreceptors*, ed. D. J. Pallot. pp. 409–414. Croom Helm, London.

Hanson, M. A., Moore, P. J. & Nijhuis, J. G. (1987). Chronic recording from the phrenic nerve in fetal sheep in utero. *Journal of Physiology*, **394**, 4P.

Hanson, M. A., Moore, P. J., Nijhuis, J. G. & Parkes, M. J. (1988). Effects of pilocarpine on breathing movements in normal, chemodenervated and brainstem-transected fetal sheep. *Journal of Physiology*, **400**, 415–24.

Harada, Y., Kuno, M. & Wang, Y. Z. (1985a). Differential effects of carbon dioxide and pH on central chemoreceptors in the rat respiratory center in vitro. *Journal of Physiology*, **368**, 679–93.

Harada, Y., Wang, Y. Z. & Kuno, M. (1985b). Central chemosensitivity to H^+ and CO_2 in the respiratory center in vitro. *Brain Research*, **333**, 336–9.

Heywood, P., Moosavi, S. & Guz, A. (1992). CO_2 sensitivity and breathing at rest and during excercise in human subjects with unilateral brainstem lesions. *Journal of Physiology*, **459**, 353P.

Hohimer, A. R., Bissonnette, J. M., Machida, C. M. & Horowitz, B. (1985a). The effect of carbonic anhydrase inhibition on breathing movements and electrocortical activity in fetal sheep. *Respiration Physiology*, **61**, 327–34.

Hohimer, A. R., Bissonnette, J. M., Richardson, B. S. & Machida, C. M. (1983). Central chemical regulation of breathing movements in fetal lambs. *Respiration Physiology*, **52**, 99–111.

Hohimer, A. R., Richardson, B. S., Bissonnette, J. M. & Machida, C. M. (1985b). The effect of indomethacin on breathing movements and cerebral blood flow and metabolism in the fetal sheep. *Journal of Developmental Physiology*, **7**, 217–28.

Honda, Y. & Natsui, T. (1967). Effect of sleep on ventilatory response to CO2 in severe hypoxia. *Respiration Physiology*, **3**, 220–8.

Hooker, D. R., Wilson, D. W. & Connett, H. (1917). The perfusion of the mammalian medulla: the effect of carbon dioxide and other substances on the respiratory and cardiovascular centers. *American Journal of Physiology*, **43**, 351–61.

Jansen, A. H. & Chernick, V. (1974). Cardiorespiratory response to central cyanide in fetal sheep. *Journal of Applied Physiology*, **37**, 18–21.

Jansen, A. H., Ioffe, S., Russell, B. J. & Chernick, V. (1981). Effect of carotid chemoreceptor denervation on breathing in utero and after birth. *Journal of Applied Physiology*, **51(3)**, 630–3.

Jensen, A. & Berger, R. (1991). Fetal circulatory responses to oxygen lack. *Journal of Developmental Physiology* **16**, 181–207.

Johnson, G. R. (1989). Erythropoietin. *British Medical Bulletin*, **45**, 506–14.

Johnston, B. M., Moore, P. J., Bennet, L., Hanson, M. A. & Gluckman, P. D. (1990). Almitrine mimics hypoxia in fetal sheep with lateral pontine lesions. *Journal of Applied Physiology*, **69**, 1330–5.

Joseph, S. A. & Walker, D. W. (1990). Catecholamine neurons in fetal brain: effects on breathing movements and electrocroticogram. *Journal of Applied Physiology*, **69**, 1903–11.

Keesey, R. E., Corbett, S. W., Hirvonen, M. D. & Kaufman, L. N. (1984). Heat production and body weight changes following lateral hypothalamic lesions. *Physiology & Behaviour*, **32**, 309–17.

Kiley, J. P., Eldridge, F. L. & Millhorn, D. E. (1985). The roles of medullary extracellular and cerebrospinal fluid pH in control of respiration. *Respiration Physiology*, **59**, 117–30.

Kimura, H., Hayashi, F., Yoshida, A., Watanabe, S., Hashizume, I. & Honda, Y. (1984). Augmentation of CO_2 drives by chlormadinone acetate, a synthetic progesterone. *Journal of Applied Physiology*, **56**, 1627–32.

Kitterman, J. A., Liggins, G. C., Clements, J. A. & Tooley, W. H. (1979). Stimulation of breathing movements in fetal sheep by inhibitors of prostaglandin synthesis. *Journal of Developmental Physiology*, **1**, 453–66.

Kitterman, J. A., Liggins, G. C., Fewell, J. E. & Tooley, W. H. (1983). Inhibition of breathing movements in fetal sheep by prostaglandins. *Journal of Applied Physiology*, **54**, 687–92.

Konig, S. A. & Seller, H. (1991). Historical development of current concepts on central chemosensitivity. *Archives Italiennes de Biologie*, **129**, 223–37.

Koos, B. J. (1982). Central effects on breathing in fetal sheep of sodium meclofenamate. *Journal of Physiology*, **330**, 50–1P.

Koos, B. J. (1985). Central stimulation of breathing movements in fetal lambs by prostaglandin synthetase inhibitors. *Journal of Physiology*, **362**, 455–66.

Koos, B. J., Chao, A. & Doany, W. (1992). Adenosine stimulates breathing in fetal sheep with brainstem section. *Journal of Applied Physiology*, **72**, 94–9.

Koos, B. J. & Matsuda, K. (1990). Fetal breathing, sleep state, and cardiovascular responses to adenosine in sheep. *Journal of Applied Physiology*, **69**, 489–95.

Koos, B. J., Matsuda, K. & Power, G. G. (1988). Fetal breathing and sleep state responses to graded carboxyhemoglobinemia in sheep. *Journal of Applied Physiology*, **65**, 2118–23.

Koos, B. J., Matsuda, K. & Power, G. G. (1990). Fetal breathing and cardiovascular responses to graded methemoglobinemia in sheep. *Journal of Applied Physiology*, **69**, 136–40.

Koos, B. J. & Sameshima, H. (1988). Effects of hypoxaemia and hypercapnia on breathing movements and sleep state in sinoaortic-denervated fetal sheep. *Journal of Developmental Physiology*, **10**, 131–44.

Koos, B. J., Sameshima, H. & Power, G. G. (1986). Fetal breathing movement, sleep state and cardiovascular responses to an inhibitor of mitochondrial ATPase in sheep. *Journal of Developmental Physiology*, **8**, 67–75.

Koos, B. J., Sameshima, H. & Power, G. G. (1987). Fetal breathing, sleep state, and cardiovascular responses to graded anemia in sheep. *Journal of Applied Physiology*, **63**, 1463–8.

Lardy, H. A., Tousky, P. W. & Johnson, D. C. (1965). Antibiotics as tools for metabolic studies. IV. Comparative effectiveness of oligomycins A,B,C and rutamycin as inhibitors of phosphoryl transfer reactions in mitochondria. *Biochemistry*, **4**, 552–60.

Laubie, M. & Schmitt, H. (1980). Long-lasting hyperventilation induced by almitrine: evidence for a specific effect on carotid and thoracic chemoreceptors. *European Journal of Pharmacology*, **61**, 125–36.

Le Gallois, C. J. J. (1812). *Experiences sur le principe de la vie notamment sur celui des mouvements du coeur, et sur le siège de ce principe*. D'Hantel, Paris.

Lee, D. S., Choy, P., Davi, M. et al. (1989). Decrease in plasma prostaglandin E2 is not essential for the establishment of continuous breathing at birth in sheep. *Journal of Developmental Physiology*, **12(3)**, 145–51.

Lehmann, C. (1888). Uber den einfluss von Alkali and Sanre auf die erregung des athemzentrums. *Pflugers Archiv*, **42**, 284–302.

Loeschcke, H. H. (1982). Central chemosensitivity and the reaction theory. *Journal of Physiology*, **332**, 1–24.

Loeschcke, H. H. & Fukuda, Y. (1979). A cholinergic mechanism involved in the neuronal excitation by H+ in the respiratory chemosensitive structures of the ventral medulla oblongata of rats in vitro. *Pflugers Archiv*, **379**, 125–35.

Loeschcke, H. H., De Lattre, J., Schlaefke, M. E. & Trouth, C. O. (1979). Effects on respiration and circulation of electrically stimulating the ventral surface of the medulla oblongata. *Respiration Physiology*, **10**, 184–97.

Long, W. A. (1988). Prostaglandins and control of breathing in newborn piglets. *Journal of Applied Physiology*, **64**, 409–18.

Lumsden, T. (1923). Observations on the respiratory centres in the cat. *Journal of Physiology*, **57**, 153–60.

Lundell, B. P. W., Sonesson, S. -E. & Sundell, H. (1989). Cerebral blood flow following indomethacin administration. *Developmental Pharmacology and Therapeutics*, **13**, 139–44.

Maloney, J. E., Adamson, T. M., Brodecky, V., Cranage, S., Lambert, T. F. & Ritchie, B. C. (1975). Diaphragmatic activity and lung liquid flow in the unanaesthetized sheep. *Journal of Applied Physiology*, **39(3)**, 423–8.

Martin-Body, R. L. & Johnston, B. M. (1988). Central origin of the hypoxic depression of breathing in the newborn. *Respiration Physiology*, **71**, 25–32.

Martin-Body, R. L., Robson, G. J. & Sinclair, J. D. (1985). Respiratory effects of sectioning the carotid sinus, glossopharyngeal and abdominal vagus nerves in the awake rat. *Journal of Physiology*, **361**, 35–45.

Massik, J., Jones, M. D., JR., Miyabe, M. et al. (1989). Hypercapnia and response of cerebral blood flow to hypoxia in newborn lambs. *Journal of Applied Physiology*, **66**, 1065–70.

McQueen, D. S. & Ribeiro, J. A. (1981). Effect of adenosine on carotid chemoreceptor activity in the cat. *British Journal of Pharmacology*, **74**, 129–36.

Miescher-Rusch, F. (1885). Bemerkungen zur lehre von den athembewegungen. *Archives of Anatomy and Physiology*, 355–80.

Miles, R. (1983). Does low pH stimulate central chemoreceptors located near the ventral medullary surface? *Brain Research*, **271**, 249–53.

Millhorn, D. E. & Eldridge, F. L. (1986). Role of ventrolateral medulla in regulation of respiratory and cardiovascular systems. *Journal of Applied Physiology*, **61**, 1249–63.

Mitchell, R. A., Loeschcke, H. H., Massion, W. H. & Severinghaus, J. W. (1963a). Respiratory responses mediated through superficial chemosensitive areas on the medulla. *Journal of Applied Physiology*, **18**, 523–33.

Mitchell, R. A., Loeschcke, H. H., Severinghaus, J. W., Richardson, B. W. & Massion, W. H. (1963b). Regions of respiratory chemosensitivity on the surface of the medulla. *Annals of the New York Academy of Sciences*, **109**, 661–81.

Molteni, R. A., Melmed, M. H., Sheldon, R. E., Jones, M. D. & Meschia, G. (1980). Induction of fetal breathing by metabolic acidemia and its effect on blood flow to the respiratory muscles. *American Journal of Obstetrics and Gynaecology*, **136**, 609–20.

Moore, P. J., Hanson, M. A. & Parkes, M. J. (1989a). Almitrine inhibits breathing movements in fetal sheep. *Journal of Developmental Physiology*, **11(5)**, 277–81.

Moore, P. J., Parkes, M. J., Nijhuis, J. G. & Hanson, M. A. (1989b). The incidence of breathing movements of fetal sheep in normoxia and hypoxia after peripheral chemodenervation and brain-stem transection. *Journal of Developmental Physiology*, **11(3)**, 147–51.

Moore, P. J., Parkes, M. J., Noble, R. & Hanson, M. A. (1991). Reversible blockade of the secondary fall of ventilation during hypoxia in anaesthetized newborn sheep by focal cooling in the brain stem. *Journal of Physiology*, **438**, 242P.

Mottershead, J. P., Nye, P. C. G. & Quirk, P. G. (1988). The effects of almitrine on electron transport in mitochondria isolated from rat liver. *Journal of Physiology*, **396**, 91P.

Murai, D. T., Clyman, R. I., Mauray, F. E., Lee, C. C. & Kitterman, J. A. (1984). Meclofenamate and prostaglandin E2 affect breathing movements independently of glucose concentrations in fetal sheep. *American Journal of Obstetrics and Gynaecology*, **150**, 758–64.

Murai, D. T., Lee, C. C., Wallen, L. D. & Kitterman, J. A. (1985). Denervation of peripheral chemoreceptors decreases breathing movements in fetal sheep. *Journal of Applied Physiology,* **59**, 575–9.

Murai, D. T., Wallen, L. D., Lee, C. C., Clyman, R. I., Mauray, F. & Kitterman, J. A. (1987). Effects of prostaglandins on fetal breathing do not involve peripheral chemoreceptors. *Journal of Applied Physiology,* **62**, 271–7.

Murata, Y. Martin, C. B. Miyake, K. Socol, M. & Druzin, M. (1981). Effect of catecholamine on fetal breathing activity in rhesus monkeys. *American Journal of Obstetrics and Gynaecology,* **139**, 942–7.

Nattie, E. E., Mills, J. W., Ou, L. C. & St John, W. M. (1988). Kainic acid on the rostral ventrolateral medulla inhibits phrenic output and CO_2 sensitivity. *Journal of Applied Physiology,* **65**, 1525–34.

Noble, R. (1991). Concepts of neural control applied to the developing brainstem. In *The Fetal and Neonatal Brainstem*, ed. M. A. Hanson. pp. 48–58. Cambridge University Press, Cambridge, UK.

Parkes, M. J., Bamford, O. S., Dawes, G. S., Hofmeyr, G. J., Gianopoulos, J. G. & Quail, A. W. (1984). The effects of removal of cerebellum, brain stem transection, and discrete lesions in fetal lambs. *Proceedings of the Society for the Study of Fetal Physiology*, Oxford, p. 9.

Paton, J. F. R. & Spyer, K. M. (1992). Cerebellar cortical regulation of circulation. *News in Physiological Sciences,* **7**, 124–9.

Patrick, J., Challis, J. R. G. & Cross, J. (1987*a*). Effects of maternal indomethacin administration on fetal breathing movements in sheep. *Journal of Developmental Physiology,* **9**, 295–300.

Patrick, J., Challis, J. R. G., Cross, J., Olson, D. M., Lye, S. J. & Turliuk, R. (1987*b*). The relationship between fetal breathing movements and prostaglandin E2 during ACTH-induced labour in sheep. *Journal of Developmental Physiology,* **9**, 287–94.

Pfluger, E. (1868). Ueber die Ursache der athembewegung, sowie die Dyspnoe und der Apnoe. *Pflugers Archiv,* **1**, 61–106.

Redgate, Z. S. & Gellhorn, E. (1958). Respiratory activity and the hypothalamus. *American Journal of Physiology,* **193**, 189–94.

Ridderstrale, Y. & Hanson, M. A. (1985). Histochemical studies of the distribution of carbonic anhydrase in the cat brain. *Acta Physiologica Scandinavica,* **124**, 557–64.

Rigatto, H., Hasan, S. U., Jansen, A. H., Gibson, D. A., Nowaczyk, B. J. & Cates, D. (1988). The effect of total peripheral chemodenervation on fetal breathing and on the establishment of breathing at birth in sheep. In *Fetal and Neonatal Development*, ed. C. T. Jones. pp. 613–21. Perinatology Press, New York.

Robin, E. D., Whaley, R. D., Crump, C. H. & Travis, D. M. (1958). Alveolar gas tensions, pulmonary ventilation and blood pH during physiologic sleep in normal subjects. *Journal of Clinical Investigations,* **37**, 981–89.

Roumy, M. & Leitner, L. M. (1981). Stimulant effect of almitrine (S 2620) on the rabbit carotid chemoreceptor afferent activity. *Bulletin Européen de Physiopathogie Respiratoire,* 255–9.

Schlaefke, M. E. (1981). Central chemosensitivity: A respiratory drive. *Reviews of Physiology, Biochemistry and Pharmacology,* **90**, 171–244.

Schlaefke, M. E., See, W. R. & Loeschcke, H. H. (1970). Ventilatory response to alterations of H+ ion concentration in small areas of the ventral medullary surafce. *Respiration Physiology*, **10**, 198–212.

Schlaefke, M. E., See, W. R., Herker-See, A. & Loeschcke, H. H. (1979). Respiratory response to hypoxia and hypercapnia after elinination of central chemosensitivity. *Pflugers Archiv*, **381**, 241–8.

Schwieler, G. H. (1968). Respiratory regulation during postnatal development in cats and rabbits and some of its morphological substrate. *Acta Physiologica Scandinavica*, **72**, Suppl. 04–Suppl1-123.

Seller, H., Konig, S. & Czachurski, J. (1990). Chemosensitivity of sympathoexcitatory neurones in the rostroventrolateral medulla of the cat. *Pflugers Archiv*, **416**, 735–41.

Skatrud, J. B., Dempsey, J. A. & Kaiser, D. G. (1978). Ventilatory response to medroxyprogesterone acetate in normal subjects: time conrse and mechanism. *Journal of Applied Physiology*, **44**, 939–44.

Smith, J. A., Li, F. & Noble, R. (1992). The effect of mild hypoxia on discharge frequency of hypoglossal motoneurones in anaesthetized neonatal kittens. *Journal of Physiology*, **459**, 143P.

Snyder, F. F. (1949). *Obstetric Analgesia and Anaesthesia: Their Effects upon Labor and the Child*. W. B. Saunders Co., Philadelphia.

Spode, R. & Schlaefke, M. E. (1975). Influence of muscular exercise on respiration after central and peripheral chemodenervation. *Pflugers Archiv*, **359**, R49.

St John, W. M. (1986). Diffuse pathways convey efferent activity from rostral pontile pneumotaxic centre to medullary respiratory regions. *Experimental Neurolology*, **94**, 155–65.

Suguihara, C., Bancalari, E. & Hehre, D. (1990). Brain blood flow and ventilatory response to hypoxia in sedated newborn piglets. *Pediatric Research*, **27**, 327–31.

Suzuki, A., Nishimura, M., Yamamoto, H., Miyamoto, K., Kishi, F. & Kawakami, Y. (1989). No effect of brain blood flow on ventilatory depression during sustained hypoxia. *Journal of Applied Physiology*, **66**, 1674–8.

Tenney, S. M. & Ou, L. C. (1977). Ventilatory response of decorticate and decerebrate cats to hypoxia and CO_2. *Respiration Physiology*, **29**, 81–92.

Tzagoloff, A. (1982). *Mitochondria*. Plenum Press, New York.

Wallen, L. D., Murai, D. T., Clyman, R. I., Lee, C. H., Mauray, F. E. & Kitterman, J. A. (1986). Regulation of breathing movements in fetal sheep by prostaglandin E2. *Journal of Applied Physiology*, **60**, 526–31.

Wallen, L. D., Murai, D. T., Clyman, R. I., Lee, C. H., Mauray, F. E. & Kitterman, J. A. (1988). Effects of meclofenamate on breathing movements in fetal sheep before delivery. *Journal of Applied Physiology*, **64**, 759–66.

Watanabe, T. Kumar, P. & Hanson, M. A. (1992) Comparison of respiratory responses to CO_2 and hypoxia in neonatal kittens. *Journal of Physiology*, **459**, 141P.

Watchko, J. F., Klesh, K. W., O'Day, T. L., Weiss, M. G. & Guthrie, R. D. (1989). Genioglossal recruitment during acute hypoxia and hypercapnia in kittens. *Pediatric Pulmonology*, **7**, 235–43.

Wennergren, G. & Wennergren, M. (1980). Respiratory effects elicitated in newborn animals via central chemoreceptors. *Acta Physiologica Scandinavica,* **108**, 309–11.

Williams, B. A. & Hanson, M. A. (1989). The effect of decerebration and brain-stem transection on the ventilatory response to acute hypoxia in normoxic and chronically hypoxic newborn rats. *Journal of Physiology,* **414**, 25P.

Wolsink, J. G., Berkenbosch, A., Degoede, J. & Olievier, C. N. (1991). Ventilatory sensitivities of peripheral and central chemoreceptors of young piglets to inhalation of CO_2 in air. *Pediatric Research,* **30**, 491–5.

7

Neonatal respiratory mechanics

JACOPO P. MORTOLA

Introduction

In mammals, diffusion of gases across the skin is of minimal importance for gas exchange; hence, pulmonary ventilation provides the key mechanism for the maintenance of aerobic metabolism. The coupling between ventilation and metabolic rate is achieved via the continuous integration of peripheral information and the generation of appropriate responses (see Chapters 5 & 6). Ultimately, the translation of the neural output into ventilation is constrained by the mechanical properties of the respiratory structures. In fact, once the respiratory muscles are activated, the *force* generated depends on their intrinsic mechanical characteristics (Force–length & Force–velocity relationships). The muscle force will produce a *pressure* the magnitude of which depends on the geometrical characteristics of the muscle itself and of the structure to which it is applied. Finally, the pressure will translate into *flow* according to the mechanical impedance of the respiratory system, with the pressure being dissipated against the elastic properties of the respiratory system to increase lung volume, and against the flow-resistive properties to generate flow.

The goal of this chapter is to summarize the aspects governing the translation of neural output into force, pressure and flow in the neonatal respiratory system, by examining the mechanical contributions of the structures which participate in these processes. Emphasis is given to the human neonate, but comparison with other species will be included when the information from human studies is incomplete. References have been kept to a minimum, with almost absolute preference to general recent reviews; in these, the interested reader will find references to more specialized articles.

Basic concepts and terminology

At the resting volume (V_r), by definition, the respiratory system tends neither to inflate, nor to deflate, and its recoil pressure (P_{recoil}) is nil.

Inflation of the respiratory system above V_r occurs whenever the inflating pressure (P_{tot}) exceeds P_{recoil}. P_{tot} could be generated intrinsically by the inspiratory muscles during spontaneous breathing, or extrinsically, as during artificial ventilation. In the former case, P_{tot} equals the pressure generated by the inspiratory muscles ($P_{musinsp}$), in the latter case $P_{musinsp}$ = 0.

The direction of the change in lung volume depends on the P_{tot}-P_{recoil} difference; with P_{tot} > or < than P_{recoil}, lung volume, respectively increases or decreases (hence flow $\dot{V} \neq 0$), until the equality between P_{tot} and P_{recoil} is re-established ($\dot{V} = 0$)[1]. From the above, it follows that the operational mode of the respiratory system can be defined as

(a) *Active*: $P_{musinsp} > 0$, or *Passive*: $P_{musinsp} = 0$, and
(b) *Static*: Ptot=Precoil ($\dot{V} = 0$), or *Dynamic*: $P_{tot} \neq$ Precoil ($\dot{V} \neq 0$).

In adult humans, during spontaneous breathing in resting conditions, expiration is a passive–dynamic event, since the respiratory muscles are usually inactive; on the other hand, a forced expiration is an active–dynamic process. Breath-holding is active–static, while during relaxation against closed glottis at end-inspiration (a phenomenon very common in the early hours after birth) the respiratory system is in passive–static mode.

For any given $P_{tot} - P_{recoil}$ difference, the magnitude of the volume change depends on the elastic resistance offered by the respiratory system, where elastic resistance (E) is defined as the change in P_{tot} required for a unitary change in volume *in static conditions* ($E = \Delta P_{tot(static)}/\Delta V$); its reciprocal is compliance ($C = \Delta V/\Delta P_{tot(static)}$). The time T_I required for the inflation to volume V, and therefore the $\dot{V}$ ($\dot{V} = V/T_I$) depends on the flow resistance (R) offered by the respiratory system, where R is defined as the fraction of P_{tot} required for unitary change in $\dot{V}$. The previous statements are described by the equation of motion of the respiratory system[2]

$$P_{tot} = E \cdot V + R \cdot \dot{V}. \qquad (1)$$

---

[1] P_{tot} here indicates an *inflatory* pressure. If P_{tot} was deflatory, $P_{tot} > P_{recoil}$ would result in deflation below V_r; this, for example, can occur during the expiratory phase of exercise-induced hyperventilation, where deflatory P_{tot} results from activation of the expiratory muscles.

[2] An additional component of P_{tot} is required to accelerate the gas, its magnitude depending on the inertia of the gas and of the respiratory structures. During resting breathing, it is usually small and, for simplicity, neglected. However, during rapid changes of $\dot{V}$, as during high frequency ventilation, the pressure losses due to inertia can represent an important fraction of P_{tot}.

Table 7.1. *Common abbreviations, specifiers and units*

ab	Abdomen	
C (C_L, C_{rs}, C_w)	Compliance (of lungs, resp.system, chest wall)	ml cm H_2O^{-1}
$C_{Lspecific}$	Specific lung compliance, C_L/V	cm H_2O^{-1}
E	Elastance $(=1/C)$	cm H_2O ml^{-1}
FRC	Functional residual capacity[1]	ml
P	Pressure	cm H_2O
P_{ab}	Transabdominal pressure	cm H_2O
P_{ao}	Pressure at the airways opening	cm H_2O
P_{di}	Transdiaphragmatic pressure	cm H_2O
P_{el}	Elastic pressure[2]	cm H_2O
P_L	Transpulmonary pressure	cm H_2O
P_{mus}	Pressure generated by muscles	cm H_2O
$P_{musinsp}$	Pressure generated by the inspiratory muscles	cm H_2O
P_{pl}	Pleural surface pressure	cm H_2O
P_{res}	Resistive pressure[3]	cm H_2O
P_{tot}	Total pressure moving the respiratory system	cm H_2O
R (R_L, R_{rs}, R_w)	Resistance (of lungs, resp.system, chest wall)	cm H_2O ml^{-1} s^{-1}
rc	Rib cage	
T_I	Inflatory (or inspiratory) time	s
T_E	Deflatory (or expiratory) time	s
V	Volume	ml
$\dot{V}$	Flow	ml s^{-1}
V_r	Relaxation (or resting) volume	ml
V_T	Tidal volume	ml
τ $(\tau_L, \tau_{rs}, \tau_w)$	Passive time constant (lungs, resp. system, chest wall)	s
$\tau_{rs(exp)}$	Expiratory time constant of the resp. system	s

[1] or end-expiratory level. [2] P_{el} equals $P_{tot(stat)}$.
[3] $P_{res} = P_{tot} - P_{el}$.
All volumes are measured in BTPS.

Table 7.1 summarizes the terminology used above, and also includes common glossary and units adopted in the text. A brief summary of the average values of some parameters pertinent to respiratory mechanics in the newborn infant is provided in Table 7.2; a much more comprehensive collection is provided elsewhere (Polgar & Weng, 1979; Mortola, 1992).

Table 7.2. *Average values of some parameters pertinent to respiratory mechanics*

	Newborn infant	Adult man
C_L ml cm H_2O^{-1} kg^{-1}	1.2	2.4
C_{rs} ml cm H_2O^{-1} kg^{-1}	1.0	1.20
C_w/C_L	5	1
R_{rs} cm H_2O ml^{-1} s kg	0.21	0.4
R_L cm H_2O ml^{-1} s kg	0.15	0.34
FRC ml/kg	30	30
FRC–V_r ml/kg	3	0
τ_{rs}	0.2	0.5
$\dot{V}_E$ ml min^{-1} kg^{-1}	310	90
V_T ml/kg	7	7
f breaths/min	45	13

Values are derived from averages of several studies, but variations can be very large, especially in the newborn period, during which the values of all the above variables have rapid postnatal changes. Abbreviations as in Table 7.1.

Passive respiratory mechanics

The lungs

The process of lung development is characterized by formation of primitive airways which gradually branch into more peripheral structures. At birth, in most mammals including humans, this process is not complete, and only a small portion of the adult population of alveoli is present (see Chapter 1). An obvious functional implication would be that the pulmonary dead space is large with respect to the gas exchange volume, although this has not been conclusively documented owing to the difficulties of an accurate measurement of dead space at this age.

The mass of the newborn lung is a larger fraction of body weight than in the adult, but the pulmonary elastin and collagen contents are low, which has some bearing on the mechanical behaviour of the lung. Lung air volume (per unit of weight of lung tissue) and lung recoil (P_L, the collapsing pressure developed by the lung) are low in the newborn, and gradually increase with postnatal development as the pulmonary elastin content increases. The answer to the question of how the newborn's lung compliance (C_L) compares to that of the adult depends on which parameter is used for normalization. When it is compared per unit of lung weight, C_L is found to be smaller in newborns, but the opposite emerges when body weight is used as the normalizing parameter, because of the above mentioned differences in lung weight–body weight ratio with growth. C_L normalized by lung volume (often referred to as $C_{Lspecific} = C_L/V$) is less in newborns than in adults. This is probably due to the smaller volume of the air spaces per unit of lung mass rather than to a lower tissue distensibility. In fact, stress relaxation[3], which reflects the pulmonary viscous properties and contributes to the pulmonary distensibility, is actually very pronounced in the newborn lung, and more important than in the adult. Such plastic behaviour of the neonatal pulmonary tissue tends to decrease the efficiency of the respiratory system, because it lowers the recoil during deflation, favouring air trapping. During inflation, the pulmonary viscous properties contribute, together with the asynchronous behaviour of peripheral lung units, to the phenomenon of the decrease in C_L with the increase in the frequency of ventilation (often referred to as the frequency-dependence behaviour of C_L), which is quite common in the normal infant, unlike the adult.

The specific compliance of the trachea and main bronchi, measured in isolated specimens, has been found to be particularly high in the newborn infant; this mechanical characteristic, coupled to the low lung recoil, can contribute to the dynamic airway compression and air trapping during forced expiration.

Coupling between lung and chest

As in the adult, the passive mechanical behaviour of the respiratory system in the newborn infant reflects the net balance of the forces acting on the lung and on the chest wall[4]. In the adult man, the compliance of these two units (C_L & C_w) is similar, almost equally contributing to that of the respiratory system (C_{rs}). On the other hand, in the newborn C_w is about five times higher than C_L[5] (Polgar & Weng, 1979); indeed, the P–V curve of the respiratory system is similar to that of the lung alone, suggesting that, at least over a large range of V, the passive mechanical

---

[3] Stress relaxation of the pulmonary tissue can be measure in liquid-filled lungs or in pulmonary tissue strips. In the former case, it is the time dependent change in P_L *at zero V* after a step change in V. In the latter case, it is the time dependent change in force *at constant length* after a step change in length.

[4] Chest wall is functionally, rather than anatomically, defined as comprising any structure outside the lung that moves during passive changes in lung volume.

[5] Since $1/C_{rs} = 1/C_L + 1/C_w$, $1/1 + 1/5 = 1.2$, i.e. C_{rs} is about 83% of C_L.

behaviour of the chest wall contributes little to the static properties of the neonatal respiratory system. This fact lends itself to a useful practical implication, which is that measurements of passive respiratory mechanics are much easier to perform than measurements of lung mechanics (Mortola, 1992); these often require the subject's cooperation and the application of techniques, such as use of the oesophageal balloon for estimation of pleural pressure, which in infants are not as reliable as in adults.

A very flexible chest wall is a structural necessity during the passage through the birth canal. Postnatally, C_w gradually drops, because of geometrical changes which accompany lung aeration, and, over a longer time frame, because of the progressive stiffening of the cartilaginous structures. The high $C_w - C_L$ ratio implies that the relaxation volume of the newborn's respiratory system (V_r) and the corresponding P_L are low, as is found in infants and many other species at birth (Mortola, 1987). A low V_r is not a desirable arrangement, neither from the view-point of mechanical efficiency nor from that of gas exchange. The active solutions of the infant to this structural problem are discussed later in this chapter.

Airflow resistance

Airflow resistance (R) was above defined as the ratio between the resistive P and $\dot{V}$. The former equals the difference between P_{tot} and the elastic pressure component $(E \cdot V)$, as apparent from a rearrangement of eqn. 1:

$$R = (P_{tot} - E \cdot V)/\dot{V} \qquad (2)$$

In infants during artificial ventilation (with $P_{musinsp} = 0$, i.e. by definition, in passive mode), P_{tot} can be easily measured as the pressure generated by the ventilator at the airway opening (P_{ao}, Fig. 7.1); as expected, an increase in Pao (between the two dotted vertical lines) generates an inflow and an increase in V, until $P_{ao} = P_{recoil}$ (dotted line d); at this point in time (end-inflation) the system is in static mode ($\dot{V} = 0$), hence $R = 0$, and E_{rs} can be easily measured from eqn. 1 as $\Delta P_{ao}/\Delta V$. If one assumes that E_{rs}, as measured at end inflation, remains constant throughout the inflation, it follows that eqn. 2 can be solved for R_{rs} at any time. Fig. 1 presents three graphical examples of this solution for the computation of R_{rs}, at mid-inflation (A), as the average value during the whole inflation

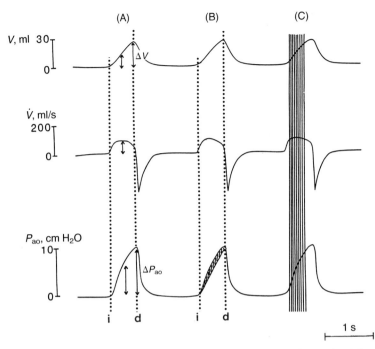

Fig. 7.1. Schematic records of the changes in lung volume (V, top), airflow ($\dot{V}$, middle), and pressure at the airways opening (P_{ao}, bottom) during artificial ventilation. A,B, and C represent three methods for measurements of respiratory system resistance (R_{rs}). i,d indicate beginning of inflation and deflation, respectively. For simplicity, Pao at the end of the cycle (end-expiratory pressure, PEEP) is set $= 0$, although this is often not the case (Mortola, 1992).

(B), or at fixed time intervals during the inflation (C) (Mortola, 1992). The numerical results are not necessarily the same since airflow resistance depends on numerous factors which can change during the breathing cycle, including lung volume itself (Mortola, 1987).

In infants during spontaneous breathing, a simple approach to the computation of R_{rs} is its measurement during expiration. As soon as the inspiratory muscles relax at the onset of expiration ($P_{musinsp} = 0$), $P_{recoil} >$ P_{tot} and the respiratory system deflates. In fact, under these conditions, P_{recoil} is the pressure generating expiratory flow, the magnitude of which depends on R_{rs}. Hence, one analytical approach for the measurement of R_{rs} could be to compute P_{recoil} at any chosen V during expiration ($P_{recoil} = E_{rs} \cdot V$) and divide it by the corresponding expiratory $\dot{V}$. In the spontaneously breathing infant, however, this approach could result in

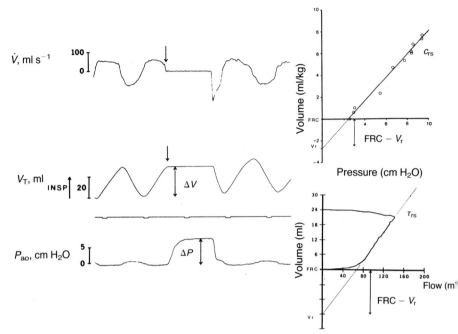

Fig. 7.2. Records of airflow ($\dot{V}$,top), tidal volume (V_T,middle) and pressure at the airways opening (P_{ao}, bottom) in an infant during spontaneous breathing. Time mark = 1 s. At the end of the second inspiration (arrow at top) the airways have been occluded to trigger the Hering–Breuer reflex. From the $\dot{V}$ and P_{ao} values of this and other occlusions at various V_T, the P_{ao}–V relation at top right is constructed. Its slope represents the compliance of the respiratory system (C_{rs}), and the intercept on the y-axis is the dynamic elevation of the end-expiratory level above the resting volume (FRC–V_r difference). The linear portion of the expiratory V–$\dot{V}$ curve following occlusion release represents the time constant of the respiratory system (τ_{rs}) (Mortola, 1987).

incorrect values for two reasons, the often substantial dynamic elevation of the end-expiratory level above V_r (FRC-V_r difference), and the prolonged post-inspiratory activity of the inspiratory muscles (Mortola, 1987). To circumvent these problems, the measurement is more properly performed after a brief artificial interruption of the expiratory flow. As breathing is commonly recorded with a pneumotachograph connected to a face mask, brief occlusions can be easily performed at different times during expiration (Fig. 7.2). The manoeuvre triggers the Hering–Breuer inspiratory inhibitory reflex, and therefore the relaxed conditions required for appropriate measurements; E_{rs} is computed from the occlusions data (top panel at right), and R_{rs} can be measured during the expiration following the occlusion release. If R_{rs} was constant for a large portion of expiration, then a plot of expiratory $\dot{V}$ against expired V yields a linear relationship, the slope of which represents the passive time constant of the respiratory system ($\tau_{rs} = C_{rs} \cdot R_{rs}$, bottom panel at right).

Although the above-mentioned measurements of passive mechanics of the respiratory system often provide the essential information, a more detailed analysis of the lung and chest wall properties would be desirable in some clinical conditions. However, the partitioning of neonatal passive mechanics into its various components, as well as forced expiratory manoeuvres, often relies on important assumptions and the results need a very critical interpretation; hence, they are usually adopted only for research purposes (England, 1988; Wohl, 1991).

The respiratory muscles

Among mammals, respiratory muscle mass is a fixed proportion of body mass, irrespective of species and age; the diaphragm weight, for example, is about 0.35% of body weight in both newborns and adults (Mortola, 1987). If one considers that the force of a muscle is proportional to its cross-sectional area, and that the pressure generated is the ratio between the force and the surface area on which it is applied, the proportionality between respiratory muscle mass and body mass offers the potential for similar values of inspiratory and expiratory pressures irrespective of age. In other words, the smaller respiratory muscles of the newborn generate much less force than those of the adult, but because this force is applied on a proportionally smaller chest the resulting inflating pressure is similar. Indeed, during resting breathing both newborns and adults inflate their lungs with similar swings in P_L (5–7 cm H_2O); during the first inspiration at birth, the muscles generate very high inspiratory P, between 30 and 100 cm H_2O, and the values of maximal expiratory P developed by children are close to those of adults (Mortola, 1987). The similarity in muscle mass–body weight between newborns and adults, and during growth within a given species, despite the remarkable differences in breathing rate and respiratory mechanical properties, suggests that changes in the work-load of the respiratory muscles are not met by changes in muscle mass but by changes in fibre composition and biochemical properties.

The question of the mechanisms which permit the respiratory muscles to work without fatigue, despite their repetitive contractions, has attracted a considerable amount of interest during the last 20 years. As various morphological, biochemical and functional features of the respiratory muscles were becoming known, they were also often compared among different age groups, and more specifically between newborns and adults (Nichols, 1991; Haddad & Bazzy-Asaad, 1991). At various times, several age-related differences have been reported, and some have been quickly interpreted as indicating that the respiratory muscles of the newborn are more prone to fatigue than in the adult, possibly contributing to the apnoeic spells, which are certainly not uncommon in the neonatal period. It is important to stress, however, that the results presently available are still scanty and far from consistent (Mortola, 1987; Haddad & Bazzy-Asaad, 1991). For example, type I high-oxidative (fatigue-resistant) fibres would seem to be in low proportion in the human and lamb diaphragm, but they are in high concentration in the diaphragm of the newborn baboon. Changes in the frequency spectrum of the diaphragm EMG, which some believe to represent signs of muscle fatigue, were first reported in infants during chest distortion, and interpreted as indicating that the diaphragm could become overloaded. Later, however, it was shown that changes in diaphragm power spectrum can occur at any time whether the breathing pattern is irregular or not, and either before or after an apnoeic spell. The contraction time following electrical stimulation of the diaphragm was found in the kitten to be long in the early postnatal days, becoming eventually faster than in the adult cat by 2–3 weeks after birth, a biphasic pattern which has some parallel in the development of muscle fibres. Nevertheless, in the absence of more complete information, the question of the extent to which these and other neonatal characteristics make respiratory muscle fatigue a likely event in the healthy infant remains unresolved.

Low resting volume : problems and solutions

In adult humans, expiration during resting breathing is mostly a passive phenomenon, whereby the expiratory $\dot{V}$ is determined by P_{recoil}, until $P_{recoil}=0$; hence, the end- expiratory level (FRC) coincides with the passive resting volume of the respiratory system (V_r). The observations that all adult mammals have an FRC (and V_r) of considerable size, approximately proportional to their body mass (about 20–25 ml/kg), and that the establishment of FRC is one of the top priorities at birth (Mortola, 1987) are indications that, in the design of ventilatory function, complete lung deflation would not be a desirable event. In fact, by avoiding expiratory lung collapse and the high pressure required to reopen closed airways the efficiency of breathing is increased. In addition, maintenance of open airways favours a more even distribution of ventilation, hence enhancing the pulmonary gas exchange function. Finally, FRC acts as a buffer to the oscillations in alveolar, and hence arterial, gas tensions associated with the oscillatory breathing pattern. Yet mammals, including the human infant, are born with a low V_r, the unavoidable consequence of the high $C_w - C_L$ ratio (see above). The only exceptions are probably some of the most mature species, like the lamb and the piglet, born with a chest wall sufficiently stiff to oppose lung recoil effectively at a relatively high lung volume.

The newborn's solution to the potential problems of the low V_r is to maintain FRC above V_r. The FRC $- V_r$ difference, which in the full-term human infant is about 10–15 ml (or about 3 ml/kg, Fig. 7.2), is the result of co-ordinated active mechanisms which contrive to prolong the time required for expiration (conveniently expressed by the expiratory time constant, $\tau_{rs(exp)}$) with respect to the time available for deflation (expiratory time, T_E). In newborns, T_E is much shorter than in adults, because of their higher breathing rate. The importance of T_E in controlling FRC can be appreciated in the case of apnoea, even of short duration, which is invariably accompanied by a decrease in FRC toward V_r. The short T_E, however, would not by itself explain the size of the FRC–V_r difference. The second important element is the prolongation of $\tau_{rs(exp)}$ above the passive value (τ_{rs}); this is achieved mostly by partial closure of the glottis and by prolonging the activity of the inspiratory muscles during expiration. Both mechanisms, upper airway braking of expiratory flow and post-inspiratory activity of the inspiratory muscles, effectively delay the emptying of the lung, such that the next inspiration begins at an FRC larger than V_r (Mortola, 1987; Mortola & Fisher, 1988).

The integration of the neural mechanisms which contribute to the infant's FRC $- V_r$ difference is not yet completely understood. It is nevertheless important to realize that the mechanical effect of the FRC $- V_r$ difference is similar to that of a positive end-expiratory pressure (PEEP) of 2–3 cm H_2O (intercept on the x-axis in Fig. 7.2, top right); as such, it could also contribute to pulmonary fluid reabsorption during the first hours after birth (Mortola, 1987; Strang, 1991). In paralysed and intubated infants, the absence of the mechanisms normally generating the internal PEEP is effectively compensated by the addition of an external PEEP of a few cm H_2O to the expiratory line of the ventilator.

Chest wall distortion

The design of the coupling between diaphragm and chest wall is such that diaphragmatic contraction results in a rise in abdominal pressure (P_{ab}) and a reduction in pleural pressure (P_{pl}). The former not only expands the abdomen, but also helps in expanding the rib cage via the apposition region, which is the lower region of the rib cage in which the diaphragm is apposed to it without interposed lung (Fig. 7.3, top right). The direction of the diaphragmatic connection to the lower ribs also contributes to the expansion of this region. On the other hand, the drop in P_{pl}, which corresponds to an increase in P_L and therefore expands the lungs, represents a negative trans-rib cage pressure, which tends to pull the rib cage inwards. Hence, contraction of the diaphragm is expected to expand the lowermost region of the rib cage, but also to collapse the upper rib cage.

For a given diaphragmatic contraction and P_{pl}, the magnitude of the inward 'paradoxical' motion of the rib cage depends on numerous factors – the degree of upper to lower rib cage interdependence, the magnitude of the P_{ab} increase, the area of apposition, rib cage compliance, and the degree of concurrent activation of the intercostal muscles (Fig. 7.3, top right). In newborns, the high C_w must contribute to rib cage inward 'paradoxical' motion during inspiration, although the important parameter in this respect is not as much C_w as the relative compliance between rib cage and abdomen, about which no human data are as yet available. P_{ab} increases less in a compliant abdomen, and the more pronounced flattening of the diaphragm reduces the area of apposition. This area, even at end-expiration, is smaller in the newborn infant because, as in most quadrupeds, the ribs viewed from the side are more at right angles to the vertebral column than in adult man. Activation of the intercostal muscles in infants, particularly during active (REM) sleep, is only minimal. It follows, therefore, that in the newborn a large portion of potentially inspired volume (V_T) is lost because of chest distortion.

Fig. 7.3 offers an example of how to quantify the volume loss of chest distortion. The relaxation $ab - V$ line (oblique line) can be constructed with multiple airway occlusions, and is extrapolated to the ab value of end-inspiration; the extrapolated V on the relaxation $ab - V$ relationship represents the V at which the system could have been inflated to, if diaphragmatic contraction, and abdominal expansion, was not accompanied by distortion. The volume of distortion is the difference between the extrapolated passive V and V_T ($V_{pass} - V_T$, Fig. 7.3); in infants during resting breathing the volume of distortion is almost as large as V_T itself.

The question of whether the lack of intercostal compensation to diaphragmatic distortion is dictated by some structural or functional limitations does not have a clear answer. In infants, intercostal activity can increase whenever a large V_T is required, as during crying, sighing or hypercapnic conditions. On the other hand, the fine neural loops controlling the activity of the muscle α-fibres via the proprioceptors do not seem to be as effective as in adults (Mortola, 1987). Therefore, in the newborn, there could be a functional basis for the lower intercostal compensation against the P collapsing the rib cage during inspiration.

Passive versus active mode

An important functional question is whether or not the mechanical properties measured during passive conditions reflect the mechanical constraints confronting the respiratory muscles during spontaneous (active) breathing. The information presented in the earlier sections suggests that the answer to this question will be negative. In inspiration, the effective C_{rs} is less than apparent from passive measurements, because a substantial portion of muscle force and potential inflation pressure is dissipated in the volume of distortion. Other factors, including the intrinsic mechanical properties of the respiratory muscles and the lung stress relaxation, contribute to a dynamic stiffening of the respiratory system. In expiration, the upper airway control of expiratory flow, coupled to the post-inspiratory activity of the inspiratory muscles, effectively prolongs the expiratory R_{rs}, hence τ_{rs}. It follows, therefore, that in active conditions the effective behaviour of the respiratory system departs substantially from that estimated under passive conditions.

Several approaches have been suggested to estimate the magnitude of the active–passive difference, each based on a number of assumptions (Mortola, 1987). In inspiration, a tentative estimate would be that the force of the newborn's respiratory muscles to generate V_T needs to be about twice what would be expected on the basis of passive measurements. In expiration, a visual impression of the passive–active difference can be obtained by comparing the passive expiratory flow-volume curve, obtained as described earlier (Fig. 7.2, bottom right), with the expiratory flow–volume curve during resting breathing; most commonly, the two curves do not coincide, the resting curve being to the left of the passive

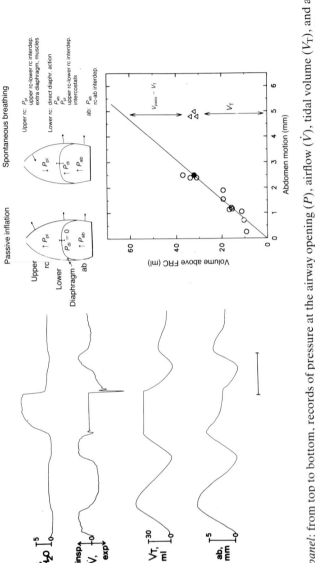

Fig. 7.3. *Left panel*: from top to bottom, records of pressure at the airway opening (*P*), airflow (*V̇*), tidal volume (*V*$_T$), and antero-posterior motion of the abdomen (ab) in an infant during spontaneous breathing. Horizontal bar = 1 s. At the end of the second inspiration the airways have been occluded to trigger the Hering–Breuer reflex, similarly to that shown in Fig. 7.2. Once *P* reaches a plateau, the system is relaxed, i.e. it is in static passive mode. From the passive *V* and *ab* values of this and other occlusions, the *ab-V* relation can be constructed (graph at *bottom right*). The filled symbol refers to the occlusion shown in the record. The slope of the line represents the passive *ab-V* curve. Triangles represent the *ab-V* values of three breaths at end-inspiration (static active mode). At the same *ab*, the *V* difference between the passive curve and end-inspiration represents the *V* lost due to distortion (*V*$_{pass}$ − *V*$_T$). The diagrams at the *top right* summarize the pressures applied to the chest wall and its components, rib cage (rc) and abdomen (ab) during passive inflation and active inspiration. The arrows indicate the expected direction of motion in absence of activity of extra-diaphragmatic muscles. Abbreviations as in Table 7.1.

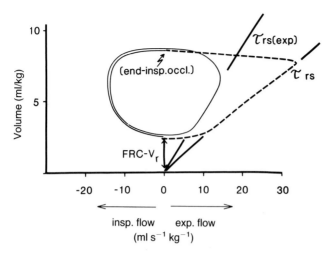

Fig. 7.4. Schematic representation of the infant's flow–volume relationship in active and passive modes. Positive flows indicate expiration, negative flows indicate inspiration. Resting breathing is illustrated by the thin line of the continuous loop. The tangent to the line is the expiratory time constant $\tau_{rs(exp)}$. At end-inspiration the airways are briefly occluded to promote muscle relaxation; the slope of the flow–volume curve during the deflation following the occlusion release (dashed line) is the passive time constant of the respiratory system τ_{rs}, which is normally shorter than $\tau_{rs(exp)}$. FRC-V_r, difference between end-expiratory level and resting volume of the respiratory system.

curve (Fig. 7.4). This indicates that the expiratory time constant $\tau_{rs(exp)}$, which, at any flow, is the tangent to the curve, is longer than τ_{rs}, a phenomenon reflecting the active prolongation in R_{rs} mentioned above.

Concluding remarks

Most of the mechanical aspects of the respiratory system in the newborn have by now been explored in the human infant and in many other species, and the major developmental changes and differences from the adult have been defined. This research has provided two important by-products. First, we now have a battery of simple and relatively inexpensive techniques which can be easily applied as part of the clinical assessment of the human infant. Nevertheless, their correct application as useful clinical tools and the proper interpretation of the results require complete critical awareness of the premises and of the assumptions on which each technique is based. Secondly, studies on newborns, possibly more than on adults, have helped us to realize that the mechanical behaviour of the respiratory system varies remarkably depending upon the conditions that we are examining. The classic approach to passive mechanics is useful, in that the results provide us with functional values about the morphological structure of the respiratory system. Yet the information on passive mechanics provides only the background to understanding the overall mechanical behaviour under active conditions. Numerous neural mechanisms effectively modify the passive mechanical properties, in an effort to integrate them with the metabolic and ventilatory requirements of the organism.

References

England, S. J. (1988). Current techniques for assessing pulmonary function in the newborn infant: advantages and limitations. *Pediatric Pulmonology*, **5**, 48–53.

Haddad, G. G. & Bazzy-Asaad, A. R. (1991). Respiratory muscle function: implications for ventilatory failure. In *Basic Mechanisms of Pediatric Respiratory Disease, Cellular and Integrative,* ed. V. Chernick & R. B. Mellins. Chap. 9, pp. 100–13. B. C. Decker Inc, Philadelphia.

Mortola, J. P. (1987). Dynamics of breathing in newborn mammals. *Physiological Reviews*, **67**, 187–243.

Mortola, J. P. (1992). Measurements of respiratory mechanics. In *Fetal and Neonatal Physiology*, ed. R. A. Polin & W. W. Fox. Vol. 1, chapter 77, pp. 813–822. Saunders Co, Philadelphia.

Mortola, J. P. & Fisher, J. T. (1988). Upper airway reflexes in newborns. In *Respiratory Function of the Upper Airway*, ed. O. P. Mathew & G. Sant'Ambrogio. Lung Biology in Health and Disease Series. Vol 35, pp. 303–57. Marcel Dekker Inc, New York.

Nichols, D. G. (1991). Respiratory muscle performance in infants and children. *Journal of Pediatrics*, **118**, 493–502.

Polgar, G. & Weng, T. R. (1979). The functional development of the respiratory system. From the period of gestation to adulthood. *American Review of Respiratory Disease*, **120**, 625–95.

Strang, L. B. (1991). Fetal lung liquid: secretion and reabsorption. *Physiological Reviews*, **71**, 991–1016.

Wohl, M. E. B. (1991). Lung mechanics in the developing human infant. In *Basic Mechanisms of Pediatric Respiratory Disease, Cellular and Integrative*, ed. V. Chernick & R. B. Mellins. pp. 89–99. B. C. Decker Inc, Philadelphia.

8

Breathing during sleep in fetus and newborn

MONIQUE BONORA and MICHÈLE BOULÉ

Introduction

For many years, the standard experimental model for fetal research was the acutely exteriorized ovine fetus, a preparation first used in 1927 by Huggett and later refined by Barcroft and Barron (1937–1938). Because of possible doubts about the physiological normality of acute studies on exteriorized fetuses, fetal breathing movements (FBM) observed in these experiments have not been accepted generally as being normal physiological events. During the last few decades, chronic animal experiments and human fetal observations performed in utero have facilitated research into fetal breathing and have established (Dawes et al., 1972), that the normal fetus makes respiratory movements in utero. These breathing movements which are a universal phenomenon of fetal mammals, appear to be intimately related to behavioural states and are necessary for lung development. The present knowledge of fetal respiratory control in relation to behaviour and sleep will be briefly reviewed here. More detailed reviews of the control of fetal breathing are given in Chapters 5 and 6. The bulk of this chapter is concerned with the control of neonatal breathing in sleep.

Fetus

Development of fetal behavioural states

As in newborn babies, three different types of behaviour corresponding to wakefulness, quiet sleep and active or paradoxical sleep have been described in near term fetal sheep (Ruckebusch, 1972; Dawes et al., 1972; Ioffe et al., 1980a). These different behavioural states were determined by assessment of electrocorticogram (ECoG), analysis of eye movements (lateral rectus EMG) and nuchal muscle activity. High voltage slow wave activity was considered as quiet sleep or 'NREM sleep' and low voltage fast electrocortical activity accompanied by eye move-

ments and absence of nuchal muscle activity was regarded as paradoxical
or 'REM sleep'. The same ECoG activity with no eye movements but
with muscle tone was interpreted as 'wakefulness' (Ruckebush, 1972;
Dawes et al., 1972; Ioffe et al., 1980a). However, when behavioural
states were observed through a double-walled plexiglas window, the state
of wakefulness with eyes open as observed postnatally was never seen in
the fetus (Rigatto, Moore & Cates, 1986).

In the fetal lamb (term 145 days), the ECoG has been studied from 95
days gestation. Up to 106 days, although electrocortical activity has been
observed, there was no evidence of episodic changes in ECoG between
high and low voltage activity. Between 107 days and 120 days (0.7–0.8
term of gestation), brief episodes of high and low voltage ECoG activity
were observed and after 120 days gestation, the alternating periods of
high and low voltage activity were clearly definable (see Clewlow et al.,
1983). Two weeks prepartum, fetal lambs have been shown to spend
about 40% of the time in REM sleep and 54% in NREM sleep. The mean
durations of REM and NREM sleep periods were 16 min and 21.5 min,
respectively (Ruckebusch, Gaujoux & Eghbali, 1977; Ioffe et al., 1980b).
In the younger fetus when ECoG activity is not yet differentiated, the
presence of eye movements and lack of nuchal muscle tone have been
used to identify REM sleep state (Ioffe, Jansen & Chernick, 1987).

In near term human fetuses, Nijhuis et al., (1982) have determined
behavioural states similar to those of newborn infants (Prechtl, 1974)
using real time ultrasonic imaging and a fetal heart rate measurement
technique. By using the same technique, Arduini et al.,. (1986) have
described quiet and active phases. The quiet phases, characterized by the
absence of gross body and eye movements and low heart rate variability
(<10 beats/min), have been identified as NREM sleep periods, while the
active phases with rapid eye movements were considered as REM sleep
periods (active phases occupying 73% and quiet phases 26% of the time).
Also, it has been proposed that the active phases, in which there were
only intermittent eye movements, correspond to the waking state
(Arduini et al., 1986). These phases were clearly detected from 28 weeks
of gestation but well-defined fetal behavioural states were observed only
after 36 weeks gestation.

Development of fetal breathing during sleep

Most of the work in which fetal breathing movements were studied in
relation to behavioural states was performed on chronically instrumented

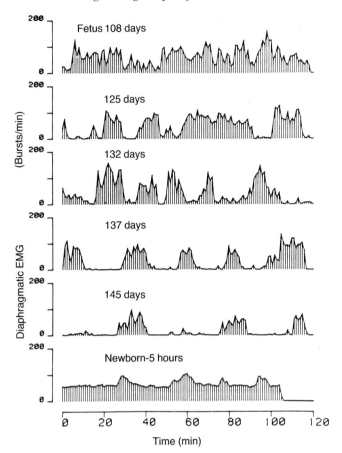

Fig. 8.1. Analysis of diaphragmatic electromyogram (EMG) activity from sheep fetus at five different gestational ages and as a newborn. Rate of respiratory activity is shown on ordinate for each minute of 2 h recording period (newborn record only 105 min duration). Gestational age (days) is displayed on each graph, as is post-delivery time (h) for newborn. Note increasing duration of periods of diaphragmatic quiescence as gestation proceeds and significant change in respiratory pattern after delivery. (From Bowes et al., 1981.)

fetal lambs in utero. FBM were assessed from tracheal pressure changes (Dawes et al., 1972; Boddy et al., 1974; Ioffe et al., 1980a) and by diaphragmatic electromyogram (EMG) activity (Bowes et al., 1981) (Fig. 8.1, Fig. 8.2). In the human fetus, FBM have been recorded by real time two-dimensional B mode ultrasound imaging (Nijhuis et al., 1983; Arduini et al., 1986).

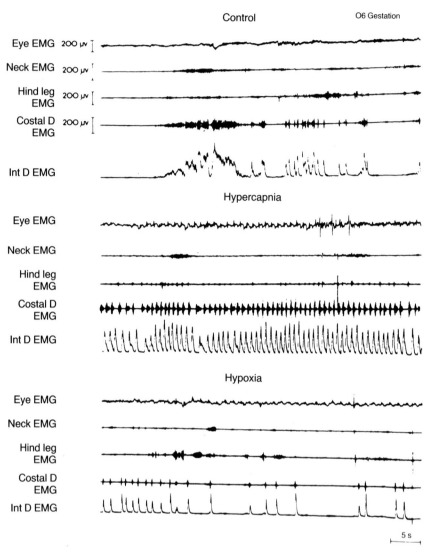

Fig. 8.2. Sheep fetus at 0.6 gestation (87–100 days) showing recordings made during control, hypercapnia and hypoxaemia of EMGs of eye muscle, extensor muscle of neck, hind limb and costal diaphragm (raw and integrated signals shown). (From Ioffe et al., 1987.)

Although FBM have been observed in fetal lambs as early as 40 days gestation, chronic experiments have been performed only from 70 days gestation. Up to 108 days, when the ECoG is still undifferentiated, FBM are reported to be continuous even if their rate is very low

(Maloney, Bowes & Wilkinson, 1980; Bowes et al., 1981; Clewlow et al., 1983). During the last third of gestation, the periods of absent FBM become progressively longer until the pattern described in the near term fetus is established. In the near term fetal lamb, FBM are characterized by their 'episodic' nature as they occur for 30–40% of the time and only during REM sleep. Apnoeic periods were also observed in REM sleep over 17 to 35% of the recording time (Dawes et al., 1972; Boddy et al., 1974; Jansen et al., 1982). FBM have also been described as 'rapid and irregular' in frequency (60 to 240/min) and depth. Short bursts of very rapid breathing may alternate with episodes of slow and regular breathing or with pauses of various length independent of the fetal blood gases (Dawes et al., 1972).

In human fetuses, FBM studies have shown conflicting results. According to Nijhuis et al. (1983), between 37 and 41 weeks gestation FBM were observed in states equivalent to both REM and NREM sleep, but a pattern of more regular breathing was concomitant with NREM sleep. In contrast, Arduini et al. (1986) have found that after 38 weeks, FBM were almost exclusively observed in a state equivalent to REM sleep.

Newborn

Determination of behavioural states

In the newborn, the different behavioural states are usually determined as in adults, by observation of behaviour and polygraphic recordings of electroencephalogram (EEG), muscle tone, eye movements, breathing and heart rate. Because the EEG is undergoing major developmental changes in preterm and full-term infants, as it does in some immature animals up to the age of 2–3 weeks (Jouvet-Mounier, Astic & Lacote, 1970; Anders & Keener, 1985), an accurate assessment of the different states of vigilance has been made essentially by examining the electromyogram of the neck or submental muscle combined with several behavioural observations (Prechtl, 1974). The different behavioural states have also been distinguished by using a non-invasive technique based on the recording of total body and respiratory movements with a static charge sensitive bed (Hilakivi & Hilakivi, 1986).

The states of vigilance are divided into active sleep (or REM sleep), quiet sleep (or non-REM sleep), transitional sleep (a mixture of active and quiet sleep characteristics in immature infants), and wakefulness (sometimes separated into alert & quiet). 'REM sleep' is essentially characterized by low voltage fast EEG, rapid eye movements, absence of tonic muscle activity with twitches and irregular breathing, 'NREM sleep' by high voltage slow EEG or 'tracé alternant', moderate EMG activity, no eye movements and regular breathing, and 'wakefulness' by a similar EEG as during REM sleep, tonic muscle activity and no eye movements.

The percentage of time spent in each sleep–wake state depends on the given species and the gestational and postnatal age. Except for the first day after birth, when the average duration of REM sleep is shorter than on the following days (Jouvet-Mounier et al., 1970; Prechtl, 1974), a full-term infant spends an average of 50% of the time in REM sleep (Roffwarg, Muzio & Dement, 1966; Anders & Keener, 1985), whereas in a preterm infant the percentage of time in REM sleep is approximately 58% at 36–38 weeks (Roffwarg et al., 1966; Parmelee et al., 1967). With advancing postnatal age, the proportion of REM sleep diminishes, an adult-like sleep pattern occurring only later in the first year of infant life (Anders & Keener, 1985). Conversely, the percentage of time spent in wakefulness increases with maturation while the amount of NREM sleep (quiet and transitional sleep being combined together) is relatively unchanged (Roffwarg et al., 1966; Hilakivi & Hilakivi, 1986; Scott, Inman & Moss, 1990).

In animals, the distribution of sleep–wakefulness in a given species depends on the degree of maturity of its central nervous system. The more immature the animal is at birth, the greater is the time spent in REM sleep in early life. Indeed, newborn rats spend 70% of the time in REM sleep in the first week of life, whereas some precocial animal species such as lambs or guinea-pigs show a sleep staging already qualitatively similar to the adult spending only 7–8% of sleep time in REM during the first 5 postnatal weeks (Jouvet-Mounier et al., 1970; Ball et al., 1989).

The sleep–wake pattern also differs from that of adults, in as much as the duration of each state during a cycle is shorter in the newborn than in the adult; moreover, in the newborn REM sleep periods often occur immediately after wakefulness, while in the adult REM periods only occur after a consistent period of NREM sleep. Other factors have been shown to influence the incidence and duration of sleep epochs, such as the type of feeding or the environmental temperature. It has been found that breast-fed infants have significantly fewer REM epochs when compared to formula-fed infants (Steinschneider & Weinstein, 1983). In preterm infants, Brück, Parmelee & Brück (1962) reported that when ambient temperature was increased to 35°C, the cyclical pattern of REM and NREM sleep was apparently unchanged, while when ambient temperature was below the thermoneutral range of 32°–34°C, the total length of NREM sleep was shortened. Similarly, in young lambs, exposure to a cool environment (10–15°C) did not change the pattern of NREM sleep, but REM sleep was significantly altered with a reduction of total REM sleep time owing to the decrease in both the number and length of REM sleep episodes (Ball et al., 1989), or with shortened but more frequent REM sleep episodes (Berger, Horne & Walker, 1989). The abbreviation of the REM epochs in cool temperatures induced by arousal may be considered as an important mechanism in controlling respiratory activity, especially in infants suffering from prolonged sleep apnoea.

Resting ventilation during sleep

The respiratory activity of newborn infants and animals is measured by using several methods such as a trunk plethysmograph (Cross, 1949), body plethysmograph based on a barometric method (Drorbaugh & Fenn, 1955), face mask connected to a pneumotachograph, nasal prongs and a hot-wire anemometer (Godal et al., 1976), nose piece and screen flowmeter (Rigatto & Brady, 1972a), magnetometers or more recently respiratory inductance plethysmography (Respitrace) (Duffty et al., 1981).

The respiratory pattern has long been considered as one of the important criteria for assessing behavioural state (Pretchl, 1974), breathing being generally regular during NREM sleep and irregular during REM sleep. Nevertheless, brief episodes of regular breathing are also present in REM sleep and periodic changes in breathing with regular oscillations in tidal volume and respiratory frequency have been detected in both sleep states (Hathorn, 1979). These oscillations have a similar length ($\sim$10 s) in both states, but their amplitude is greater and their occurrence is more irregular during REM sleep. The oscillations in V_T tend to be 'in phase' with the oscillations in f, while during NREM sleep changes in V_T and f are mostly 'out of phase' leading to more stable ventilation in this sleep state (Hathorn, 1979).

Regardless of the state of consciousness, resting ventilation progressively increases as maturation proceeds. This has been found in preterm and term infants (Haddad et al., 1979; Fisher et al., 1982), in premature and term primates (Guthrie et al., 1981), in kittens and rabbit pups (Wyszogrodski, Thach & Milic-Emili, 1978; Marlot et al., 1984) (Fig.

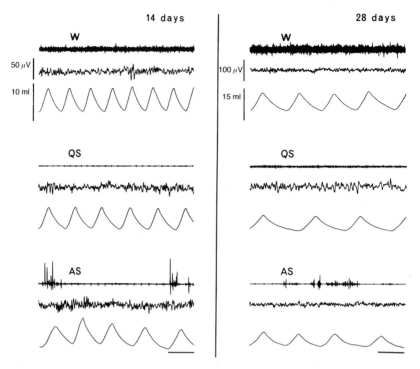

Fig. 8.3. Neurophysiological and respiratory records in 2 kittens, 14 and 28 days old respectively. For each kitten, typical records are shown in wakefulness (W), quiet sleep (QS), and active sleep (AS). For each state of consciousness: *upper trace*, EMG of neck muscles; *middle trace*, EEG; *lower trace*, tidal volume. Time scale, 1 s. (From Marlot et al., 1984.)

8.3). Concomitantly, PaO_2 increases and P_aCO_2 decreases with advancing postnatal age (Guthrie et al., 1980) (Fig. 8.4). The increased $\dot{V}_\epsilon$ is due to a progressive rise in V_T which is more important than the fall in f. When $\dot{V}_\epsilon$ and V_T are normalized to body weight, similar maturational changes are observed in premature and term primates between day 2 and day 21 (Guthrie et al., 1980) (Fig. 8.4), whereas in rabbit pups V_T/kg increases but $\dot{V}_\epsilon/kg$ does not change during the first week after birth (Wyszogrodski et al., 1978). The decrease in frequency with age is due to the prolongation of both T_I and T_E in the two sleep states.

The profound influences of sleep states on eucapnic ventilation and respiratory control have only been recently recognized and thoroughly studied. In some studies in preterm and term infants, $\dot{V}_\epsilon$ has been shown to increase slightly (approximately 20%) in REM sleep as compared to NREM sleep (see, for example, Davi et al., 1979). Such increased $\dot{V}_\epsilon$ was

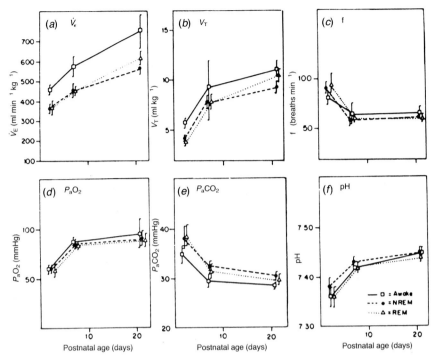

Fig. 8.4. Relationship of various respiratory variables with sleep state and postnatal age in monkeys when breathing room air. Each point represents mean ± SE for each variable. (*a*): minute volume/kg; (*b*): tidal volume/kg; (*c*): respiratory frequency; (*d*): arterial PO_2; (*e*): arterial PCO_2; (*f*): pH (from Guthrie et al., 1980).

caused mainly by an increase in f while V_T was unchanged or slightly decreased. When transcutaneous blood gas measurements were performed with electrodes heated to 42 or 44 °C, it was found that both $tcPO_2$ and $tcPCO_2$ were lower in REM than in NREM sleep. While the decrease in $tcPCO_2$ is relevant to the increased $\dot{V}_\epsilon$ reported in REM sleep, no satisfactory explanation has been found concerning the simultaneous decrease in $tcPO_2$ (Martin, Herrell & Pultusker, 1981). In contrast, other studies did not find any difference in $\dot{V}_\epsilon$ between REM and NREM sleep in term infants less than 3 months of age (Fagenholtz, O'Connell & Shannon, 1976; Haddad et al., 1979), premature or term primates (Guthrie et al., 1980, 1981), rabbits (Wyszogrodski et al., 1978) or kittens (Marlot et al., 1984) and when arterial blood gas tensions were measured, they did not differ between REM and NREM sleep (Guthrie et al., 1981). In some of these studies, complementary changes in V_T and f were observed (Haddad et al., 1979) whereas, in others, the two components of the breathing pattern were not affected by sleep state (Guthrie et al., 1980, 1981; Marlot et al., 1984).

The discrepancies among the different studies of the effect of sleep state on eucapnic $\dot{V}_\epsilon$ may have several explanations, e.g. the different methods used to record respiration, ($\dot{V}_\epsilon$ & behavioural state may be affected by face mask or nasal prongs), criteria used to identify sleep states, the selection and number of respiratory cycles analysed or species differences.

In a few studies which have investigated the ventilatory changes between wakefulness and sleep in newborns, it appears that $\dot{V}_\epsilon$ is always greater during wakefulness than during either NREM or REM sleep (Guthrie et al., 1980; Schulze et al., 1981; Marlot et al., 1984). This increased $\dot{V}_\epsilon$ was due to a larger V_T in the primate infant and to a larger f in kittens during wakefulness as compared to either sleep state. The magnitude of the rise in $\dot{V}_\epsilon$ and changes in breathing pattern during wakefulness as compared to sleep probably depends on the degree of alertness, the awake state showing alternately active or quiet periods with consequent changes in respiratory activity.

Periodic Breathing

Periodic breathing is observed primarily during REM sleep in premature newborns and is characterized by episodes of ventilatory effort lasting usually more than 20 seconds, regularly interrupted by apnoeic periods of 2–10 seconds (Chernick, Heldrich & Avery, 1964; Hoppenbrouwers et al., 1977). Dramatic changes in heart rate are not seen during apnoeic periods in contrast to apnoeic *spells* which, although similar to periodic breathing in being frequently seen in premature infants, are characterized by longer apnoeic periods occurring at irregular intervals and are accompanied by marked bradycardia.

The proportion of newborn infants which experience periodic breathing varies inversely with birth weight (94.5% at <2.5 kg vs 36.1% at >2.5 kg), with gestational age (86.5% at <37 weeks vs 41% at >37 weeks), and with postnatal age (78% at 0–2 weeks vs 29% at 39–52 weeks) (Bouterline-Young & Smith, 1950; Fenner et al., 1973; Kelly et al., 1985). The time spent in periodic breathing decreases with gestational age (14% at 31–34 weeks vs 0.7% near term: Hoppenbrouwers et al., 1977) but, in premature infants who reach normal term, the time spent in periodic breathing remains high (Curzi-Dascalova, Christova-Guerguieva & Korn, 1981).

Periodic breathing produces slight hyperventilation (Lee et al., 1987) which could be the result of simultaneous increases in tidal volume and respiratory rate which occur in oscillatory cycles (Hathorn, 1978). These oscillations may lead to unstable alveolar ventilation. At the start of cycles of periodic breathing, 80% of infants have a complete obstruction at the level of the pharynx, suggesting that there is an imbalance between the central drive to the diaphragm and to the muscles of the upper airway (Miller et al., 1988). Periodic breathing occurs in REM sleep (Hoppenbrouwers et al., 1977) so with increasing postnatal age the reduction in the amount of REM sleep would be related to decreasing time spent in periodic breathing and thus to more efficient ventilation.

Periodic breathing, because it is not associated with significant hypoxia or bradycardia (Fenner et al., 1973), is considered generally to be a benign and transient disturbance in the breathing pattern of premature infants. However, since it shares characteristics with apnoeic *spells* (e.g. decreased incidence with increasing chemical drive; dependence on maturation) some investigators have suggested that periodic breathing may be a 'marker' for increased risk of SIDS (Kelly et al., 1980).

Ventilatory responses to chemical stimuli during sleep

The influence of sleep on the regulation of breathing during the newborn period has been scarcely studied although it is universally recognized that sleep profoundly affects the regulation of respiratory activity. However, before reviewing the studies on the ventilatory responses to chemical stimuli which take sleep into consideration, we will consider the influence of gestational age and postnatal age on these responses.

Ventilatory response to hypercapnia

Newborns, either human or animal, respond to CO_2 by a sustained increase in $\dot{V}_\epsilon$ (for review see Steele, 1986; Saetta & Mortola, 1987; Mortola & Rezzonico, 1988). A brisk increase in $\dot{V}_\epsilon$ mediated by the peripheral chemoreceptors appears within 3–5 s and a secondary increase in $\dot{V}_\epsilon$ mediated by the central chemoreceptors begins 25–30 s later (Carroll, Canet & Bureau, 1991). Immediate hyperventilation results from an increase in both V_T and f (Martin et al., 1985), while the late response is related to a rise in tidal volume, respiratory frequency remaining essentially unchanged.

The sustained ventilatory response to CO_2 has been often studied in terms of sensitivity to CO_2 characterized by the CO_2 response curve (changes in minute $\dot{V}_\epsilon$ per body weight/changes in P_aCO_2). The magnitude of the response to CO_2 has been found to depend on the gestational and postnatal age. Several studies have shown that, in newborn infants, the sensitivity to CO_2 increases with increasing gestational age (Rigatto, Brady & de la Torre Verduzco, 1975b; Krauss et al., 1975; Frantz et al., 1976a; Moriette et al., 1985), while others found no difference between premature and term infants or primates (Davi et al., 1979; Guthrie et al., 1981). Such discrepancy may result from the degree of immaturity studied or species differences.

The influence of postnatal age on the ventilatory response to CO_2 has also been examined in neonates as compared to adults of the same species. It has been shown that the slope of the CO_2 response curve is similar to that of adult subjects although the curve is slightly shifted to the left in neonates due to lower resting CO_2 levels (Avery et al., 1963; Rigatto et al., 1975b). On the other hand, the sensitivity to CO_2 has been found to increase in preterm infants within the first postnatal month (Rigatto et al., 1975b; Krauss et al., 1975) and in both premature and full-term primates from birth up to 21 days postnatally (Guthrie et al., 1980, 1981). On the contrary, in puppies, the percentage change in $\dot{V}_\epsilon$ in response to CO_2 does not change between 2 weeks and 4 months of age (Haddad et al., 1980), but comparisons with other studies are difficult since the authors did not measure the CO_2 response curve and the level of inspired CO_2 used is quite low (2%). In addition, the increased $\dot{V}_\epsilon$ in response to CO_2 could be slightly diminished by the relative hypoxaemia present in the early life of some neonates breathing room air (Guthrie et al., 1981).

In the last decade, several groups of investigators have studied the influence of sleep state on the ventilatory response to CO_2. The magnitude of the transient ventilatory response to CO_2 is not different in REM and NREM sleep, although there was a greater variability during REM sleep as compared to NREM sleep (Anderson et al., 1983) and the transient increase in f is only observed during NREM sleep (Martin et al., 1985). The effect of sleep state on the sustained ventilatory response to CO_2 seems to depend on the technique used. When the rebreathing technique described by Read (1967) is used, there is a consensus emerging that the ventilatory response to CO_2 of the human newborn is reduced during REM sleep and is more variable and irregular than during NREM sleep (Bryan et al., 1976; Hagan & Gulston, 1981; Honma et al., 1984; Moriette et al., 1985; Carlo, Martin & Difiore, 1988; Cohen, Xu & Henderson-Smart, 1991). While V_T has been found to increase in both sleep states, f tended to decrease during REM sleep and to increase during NREM sleep. These results are similar to that found in adult humans and dogs with the same rebreathing method (Phillipson et al., 1977). In contrast, when a steady-state method is used, infants and primates up to 3 weeks of age respond to CO_2 by a similar increase in $\dot{V}_\epsilon$ or diaphragmatic EMG in both sleep states primarily owing to a rise in V_T (Fagenholz et al., 1976; Davi et al., 1979; Haddad et al., 1980; Guthrie et al., 1980, 1981; Anderson et al., 1983; Martin et al., 1985). However, the ventilatory response to hypercapnia could became sleep-state dependent with advancing age since monkeys aged more than 3 weeks show less sensitivity to CO_2 in REM than in NREM sleep (Guthrie et al., 1981).

It is possible that the different methodology used has influenced the results. With the steady-state method, a steady $\dot{V}_\epsilon$ is not always reached within the usual test duration (4– 5min). With the rebreathing method, based on rising CO_2 levels, experiments are often conducted under hyperoxic conditions (40%) which lead to a combined effect of raised PO_2 and PCO_2 on $\dot{V}_\epsilon$. When rebreathing is performed under normoxic conditions, there is still a reduced ventilatory response to CO_2 during REM sleep as compared to NREM sleep, but because peripheral chemo-receptor drive is not reduced by hyperoxia, the magnitude of the response is greater in both sleep states than in hyperoxic hypercapnia (Cohen & Henderson-Smart, 1991). Finally, if the ventilatory response to CO_2 is only reduced during 'phasic' but not during 'tonic' REM sleep as in adults (Phillipson et al., 1977), the different methods used may affect the response to CO_2 via a change in REM state.

Changes in $\dot{V}_\epsilon$ and breathing pattern may also depend, in a given sleep state, on whether the baseline respiration is regular or periodic. The administration of CO_2 in low concentrations (0.5–1.5%) induces an increase in P_aCO_2 and $\dot{V}_\epsilon$ in both sleep states, but this effect is due to an increase in V_T when control breathing is regular, and to an increase in f when control breathing is periodic (Kalapesi et al., 1981). In general, low levels of inspired CO_2 tend to make breathing regular (Chernick & Avery, 1966; Fenner et al., 1973; Rigatto et al., 1980; Kalapesi et al., 1981) and such changes produced by CO_2 could mimic the spontaneous ventilatory changes occurring during a particular sleep state.

Ventilatory response to hyperoxia

The administration of high levels of O_2 induces an immediate but transient decrease in $\dot{V}_\epsilon$ (see for example Sankaran et al., 1979). In newborn infants, this response has been found to be either independent of gestational age (Rigatto et al., 1975a), slightly less (Reinstorff & Fenner, 1972) or greater (Krauss et al., 1973) in preterm than in full-term infants. Such discrepancy in the results also occurs for the influence of postnatal age on the response. For many authors, the ventilatory response to hyperoxia changes with postnatal age, very young newborns having a smaller response to O_2 than older newborns or adults (Girard, Lacaisse & Dejours, 1960; Krauss et al., 1973; Sankaran et al., 1979; Bureau & Begin, 1982; Hertzberg et al., 1990) while for others (Rigatto et al., 1975a; Fagenholz et al., 1976; Carroll & Bureau, 1987), the transient hypoventilation in response to hyperoxia is similar at different postnatal ages. This result could stem from the relative hypoxaemia present in the immediate newborn period as mentioned before since a transient hyperventilation in response to hypoxaemia may attenuate the hyperoxia-induced hypoventilation.

The immediate decrease in $\dot{V}_\epsilon$ is followed by a sustained increase after 5 min of hyperoxia (Rigatto et al., 1975a; Mortola et al., 1992). This rise of $\dot{V}_\epsilon$ may result from the transient increase in PCO_2, related to the preceding decrease in $\dot{V}_\epsilon$. The effect may also reflect a central stimulating effect of O_2, manifest in newborns with a weak peripheral drive as in carotid body-denervated adult animals (Gautier, Bonora & Gaudy, 1986).

The influence of behavioural state on the ventilatory response to hyperoxia has rarely been studied. However, it appears that the magnitude of the initial decrease and the later increase in $\dot{V}_\epsilon$ is similar in both sleep states (Bolton & Herman, 1974; Fagenholtz et al., 1976; Rigatto, 1979). Also, when preterm infants have spontaneous periodic breathing in room air during REM sleep, it has been shown that the administration of high levels of O_2 makes breathing regular, the O_2 concentration threshold for this effect decreasing with advancing postnatal age (Fenner et al., 1973).

Ventilatory response to hypoxia

In contrast to the adult, the newborn is unable to sustain an increase in $\dot{V}_\epsilon$ in response to hypoxia in early postnatal life. When placed in a moderately hypoxic environment, newborns generally respond by an immediate and brief increase in $\dot{V}_\epsilon$ followed by a progressive decline toward or even to below normoxic baseline levels. This biphasic response has been clearly shown in preterm and term humans, in piglets, monkeys, kittens and rabbits (McCooke & Hanson, 1985; for review see Steele, 1986). However, a biphasic response has also been shown in adults

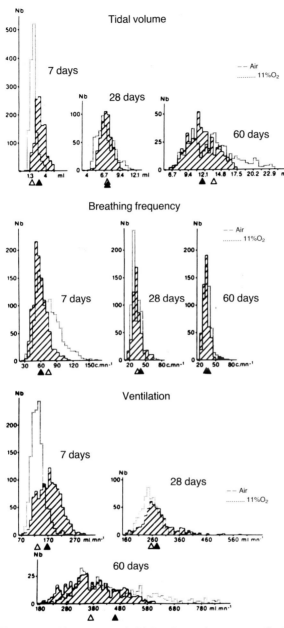

Fig. 8.5. Frequency histograms of tidal volume (*upper panel*), breathing frequency (*middle panel*; c.m n^{-1} = respiratory cycles per minute), and ventilation (*lower panel*) at three different postnatal ages in kittens breathing air (continuous line) and in hypoxia (dotted line). Mean values in air (solid triangles) and in hypoxia (open triangles) are indicated. (From Bonora et al., 1984.)

submitted to isocapnic hypoxemia although $\dot{V}_\epsilon$ rarely descend below baseline.

In infants the immediate increase in $\dot{V}_\epsilon$ in response to hypoxia is more pronounced at 37 than at 32 weeks of gestational age, while the subsequent decrease in $\dot{V}_\epsilon$ does not seem to change with increasing gestational age (Rigatto et al., 1975a).

With respect to postnatal maturation of the ventilatory response to hypoxia, the initial response does not change in preterm infants between 8 and 18 days of age when compared to adult subjects (Rigatto et al., 1975a; Sankaran et al., 1979), while it does increase in newborn monkeys, lambs and kittens during the first 2–3 weeks of postnatal life (Belenky, Standaert & Woodrum, 1979; Woodrum et al., 1981; McCooke & Hanson, 1985). Although the biphasic response to hypoxia is always present, the secondary decrease in $\dot{V}_\epsilon$ wanes progressively with increasing postnatal age (Fig. 8.5). A sustained hyperventilation is observed at various ages depending on the species, from 2 months of age in kittens to 6–10 days of age in more mature animals such as lambs (Rigatto et al., 1975a; Woodrum et al., 1981; Haddad, Gandhi & Mellins, 1982; Bureau & Begin, 1982; Bonora et al.,1984).

The influence of sleep state on the ventilatory response to hypoxia has been considered in only a few studies. In preterm infants exposed to 15% O_2 for 5 min, a sustained increase in $\dot{V}_\epsilon$ was observed during NREM sleep, while there was a progressive decrement of $\dot{V}_\epsilon$ during REM sleep, and a transient increase followed by a sustained decrease in $\dot{V}_\epsilon$ during wakefulness (Rigatto et al., 1982). In lambs (Henderson-Smart & Read, 1979a) and calves (Jeffery & Read, 1980) submitted to progressive isocapnic hypoxemia, $\dot{V}_\epsilon$ was also increased in NREM sleep but did not change in REM sleep (except at an extreme degree of hypoxemia, just preceding arousal) whereas puppies increased their $\dot{V}_\epsilon$ similarly in both sleep states (Henderson-Smart & Read, 1979a). However, this technique does not allow the measurement of a large number of breaths at any given level of hypoxia, and results are probably a mixture of transient and steady-state responses.

In studies using steady-state hypoxia, $\dot{V}_\epsilon$ decreased during NREM sleep in young monkeys, kittens and puppies, a sustained hyperventilation occurring at older ages. This decreased $\dot{V}_\epsilon$ was mainly due to a reduction in V_T in kittens and monkeys (Woodrum et al., 1981; Bonora et al., 1984; Bonora & Gautier, 1987; Bonora, Boule & Gautier, 1992), and a reduction in f in puppies (Haddad et al., 1982). During REM sleep, $\dot{V}_\epsilon$ was increased in puppies at every age during the first postnatal month of life, and in kittens from 3 weeks onward. It seems that, apart from species and age-related differences, results depend markedly on the technique used and further studies are necessary to clarify this subject.

Whilst behavioural state affects the ventilatory response to hypoxia, it appears that hypoxia produces important changes in the sleep–wakefulness pattern. In newborn kittens, hypoxia induces an increase in the percentage of time spent in wakefulness and in NREM sleep, and conversely a great decrease in REM sleep (Baker & McGinty, 1979; Bonora et al., 1984; McCooke & Hanson, 1985). This effect increases with the severity of hypoxia. The increase in NREM sleep time was due to an increase in the mean duration of NREM epochs, while the decrease in REM sleep was due both to fewer and to shorter epochs (Baker & McGinty, 1979).

In premature infants showing periodic breathing, it has been shown that mild hypoxia (17–18% O_2) significantly increases its incidence (Rigatto et al., 1972b). Similarly, in full-term infants born at altitude, a higher percentage of periodic breathing has been observed. These findings are consistent with the fact that hyperoxia inhibits periodic breathing. It appears, therefore, that hypoxaemia could play an important role in the genesis of periodic breathing.

The absence of sustained hyperventilation in response to hypoxia in the newborn has been often related to a weak peripheral chemoreceptor activity, insufficient enough to counterbalance the hypoxic inhibition originating from central nervous system. Other peripheral and central mechanisms could be involved, however, in this response, such as a reduction in dynamic lung compliance (La Framboise, Woodrum & Guthrie, 1985) or changes in the concentration of endogenous modulators of respiratory activity such as endorphins, serotonin, catecholamines, adenosine or GABA. It has also been suggested that the late decrease in $\dot{V}_e$ is due to a peripheral mechanism in the lungs or thorax since the diaphragmatic activity remains elevated at 10 min of hypoxia while the tidal volume is markedly reduced (Rigatto et al., 1988). However, it has recently been shown that the decrease in V_T is well matched to the phasic activation of the diaphragm which is also reduced by hypoxia because of the persistence of its activity throughout expiration (Bonora et al., 1992). Therefore, a central mechanism is also likely to be involved in the response to hypoxia in newborns. Indeed, a central excitatory effect of hypoxia on respiratory frequency has been shown in young immature kittens (Bonora et al., 1984) or in newborn lambs when central hypoxia was produced by the inhalation of carbon monoxide

(Bureau, Carroll & Canet, 1988). As suggested from fetal studies, a central component of the response could be located in or above the upper pons since decerebration near the pontine–midbrain junction prevented the fall in $\dot{V}_\epsilon$ in response to hypoxia (Martin-Body & Johnston, 1988).

Interaction between CO_2 and O_2

The interaction of hypercapnia with varying levels of inspired oxygen has been studied in several newborn species but the results are not consistent. In preterm infants in which the various gas concentrations were given for a short period of time, the addition of 4% CO_2 enhanced the immediate hyperventilation with 15% O_2 and reduced the immediate hypoventilation with 40% 0_2. These results suggest an interaction at the level of peripheral chemoreceptors (Albersheim et al., 1976). When the gas mixtures were given for several minutes in young infants or monkeys, the ventilatory response to CO_2 decreased with hypoxia and increased with hyperoxia. Such negative interaction between steady-state hypercapnia and hypoxia probably results from a central interaction (Rigatto, De la Torre Verduzco & Cates, 1975c; Guthrie et al., 1985). In newborn lambs (Purves, 1966), which are more mature at birth, the response to steady-state CO_2 was enhanced by hypoxia, as in adults. However, a similar response has also been observed in rats (Saetta & Mortola, 1987). In older monkeys in which $\dot{V}_\epsilon$ is stimulated by hypercapnia and hypoxia given alone, a negative interaction occurs when the stimuli are combined (Guthrie et al., 1985). These inconsistent responses may be due to the gestational age, the use of tracheostomy, or to species-related changes in metabolism during hypoxia.

Influence of sleep state on control of breathing

The control of breathing is a multifactorial system in which several components such as respiratory muscles, respiratory reflexes, peripheral chemoreceptor drive and metabolic demand are affected by the behavioural state.

Diaphragm and intercostal muscles

The respiratory activity of the diaphragm and other respiratory muscles is greatly influenced by sleep state. EMG records of the diaphragm and intercostal muscles have been performed in newborn infants by using a non-invasive technique with surface electrodes and in newborn animals by chronically implanted electrodes. In newborn infants (Hagan & Gulston, 1981; Carlo et al., 1983) and lambs (Henderson-Smart & Read, 1978; Harding, Johnson & McClelland, 1980), it has been shown that the amplitude of the phasic inspiratory activity of the diaphragm is greater in REM than in NREM sleep, while in puppies the peak diaphragmatic activity is similar in both sleep states and is greater than in wakefulness (England, Kent & Stogryn, 1985). A marked inhibition of the phasic and tonic activities of the intercostal muscles has been observed in infants and lambs during REM sleep (Prechtl, VanEykeren & O'Brien, 1977; Henderson-Smart & Read, 1978; Hagan & Gulston, 1981; Lopes et al., 1981). In newborn lambs, distinction has been made between EMG activity of external intercostals recorded laterally and the anterior intercostals, and it appears that the activity of lateral intercostals which have postural roles is completely lost during REM sleep as it is in adult cats (Duron, 1973), while the anterior intercostals maintain some activity in inspiration (Henderson-Smart & Read, 1978).

On the other hand, because newborns have a very high chest wall compliance, the diaphragm does not have a rigid support upon which to act. Therefore, a part of the diaphragmatic force is dissipated in distorting the rib cage inwards rather than producing an effective volume exchange. During REM sleep, this phenomenon is reinforced by the inhibition of tonic and phasic intercostal muscle activities. Such paradoxical breathing has also been observed by measuring thoracic and abdominal respiratory movements which are always out-of-phase during REM sleep and are essentially in-phase during NREM sleep (Knill et al., 1976; Curzi-Dascalova, 1978). The paradoxical movements of the rib cage and abdomen are common in preterm infants, even during NREM sleep (Davi et al., 1979). The stabilizing role of the intercostal muscles in this paradoxical respiration was confirmed in a quadriplegic infant suffering a birth injury of the cervical spinal cord resulting in a complete interruption of spinal pathways between the intercostal and phrenic motorneurone outflows and who showed a constant paradoxical inward movement of the rib cage during inspiration (Thach et al., 1980). Because of a stiffening of the rib cage and a decrease in the proportion of REM sleep, this phenomenon progressively diminishes with increasing gestational and postnatal age.

The excessive diaphragmatic work in infants may lead to muscle fatigue. Muller et al. (1979) suggested, after spectral frequency analysis of the diaphragmatic EMG of preterm and term infants, that diaphragmatic fatigue could occur during REM sleep when contraction of the diaphragm produces a distortion of the rib cage. This respiratory muscle fatigue could participate in the initiation of hypoventilation or apnoeas.

Abdominal muscles

Abdominal muscle activity also changes during REM sleep. EMG recording of the abdominal muscles of newborn lambs shows that their phasic or tonic activity, present during expiration in NREM sleep, is depressed throughout REM sleep. This reduction of abdominal muscle tone and abdominal pressure may play a role in permitting the paradoxical motion of the rib cage during inspiration (Henderson-Smart & Read, 1978).

Upper airway muscles

The influence of behavioural state on the neonatal larynx has been mainly examined by EMG recordings of the posterior cricoarytenoid muscle (PCA) as a laryngeal abductor muscle, cricothyroid muscle (CT) and the thyroarytenoid muscle (TA) as a laryngeal adductor muscle.

PCA has a prominent inspiratory activity with each burst of diaphragmatic activity. It has been shown in newborn puppies (see Fig. 8.6) that PCA muscle activity is greater in NREM and REM sleep than during wakefulness (England et al., 1985), while in newborn lambs, PCA and CT activities are greater in REM than in NREM sleep (Harding et al., 1980). Although these two studies show similar activity in inspiratory laryngeal muscles during REM sleep, the different results found during NREM sleep may be explained by modifications of upper airway muscle activity dependent on the head position in a given state (Bonora, Bartlett & Knuth, 1985). Expiratory laryngeal adduction which is mainly induced in newborns by TA activity does not occur during REM sleep since this muscle is not usually active during REM sleep (Harding, 1980; Harding et al., 1980; England et al., 1985). TA activity seems to increase with postnatal age in lambs, whereas it decreases with maturation in puppies (see Fig. 8.6), this latter finding being relevant to the weak activity of the adductor muscles reported in the adult animal.

The expiratory activity of the adductor muscles in newborns has been found to play a major role in expiratory airflow retardation, which aids the maintenance of an elevated functional residual capacity (FRC). Such a braking mechanism is especially important in newborns who already have a relatively low FRC because of a highly compliant chest wall (Agostoni, 1959). A rise in end-expiratory lung volume can be also provided, as in adults (Remmers & Bartlett, 1977) by a persistent EMG

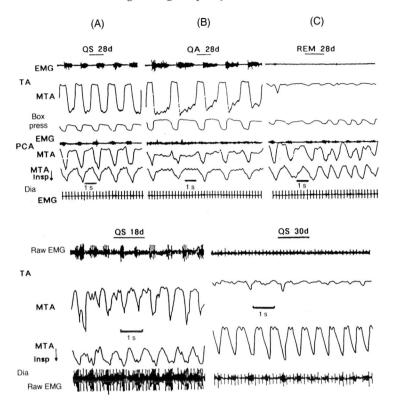

Fig. 8.6. *Upper panel*: Example of muscle activities in quiet sleep (A) quiet wakefulness (B) and REM sleep (C) in a 28 day old puppy. From the top, tracings are thyroarytenoid muscle electromyogram (EMG) and corresponding moving time average (MTA), pressure deflections from Drorbaugh-Fenn plethysmograph, posterior cricoarytenoid muscle EMG and MTA, and diaphragmatic MTA and EMG. MTAs show an increased muscle activity with a downward deflection. Time bars represent 1 s. *Lower panel*: Thyroarytenoid and diaphragmatic activities during quiet sleep in the same puppy at 18 and 30 days of age. Both post-inspiratory diaphragmatic and expiratory/thyroarytenoid activity were reduced at 30 days. However, when the puppy cried at this age, prominent TA activity was evident (not shown in Figure). Note that amplification of diaphragmatic EMG was greater at 18 days. (From England et al., 1985.)

activity of the diaphragm during expiration. This post-inspiratory diaphragmatic activity (PIA) has been indirectly evaluated in infants by calculating post-inspiratory muscle pressure (Mortola et al., 1984) and directly by recording the diaphragm EMG in newborn animals (Henderson-Smart, Johnson & McClelland, 1982; England et al., 1985; Bonora et al., 1992). During NREM sleep, PIA has been reported to be prominent, whereas during REM sleep it was either absent (Henderson-

Smart et al., 1982), reduced (Harding, Johnson & McClelland, 1979) or variable (England et al., 1985). The different results observed during REM sleep may depend on the position of electrodes in the diaphragm (Henderson-Smart et al., 1982). Nevertheless, it appears that, during REM sleep, the inhibition of laryngeal adductor activity and post-inspiratory activity of the diaphragm, together with the diminished activity of intercostal and abdominal muscles, results in the loss of expiratory braking observed in newborns (Harding et al., 1979). It should be noted that this finding is consistent with the 30% reduction of the end-expiratory lung volume found in babies during REM sleep (Henderson-Smart & Read, 1979b) and apnoeas (Lopes et al., 1981).

The influence of sleep state on upper airway muscle activities has been also studied by surface EMG recordings of genioglossus muscle activity. This muscle, which is phasically active during inspiration, is important in maintaining upper airway patency by drawing the tongue forward and out of the airway. Following imposed airway occlusion, the genioglossus EMG activity increases and this enhanced activity is independent of sleep state (Cohen & Henderson-Smart, 1989).

Finally, the newborn activates the alae nasi (AN) during inspiration, usually during periods of severe ventilatory stimulation. The onset of phasic AN activity precedes that of the DIA and this early activation of AN facilitates $\dot{V}_\epsilon$ by lowering upper airway resistance. Such AN activity has been shown to be greater during REM sleep than in NREM sleep either during resting $\dot{V}_\epsilon$ or during hypercapnia; this effect should therefore improve $\dot{V}_\epsilon$ during REM sleep (Carlo et al., 1983).

Respiratory reflexes

The Hering–Breuer inflation reflex which is due to activation of slowly adapting stretch receptors has been found to be very active in newborns at birth, in contrast to adult human (Gautier, Bonora & Gaudy, 1981); this reflex then decreases progressively within the first days of life (Cross et al., 1960). The Hering–Breuer reflex is state dependent. During NREM sleep, this vagal reflex is potent, while during REM sleep it is weak or absent (Finer, Abroms & Taeusch, 1976). Moreover, the stretch receptors are probably less stimulated when the functional residual capacity is low, i.e. during REM sleep (Henderson-Smart & Read, 1979b). The depression of the lung inflation reflex during REM sleep is relevant to the fact that proprioceptive spinal reflexes are markedly diminished during REM sleep (Lenard, Von Bernuth & Pretchl, 1968).

The load-compensatory reflexes which depend on vagal mechanisms are also quite strong at birth, although their intensity varies with sleep state. Airway occlusion produced by elastic loads (Knill et al., 1976) or with a face mask (Frantz et al., 1976b) induced a substantial reduction of the tidal volume during NREM sleep, while during REM sleep this reflex was impaired (Knill et al., 1976). It has been suggested that this effect is due to the inhibition of intercostal reflexes during REM sleep and to the operation of an intercostal-phrenic reflex (Knill & Bryan, 1976).

Arousal is considered as an important defence mechanism initiated by respiratory stimuli such as hypoxia, hypercapnia, upper airway occlusion and laryngeal stimulation. Arousal mechanisms have been previously documented in adult animals and man (Phillipson et al., 1977; Berthon-Jones & Sullivan, 1984), and have recently come under intensive investigation in newborns. During hypercapnia, arousal has been observed in newborn infants and macaque monkeys a few minutes after inhalation of 2–4% and 5% CO_2, respectively (Haddad et al., 1980; Woodrum et al., 1981). When the influence of sleep state has been examined, it appears that arousal occurs in both sleep states but the response is delayed during REM sleep compared to NREM sleep (Fewell & Baker, 1988).

Hypoxaemia causes also arousal from sleep. In newborn calves and lambs exposed to hypoxic gas mixtures, arousal has been shown to occur in both sleep states, but at a much lower SaO_2 and after a longer delay in REM than in NREM sleep (Henderson-Smart & Read, 1979a (Fig. 8.7); Jeffery & Read, 1980; Fewell & Konduri, 1989). This arousal response is impaired if lambs are exposed repeatedly to hypoxaemia, as could occur during multiple apnoeic episodes (Fewell & Konduri, 1989). Also, the addition of CO_2 to the hypoxic gas mixture enhanced the arousal response (Fewell & Konduri, 1988) resulting in a decreased delay to arousal and an increase in saturation at arousal. From several studies performed in intact and carotid-denervated newborn lambs, it has been suggested that arousal responses to respiratory stimuli could be primarily mediated by the carotid chemoreceptors (Fewell et al., 1989a,b)

These findings provide evidence that the arousal reflex which can be considered as a protective response for interrupting episodes of hypoventilation or apnoea is impaired during REM sleep and in young newborns with weak peripheral chemoreceptor drive.

Peripheral chemoreceptor drive

The peripheral chemoreceptors have been found to be tonically active in the lamb fetus. After birth, a transient abolition of their activity will occur

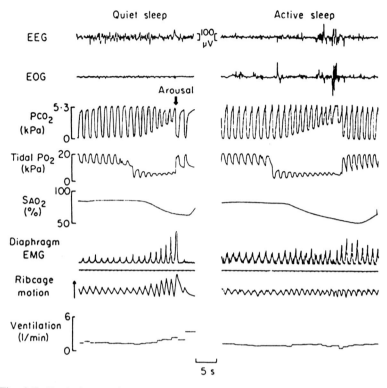

Fig. 8.7. Typical records of hypoxic tests in a lamb showing: in quiet sleep a prompt ventilatory response and arousal at an oxygen saturation (S_aO_2) of 72%; in active sleep a depressed ventilatory response and no arousal despite a fall of the S_aO_2 to 50%. In active sleep the diaphragmatic electromyogram (EMG) activity increased only at the lowest S_aO_2 levels and at this time paradoxical movements of the rib cage became more obvious and there was no ventilatory response. EOG is electro-oculogram. (From Henderson-Smart & Read, 1979a.)

because of the brisk rise in PaO_2 (physiological chemodenervation); this effect is immediately followed by a progressive resetting of the arterial chemoreceptors to a higher PaO_2 level during the first week of life (Blanco et al., 1984; Hertzberg et al., 1990). The peripheral chemoreceptor activity has been shown by recording chemoreceptor action potentials in the carotid sinus nerve (Schwieler, 1968; Blanco et al., 1984, 1988; Marchal et al., 1992) or by recording $\dot{V}_\epsilon$ in response to acute hypoxia, hyperoxia or hypercapnia or pharmacological stimulation from drugs such as cyanide (Belenky et al., 1979; Schramm & Grunstein, 1987). In newborn animals in which carotid-body denervation was performed, the immediate ventilatory response to chemical stimuli is almost completely abolished (Belenky et al., 1979; Schramm & Grunstein, 1987; Carroll & Bureau, 1987; Carroll et al., 1991), the remaining effect arising from the aortic chemoreceptors. In altricial (immature at birth) species such as rats, denervation of both carotid and aortic bodies results in severe disturbances of respiration (Hofer, 1984). Indeed, such rats have more frequent apnoeas and an atypical respiratory pattern during REM sleep (Hofer, 1985), in particular during the phasic REM periods in which respiratory irregularities are normally buffered by carotid chemoreceptors (Sullivan, Kozar & Phillipson, 1978). The carotid bodies are thus vital for $\dot{V}_\epsilon$ and arousal responses to hypoxia and hypercapnia.

Metabolism

The control of body temperature, metabolism and the regulation of breathing are intimately linked, and the postnatal development of the metabolic requirements to achieve thermoregulation should always be considered when studying the regulation of $\dot{V}_\epsilon$, particularly during hypoxaemia. Metabolic demand varies with several factors such as environmental temperature, maturity, age, size and behavioural state.

In order to minimize the influence of metabolic changes on breathing, it is generally believed that the development of control of breathing should be studied over a neutral temperature range (the environmental temperature range over which metabolism is minimal while normal body temperature is maintained). Before considering the thermoneutral range, however, it should be pointed out that the normal body temperature of newborns in their early life is generally lower than that of adults (Brück et al., 1962; Hey & Katz, 1970). Therefore, any attempt to hold neonatal body temperature at the adult value is unjustified. It has been found that the neutral thermal range for naked term babies of 3 kg at birth is between 32 and 34°C (Brück et al., 1962; Hey & Katz, 1970). However, several authors have suggested that is important to stay at the lower limit or even slightly below this thermoneutral range; most babies can maintain a normal body temperature when exposed to marked cold stress by greatly increasing heat production by shivering or non-shivering thermogenesis; in contrast, when they have to face a slight heat stress, body temperature will dramatically increase since heat loss mechanisms are not very efficient. Respiratory problems such as tachypnoea have been sometimes observed within the so-called 'thermoneutral range' (Hull,

1965; Bonora & Gautier, 1987) and more severe respiratory disturbances such as apnoea may even occur (Hey & Katz, 1970). It seems, therefore, that in newborns the neutral temperature range for *metabolism* is not necessarily the optimal environmental temperature for respiratory control. It seems appropriate therefore for babies to be maintained towards the lower end of the thermoneutral range unit or even slightly below it.

The minimal oxygen consumption measured at thermoneutrality varies with the postnatal age and the behavioural state. Except in rabbits (Hull, 1965), the minimal O_2 consumption ($\dot{V}O_2$) per kg body weight increases during the first few days after birth in most species (Mott, 1963; Spiers & Adair, 1986). The magnitude and timing of this increase in minimal $\dot{V}O_2$ depends on gestational age, rate of growth and the rise in body temperature occurring in the early newborn period (Spiers & Adair, 1986). Therefore, consideration of the oxygen consumption changes induced by warm or cold exposure should take into account the postnatal evolution of the minimal $\dot{V}O_2$. Moreover, with advancing postnatal age, the maximum $\dot{V}O_2$ increases (Mott, 1963) and the lower critical temperature at which a substantial rise in $\dot{V}O_2$ occurs, decreases (Spiers & Adair, 1986).

Sleep states have been found to affect the thermoregulatory mechanisms, as in adults (Parmeggiani, 1987). At thermoneutrality, $\dot{V}O_2$ is either similar in both sleep states (see Berger et al., 1989) or slightly greater in REM sleep than in NREM sleep (see Fleming et al., 1988). In a cool environment, different findings are reported. In lambs, $\dot{V}O_2$ increases during NREM sleep and wakefulness, but is not changed in REM sleep (Berger et al., 1989; Ball et al., 1989). In infants, however, $\dot{V}O_2$ is reported to increase to a similar degree in both sleep states in preterm babies (Darnall & Ariagno, 1982) but to increase more in REM than in NREM sleep in full-term infants (Stothers & Warner, 1978; Fleming et al., 1988). The impairment of metabolic response to cold found in lambs during REM sleep may be related to the fact that they are more mature than infants at birth; however, the different findings could also stem from the phase of REM sleep studied (only tonic in lambs) since control mechanisms may differ between tonic and phasic phases of REM sleep (Phillipson et al., 1977).

Conversely, the sleep-state pattern is affected by thermometabolism. As pointed out above, exposure to a cool environment significantly alters the REM sleep pattern, REM sleep episodes being shorter than in a warm environment (Berger et al., 1989). This finding suggests that a cool environment may reduce REM epoch duration by an arousal reflex

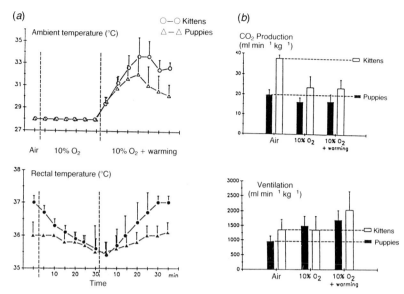

Fig. 8.8. (*a*) Effect on rectal temperature of a period of breathing 10% O_2 in newborn kittens and puppies at constant ambient temperature of 28°C, then when ambient temperature is increased. Values are mean + SD. (*b*) CO_2 production ($\dot{V}CO_2$) in newborn cats (open columns) and dogs (filled columns) during normoxia, hypoxia, and hypoxia plus warming. During hypoxia and hypoxia warming. $\dot{V}CO_2$ was significantly less than in normoxia. Values are mean values: + SD. (From Pedraz & Mortola, 1991.)

initiated to limit the extent of a fall in body temperature occurring during REM sleep (Berger et al., 1989). Indeed, at the ambient temperature of 10–15 °C, which does not induce a decrease in body temperature during wakefulness, a slight decrease in body temperature was observed during REM sleep; a slight increase occurred in a warm environment (20–25 °C). During NREM sleep, body temperature tended to decrease in both environments (Berger et al., 1989).

The changes in $\dot{V}_\epsilon$ induced by hypoxia are tightly linked to changes in metabolism (Fig. 8.8) and several reports have indicated that newborns of many species show a drop in $\dot{V}O_2$ within a few minutes of exposure to hypoxia (for review see Mortola, Okubo & Carroll, 1988; Pedraz & Mortola, 1991). This lowering of $\dot{V}O_2$ during hypoxia has been observed in both sleep states (Haddad, Gandhi & Mellins, 1981). Such an effect depends on the ambient temperature, the drop in $\dot{V}O_2$ during hypoxia being greater in a cool, than in a thermoneutral environment (Hill, 1959; Sidi et al., 1983). This result can be explained by the fact that the initial increase in $\dot{V}O_2$ induced by cold stress is decreased by a hypoxia-induced reduction in non-shivering thermogenesis (Heim & Hull, 1966). However, the fall in $\dot{V}O_2$ induced by hypoxia has been also observed at thermoneutrality (see Mortola & Rezzonico, 1988) suggesting that other mechanisms are also involved in this response.

The decrease in $\dot{V}O_2$ in hypoxia is associated with a decrease in body temperature in several species (Sidi et al., 1983; Bonora et al., 1984; Bonora & Gautier, 1987; Mortola & Rezzonico, 1988; Mortola, Rezzonico & Lanthier, 1989; Pedraz & Mortola, 1991). While the drop in temperature might be explained by decreased metabolism, the inverse effect should also be considered. But, in a recent study, it has been shown that the reduction in body temperature observed during hypoxia results from, but does not contribute to, the fall in metabolism since when external warming was applied to hypoxic kittens in order to restore body temperature to its normoxic level, the hypometabolism persisted (Pedraz & Mortola, 1991) (Fig. 8.8). As previously suggested in hypoxic adult cats (Gautier, 1986), hypoxia may decrease the set point of thermoregulation and, therefore, the low body temperature during hypoxia may represent a new normothermic level (Pedraz & Mortola, 1991). The decrease in $\dot{V}O_2$ could be considered as a strategy to protect oxygen delivery to vital organs (Mortola & Rezzonico, 1988).

Conclusions

The postnatal evolution of the control of breathing varies with multiple factors such as gestational and postnatal age, maturity at birth, species, size, methodology used and the behavioural state. However, sleep state certainly plays a crucial modulating role in the respiratory activity of the newborn. The most important features of the regulation of neonatal respiration during sleep will be summarized here in order to emphasize the issues remaining to be clarified.

With advancing postnatal age, the resting $\dot{V}_\epsilon$ and tidal volume increases while the respiratory frequency decreases. When the state of vigilance is taken into account, $\dot{V}_\epsilon$ has been found to be either similar in both sleep states or slightly increased in REM sleep as compared to NREM sleep, and always greater during wakefulness than during either REM or NREM sleep.

In response to chemical stimuli, the immediate and transient ventilatory response generally increases with both gestational and postnatal age and sleep state does not markedly affect these responses, except in preterm infants. In contrast, the enhancement of the late ventilatory response to CO_2 with gestational and postnatal age may be partially related to the reduction in the proportion of REM sleep with increasing age since the sensitivity to CO_2 has sometimes been found to be less in REM than in NREM sleep. The late ventilatory response to hyperoxia is unchanged with age and with sleep state, while the late decrease in $\dot{V_\epsilon}$ in response to hypoxia progressively disappears as maturation proceeds and a sustained hyperventilation can be elucidated a few weeks after birth. Contradictory results have been reported concerning the influence of sleep on this response, depending on the technique used.

In the neonate, the diaphragm is partly inefficient because of the very high chest wall compliance and a 'paradoxical' breathing occurs. This effect is enhanced during REM sleep because of a marked inhibition of intercostal and abdominal muscle activities. Moreover, the expiratory airflow retardation which increases the functional residual capacity is less during REM sleep since the main mechanisms providing such expiratory braking, i.e. the laryngeal adductor activity and the post-inspiratory activity of the diaphragm, are inhibited. It results in a marked decrease of the end-expiratory lung volume during REM sleep and consequently stretch receptors which are involved in the Hering–Breuer reflex are less stimulated.

The decrease in $\dot{V_\epsilon}$ during hypoxia is associated with a decrease in arterial CO_2 (see Mortola & Rezzonico, 1988). This implies that a decrease in metabolic rate represents an important factor in compensating for hypoxaemia. In fact, the drop in CO_2 production would be greater than the decrease in alveolar $\dot{V_\epsilon}$ implying that the newborn would rather hyperventilate during hypoxia. Sleep state does not greatly influence the drop in metabolic rate during hypoxia, although there may be some influence from the slightly higher $\dot{V}O_2$ in REM than in NREM sleep. However, the percentage time spent in REM sleep is known to be greatly diminished by hypoxia.

The arousal in response to hypercapnia or hypoxia which is mediated essentially by the peripheral chemoreceptors is delayed during REM sleep and occurs at a lower SaO_2. Therefore, the weakness of peripheral chemoreceptor drive in early life poses a crucial problem in elevating the arousal threshold, especially during REM sleep.

Thus, REM sleep has a pernicious influence on several mechanisms involved in the regulation of breathing, but, most of the time, newborns are able to develop compensatory responses to resist changes in the environment and to maintain homeostasis of blood gases and temperature.

References

Agostoni, E. (1959). Volume pressure relationships of the thorax and lung in the newborn. *Journal of Applied Physiology,* **14**, 909–13.

Albersheim, S., Boychuk, R., Seshia, M. M. K., Cates, D. & Rigatto, H. (1976). Effects of CO_2 on immediate ventilatory response to O_2 in preterm infants. *Journal of Applied Physiology,* **41**, 609–11.

Anders, T. F. & Keener, M. (1985). Developmental course of night time sleep–wake patterns in full-term and premature infants during the first year of life. I. *Sleep,* **8**, 173–92.

Anderson, Jr., J. V., Martin, R. J., Abboud, E. F., Dyme, I. Z. & Bruce, E. N. (1983). Transient ventilatory response to CO_2 as a function of sleep state in full-term infants. *Journal of Applied Physiology,* **54**, 1482–8.

Arduini, D., Rizzo, G., Giorlandino, C., Valensise, H., Dell'Acqua, S. & Romanini, C. (1986). The development of fetal behavioural states: a longitudinal study. *Prenatal Diagnosis,* **6**, 117–24.

Avery, M. E., Chernick, V., Dutton, R. E., & Permutt, S. (1963). Ventilatory response to inspired carbon dioxide in infants and adults. *Journal of Applied Physiology,* **18**, 895–903.

Baker, T. L. & McGinty, D. J. (1979). Sleep–waking patterns in hypoxic kittens. *Developmental Psychobiology,* 561–75.

Ball, N. J., Andrews, D. C., Vojcek, L. & Johnson, P. (1989). The effect of ambient temperature and age on sleep state and its respiratory consequences in developing lambs. *Pediatric Research,* **25**, 46A.

Barcroft, J. & Barron, D. H. (1937). The genesis of respiratory movements in the fetus of the sheep. *Journal of Physiology* (London), **88**, 56–61.

Belenky, D. A., Standaert, T. A. & Woodrum, D. E. (1979). Maturation of hypoxic ventilatory response of the newborn lamb. *Journal of Applied Physiology,* **47**, 927–30.

Berger, P. J., Horne, R. S. C. & Walker, A. M. (1989). Cardio-respiratory responses to cool ambient temperature differ with sleep state in neonatal lambs. *Journal of Physiology,* **412**, 351–63.

Berthon-Jones, M. & Sullivan, C. E. (1984). Ventilation and arousal responses to hypercapnia in normal sleeping humans. *Journal of Applied Physiology,* **57**, 59–67.

Blanco, C. E., Dawes, G. S., Hanson, M. A. & McCooke, H. B. (1984). The response to hypoxia of arterial chemoreceptors in fetal and newborn lambs. *Journal of Physiology,* **351**, 25–37.

Blanco, C. E., Hanson, M. A., Johnson, P., & Rigatto, H. (1988). Breathing pattern of kittens during hypoxia. *Journal of Applied Physiology,* **56**, 12–17.

Boddy, K., Dawes, G. S., Fisher, R., Pinter, S. & Robinson, J. S. (1974). Foetal respiratory movements, electrocortical and cardiovascular responses to hypoxaemia and hypercapnia in sheep. *Journal of Physiology,* **243**, 599–61.

Bolton, D. P. G. & Herman, S (1974). Ventilation and sleep state in the newborn. *Journal of Physiology,* **240**, 67–77.

Bonora, M., Marlot, D., Gautier, H. & Duron, B. (1984). Effects of hypoxia on ventilation during postnatal development in conscious kittens. *Journal of Applied Physiology,* **56**, 1464–71.

Bonora, M., Bartlett, Jr. D. & Knuth, S. L. (1985). Changes in upper airway muscle activity related to head position in awake cats. *Respiration Physiology*, **60**, 181–92.

Bonora, M. & Gautier, H. (1987). Maturational changes in body temperature and ventilation during hypoxia in kittens. *Respiration Physiology*, **68**, 359–70.

Bonora, M., Boule, M. & Gautier, H. (1992). Diaphragmatic and ventilatory responses to alveolar hypoxia and hypercapnia in conscious kittens. *Journal of Applied Physiology*, **72**, 203–10.

Bouterline-Young, H. J. & Smith, C. A. (1950). Respiration of the full-term and premature infant. *American Journal of Diseases in Children*, **80**, 753–66.

Bowes, G., Adamson, T. M., Ritchie, B. C., Dowling, M., Wilkinson, M. H. & Maloney, J. E. (1981). Development of patterns of respiratory activity in unanesthetized fetal sheep in utero. *Journal of Applied Physiology*, **50**, 693–700.

Brück, K., Parmelee, A. H. & Brück, M. (1962). Neutral temperature range and range of 'thermal comfort' in premature infants. *Biology of the Neonate*, **4**, 32–51.

Bryan, H. M., Hagan, R., Gulston, G. & Bryan, A. C. (1976). CO_2 response and sleep state in infants. *Clinical Research*, **24**, A689.

Bureau, M. A. & Begin, R. (1982). Postnatal maturation of the respiratory response to O_2 in awake newborn lambs. *Journal of Applied Physiology*, **52**, 428–33.

Bureau, M. A., Carroll, J. L. & Canet E. (1988). Response of newborn lambs to CO_2-induced hypoxia. *Journal of Applied Physiology*, **64**, 1870–7.

Carlo, W. A., Martin, R. J., Abboud, E. F., Bruce, E. N. & Strohl, K. P. (1983). Effect of sleep state and hypercapnia on alae nasi and diaphragm EMGs in preterm infants. *Journal of Applied Physiology*, **54**, 1590–6.

Carlo, W. A., Martin, R. J. & Difiore, J. M. (1988). Differences in CO_2 threshold of respiratory muscles in preterm infants. *Journal of Applied Physiology*, **65**, 2434–9.

Carroll, J. L., & Bureau, M. A. (1987). Quantitative analysis of the CO_2 response curve of the peripheral chemoreceptors in 2 and 10-day-old lambs. *American Review of Respiratory Disease*, **135**, A174.

Carroll, J. L., Canet, E. & Bureau, M. A. (1991). Dynamic ventilatory responses to CO_2 in the awake lamb: role of the carotid chemoreceptors. *Journal of Applied Physiology*, **71**, 2198–205.

Chernick, V., Heldrich, F. & Avery, M. E. (1964). Periodic breathing of premature infants. *Journal of Pediatrics*, **64**, 330–40.

Chernick, V. & Avery, M. E. (1966). Response of premature infants with periodic breathing to ventilatory stimuli. *Journal of Applied Physiology*, **21**, 434–40.

Clewlow, F., Dawes, G. S., Johnston, B. M. & Walker, D. W (1983). Changes in breathing, electrocortical and muscle activity in unanaesthetized fetal lambs with age. *Journal of Physiology*, **341**, 463–76.

Cohen, G. & Henderson-Smart, D. J. (1989). Upper airway muscle activity during nasal occlusion in newborn babies. *Journal of Applied Physiology*, **66**, 1328–35.

Cohen, G., Xu, C. & Henderson-Smart, D. (1991). Ventilatory response of the sleeping newborn to CO_2 during normoxic rebreathing. *Journal of Applied Physiology*, **71**, 168–74.

Cross, K. W. (1949). The respiratory rate and ventilation in the newborn baby. *Journal of Physiology*, **109**, 459–74.

Cross, K. W., Klaus, M., Tooley, W. H. & Weisser, K. (1960). The response of the newborn baby to inflation of the lungs. *Journal of Physiology*, **151**, 551–65.

Curzi-Dascalova, L. (1978). Thoracico-abdominal respiratory correlations in infants: constancy and variability in different sleep states. *Early Human Development*, **2**, 25–38.

Curzi-Dascalova, L., Christova-Gueorguieva, E. & Korn, G. (1981). Les pauses respiratoires chez les enfants prematurés et les nouveau-nés à terme normaux. *Progress in Neonatalogy*, **1**, 19–25.

Darnall, R. A. & Ariagno, R. L. (1982). The effect of sleep state on active thermoregulation in the premature infant. *Pediatric Research*, **16**, 512–14.

Davi, M., Sankaran, K., Maccallum, M., Cates, D. & Rigatto, H. (1979). Effect of sleep state on chest distortion and on the ventilatory response to CO_2 in neonates. *Pediatric Research*, **13**, 982–6.

Dawes, G. S., Fox, H. E., Leduc, B. M., Liggins, G. C. & Richards, R. T. (1972). Respiratory movements and rapid eye movement sleep in the foetal lamb. *Journal of Physiology*, **220**, 119–43.

Drorbaugh, J. E. & Fenn, W. O. (1955). A barometric method for measuring ventilation in newborn infants. *Pediatrics*, **16**, 81–6.

Duffty, P., Spriet, L., Bryan, M. H. & Bryan, A. C. (1981). Respiratory inductance plethysmography (Respitrace) – an evaluation of its use in the infant. *American Review of Respiratory Disease*, **123**, 542–6.

Duron, B. (1973). Postural and ventilatory functions of intercostal muscles. *Acta Neurobiologiae Experimentalis*, **33**, 355–80.

England, S. J., Kent, G. & Stogryn, H. A. F. (1985). Laryngeal muscle and diaphragmatic activities in conscious dog pups. *Respiration Physiology*, **60**, 95–108.

Fagenholz, S. A., O'Connell, K. & Shannon, D. C. (1976). Chemoreceptor function and sleep state in apnea. *Pediatrics*, **58**, 31–6.

Fenner, A., Schalk, U., Hoenicke, H, Wendenburg, A. & Roehling, T. (1973). Periodic breathing in premature and neonatal babies: incidence, breathing pattern, respiratory gas tensions, response to changes in the composition of ambient air. *Pediatric Research*, **7**, 174–83.

Fewell, J. E. & Baker, S. B. (1988). Arousal and cardiopulmonary response to hyperoxic hypercapnia in lambs. *Journal of Developmental Physiology*, **25**, 473–7.

Fewell, J. E. & Konduri, G. G. (1988). Repeated exposure to rapidly developing hypoxemia influences the interaction between oxygen and carbon dioxide in initiating arousal from sleep in lambs. *Pediatric Research*, **24**, 28–33.

Fewell, J. E. & Konduri, G. G. (1989). Influence of repeated exposure to rapidly developing hypoxaemia on the arousal and cardiopulmonary response to rapidly developing hypoxaemia in lambs. *Journal of Developmental Physiology*, **11**, 77–82.

Fewell, J. E., Kondo, C. S., Dascalu, V. & Filyk, S. C. (1989*a*). Influence of carotid-denervation on the arousal and cardiopulmonary responses to alveolar hypercapnia in lambs. *Journal of Developmental Physiology*, **12**, 193–9.

Fewell, J. A., Kondo, C. S., Dascalu, V. & Filyk, S. C. (1989*b*). Influence of carotid denervation on the arousal and cardiopulmonary response to rapidly developing hypoxemia in lambs. *Pediatric Research*, **25**, 473–7.

Finer, N. N., Abroms, I. F & Taeusch, H. W. (1976). Ventilation and sleep states in newborn infants. *Journal of Pediatrics*, **89**, 100–8.

Fisher, J. T., Mortola, J. P., Smith, J. B., Fox, G. S. & Weeks, S. (1982). Respiration in newborns. Developmental of the control of breathing. *American Review of Respiratory Disease*, **125**, 650–7.

Fleming, P. J., Levine, M. R., Azaz, Y. & Johnson, P. (1988). The effect of sleep state on the metabolic response to cold stress in newborn infants. In *Fetal and Neonatal Development*, ed. C. T. Jones. pp. 643–7. Perinatalogy Press: Ithaca, New York.

Frantz, III, I. D., Adler, S. M., Thach, B. T. & Taeusch, H. W. (1976*a*). Maturational effects on respiratory responses to carbon dioxide in premature infants. *Journal of Applied Physiology*, **41**, 41–5.

Frantz, III, I. D. , Adler, S. M., Abroms, I. F. & Thach, B. T. (1976*b*). Respiratory response to airway occlusion in infants: sleep state and maturation. *Journal of Applied Physiology,* **41**, 634–8.

Gautier, H. (1986). Hypoxic enigma: central effects of hypoxia on ventilatory and thermoregulatory control. In *Neurobiology of the Control of Breathing*, ed. C. von Euler & H. Lagercrantz. pp. 19–25. Raven Press, New York.

Gautier, H., Bonora, M. & Gaudy, J. H. (1981). Breuer–Hering inflation reflex and breathing pattern in anesthetized humans and cats. *Journal of Applied Physiology,* **51**, 1162–8.

Gautier, H., Bonora, M. & Gaudy, J. H. (1986). Ventilatory response of the conscious or anesthetized cat to oxygen breathing. *Respiration Physiology*, **65**, 181–96.

Girard, F., Lacaisse, A. & Dejours, P. (1960). Le stimulus O_2 ventilatoire à la période néonatale chez l'homme. *Journal de Physiologie* (Paris), **52**, 108–9.

Godal, A., Belenky, T. A., Standaert, T. A. Woodrum, D. E., Grimsrud, L. & Hodson, W. A. (1976). Application of the hot-wire anemometer to respiratory measurements in small animals. *Journal of Applied Physiology*, **40**, 275–7.

Guthrie, R. D., Standaert, T. A., Hodson, W. A. & Woodrum, D. E. (1980). Sleep and maturation of eucapnic ventilation and CO_2 sensitivity in the premature primate. *Journal of Applied Physiology,* **48**, 347–54.

Guthrie, R. D., Standaert, T. A., Hodson, W. A. & Woodrum, D. E. (1981). Development of CO_2 sensitivity: effects of gestational age, postnatal age, and sleep state. *Journal of Applied Physiology,* **50**, 956–61.

Guthrie, R. D., Laframboise, W. A., Standaert, T. A., Van Belle, G. & Woodrum, D. E. (1985). Ventilatory interaction between oxygen and carbon dioxide in the preterm primate. *Pediatric Research*, **19**, 528–33.

Haddad, G. G., Epstein, R. A., Epstein, M. A. F., Leistner, H. L., Marino, P. A. & Mellins, R. B. (1979). Maturation of ventilation and ventilatory pattern in normal sleeping infants. *Journal of Applied Physiology,* **46**, 998–1002.

Haddad, G. G., Leistner, H. L., Epstein, R. A., Epstein, M. A. F., Grodin, W. K. & Mellins, R. B. (1980). CO_2-induced changes in ventilation and ventilatory pattern in normal sleeping infants. *Journal of Applied Physiology*, **48**, 684–8.

Haddad, G. G., Gandhi, M. R. & Mellins, R. B. (1981). O$_2$ consumption during hypoxia in sleeping puppies. *American Review of Respiratory Disease*, **123**, 183.

Haddad, G. G., Gandhi, M. R. & Mellins, R. B. (1982). Maturation of ventilatory response to hypoxia in puppies during sleep. *Journal of Applied Physiology*, **52**, 309–14.

Hagan, R. & Gulston, A. G. (1981). The newborn: respiratory electromyograms and breathing. *Australian Paediatric Journal*, **17**, 230–1.

Harding, R. (1980). State-related and developmental changes in laryngeal function. *Sleep*, **3**, 307–22.

Harding, R., Johnson, P. & McClelland, M. E. (1979). The expiratory role of the larynx during development and the influence of behavioural state. In *Central Nervous Control Mechanisms in Breathing*, ed. C. Von Euler & H. Lagercrantz. pp. 353–9. Pergamon Press, New York.

Harding, R., Johnson, P. & McClelland, M. E. (1980). Respiratory function of the larynx in developing sheep and the influence of sleep state. *Respiration Physiology*, **40**, 165–79.

Hathorn, M. K. S. (1978). Analysis of periodic changes in ventilation in newborn infants. *Journal of Physiology*, **285**, 85–99.

Hathorn, M. K. S. (1979). Analysis of the depth and timing of infant breathing. In *Central Nervous Control Mechanisms in Breathing*, ed. C. von Euler and H. Lagercrantz. pp. 363–372. Pergamon Press, New York.

Heim, T. & Hull, D. (1966). The blood flow and oxygen consumption of brown adipose tissue in the new-born rabbit. *Journal of Physiology*, **186**, 42–55.

Henderson-Smart, D. J. & Read, D. J. C. (1978). Depression of intercostal and abdominal muscle activity and vulnerability to asphyxia during active sleep in the newborn. In *Sleep Apnea Syndromes*, ed. C. Guilleminot & W. C. Dement. pp. 93–117. Liss Inc, New York.

Henderson-Smart, D. J. & Read, D. J. C. (1979a). Ventilatory responses to hypoxaemia during sleep in the newborn. *Journal of Developmental Physiology*, **1**, 195–208.

Henderson-Smart, D. J. & Read, D. J. C. (1979b). Reduced lung volume during behavioral active sleep in the newborn. *Journal of Applied Physiology*, **46**, 1081–5.

Henderson-Smart, D. J., Johnson, P. & McClelland, M. E. (1982). Asynchronous respiratory activity of the diaphragm during spontaneous breathing in the lamb. *Journal of Physiology*, **327**, 377–91.

Hertzberg, T., Hellstrom, S., Lagercrantz, H. & Pequignot, J. M. (1990). Development of the arterial chemoreflex and turnover of carotid body catecholamines in the newborn rat. *Journal of Physiology*, **425**, 211–25.

Hey, E. N. & Katz, G. (1970). The optimum thermal environment for naked babies. *Archives of Disease in Childhood*, **45**, 328–34.

Hilakivi, L. A. & Hilakivi, I. T. (1986). Sleep–wake behavior of newborn rats recorded with movement sensitive method. *Behavioural Brain Research*, **19**, 241–8.

Hill, J. R. (1959). The oxygen consumption of new-born and adult mammals. Its dependence on the oxygen tension in the inspired air and on the environmental temperature. *Journal of Physiology*, **149**, 346–73.

Hofer, M. A. (1984). Lethal respiratory disturbance in neonatal rats after arterial chemoreceptor denervation. *Life Sciences*, **34**, 489–96.

Hofer, M. A. (1985). Sleep-wake state organization in infant rats with episodic respiratory disturbance following sinoaortic denervation. *Sleep*, **8**, 40–8.

Honma, Y., Wilkes, D., Bryan, M. H. & Bryan, A. C. (1984). Rib cage and abdominal contributions to ventilatory response to CO_2 in infants. *Journal of Applied Physiology,* **56**, 1211–16.

Hoppenbrouwers, T., Hodgman, J. E., Harper, R. M., Hoffman, E., Sterman, M. B. & McGinty, D. J. (1977). Polygraphic studies of normal infants during the first six months of life: III. Incidence of apnea and periodic breathing. *Pediatrics,* **60**, 418–25.

Huggett, A. St G. (1927). Foetal blood-gas tensions and gas transfusion through the placenta of the goat. *Journal of Physiology,* **62**, 373–84.

Hull, D. (1965). Oxygen consumption and body temperature of new-born rabbits and kittens exposed to cold. *Journal of Physiology,* **177**, 192–202.

Ioffe, S., Jansen, A. H., Russell, B. J. & Chernick, V. (1980a). Respiratory response to somatic stimulation in fetal lambs during sleep and wakefulness. *Pflügers Archiv,* **388**, 143–8.

Ioffe, S., Jansen, A. H., Russell, B. J. & Chernick, V. (1980b). Sleep, wakefulness and the monosynaptic reflex in fetal and newborn lambs. *Pflügers Archiv,* **388**, 149–57.

Ioffe, S., Jansen, A. H. & Chernick, V. (1987). Maturation of spontaneous fetal diaphragmatic activity and fetal response to hypercapnia and hypoxemia. *Journal of Applied Physiology,* **62**, 609–22.

Jansen, A. H., Ioffe, S., Russell, B. J. & Chernick, V. (1982). Influence of sleep state on the response to hypercapnia in fetal lambs. *Respiration Physiology,* **48**, 125–42.

Jeffery, H. E. & Read, D. J. C. (1980). Ventilatory responses of newborn calves to progressive hypoxia in quiet and active sleep. *Journal of Applied Physiology,* **48**, 892–5.

Jouvet-Mounier, D., Astic, L. & Lacote, D. (1970). Ontogenesis of the states of sleep in rat, cat, and guinea pig during the first postnatal month. *Developmental Psychobiology,* **2**, 216–39.

Kalapesi, Z., Durand, M., Leahy, F. N., Cates, D. B., Maccallum, M. & Rigatto, H. (1981). Effect of periodic or regular respiratory pattern on the ventilatory response to low inhaled CO_2 in preterm infants during sleep. *American Review of Respiratory Disease,* **123**, 8–11.

Kelly, D. H., Walker, A. M., Cahen, L. & Shannon D. C. (1980). Periodic breathing in sibling of sudden infant death syndrom victims. *Pediatrics,* **66**, 515–20.

Kelly, D. H., Stellwagen, L. M., Kaitz, E. & Shannon, D. C. (1985). Apnea and periodic breathing in normal full-term infants during the first twelve months. *Pediatric Pulmonology,* **1**, 215–19.

Knill, R. & Bryan, A. C. (1976). An intercostal-phrenic inhibitory reflex in human newborn infants. *Journal of Applied Physiology,* **40**, 352–6.

Knill, R., Andrews, W., Bryan, A. C. & Bryan, M. H. (1976). Respiratory load compensation in infants. *Journal of Applied Physiology,* **40**, 357–61.

Krauss, A. N., Tori, C. A., Soodalter, J. & Auld, P. A. M. (1973). Oxygen chemoreceptors in low birth weight infants. *Pediatric Research,* **7**, 569–74.

Krauss, A. N., Klain, D. B., Waldman, S. & Auld, P. A. M. (1975). Ventilatory response to carbon dioxide in newborn infants. *Pediatric Research,* **9**, 46–50.

LaFramboise, W. A., Woodrum, D. E. & Guthrie, R. D. (1985). Influence of vagal activity on the neonatal ventilatory response to hypoxemia. *Pediatric Research,* **19**, 903–7.

Lee, D., Caces, R., Kwiatkowski K., Cates D. & Rigatto, H. (1987). A developmental study on types and frequency distribution of short apneas (3 to 15 seconds) in term and preterm infants. *Pediatric Research*, **22**, 344–9.

Lenard, H. G., von Bernuth, H. & Prechtl, H. F. R. (1968). Reflexes and their relationship to behavioural state in the newborn. *Acta Paediatica Scandinavica*, **57**, 177–85.

Lopes, J., Muller, N. L., Bryan, M. H. & Bryan, A. C. (1981). Importance of inspiratory muscle tone in maintenance of FRC in the newborn. *Journal of Applied Physiology*, **51**, 830–4.

McCooke, H. B. & Hanson, M. A. (1985). Respiration of conscious kittens in acute hypoxia and effect of almitrine bismesylate. *Journal of Applied Physiology*, **59**, 18–23.

Maloney, J. E., Bowes, G. & Wilkinson, M. (1980). 'Fetal breathing' and development of patterns of respiration before birth. *Sleep*, **3**, 299–306.

Marchal, F., Bairam, A., Haouzi, P. et al. (1992). Carotid chemoreceptor response to natural stimuli in the newborn kitten. *Respiration Physiology*, **87**, 183–93.

Marlot, D., Bonora, M., Gautier, H. & Duron, B. (1984). Postnatal maturation of ventilation and breathing pattern in kittens : influence of sleep. *Journal of Applied Physiology*, **56**, 321–5.

Martin, R. J., Herrell, N. & Pultusker, M. (1981). Transcutaneous measurement of carbon dioxide tension : effect of sleep state in term infants. *Pediatrics*, **67**, 622–5.

Martin, R. J., Carlo, W. A., Robertson, S. S., Day, W. R. & Bruce, E. N. (1985). Biphasic response of respiratory frequency to hypercapnea in preterm infants. *Pediatric Research*, **19**, 791–6.

Martin-Body, R. L. & Johnston, B. M. (1988). Central origin of the hypoxic depression of breathing in the newborn. *Respiration Physiology*, **71**, 25–32.

Miller, M. J., Waldemar, A. C., Difiore, J. M. & Martin, R. J. (1988). Airway obstruction during periodic breathing in premature infants. *Journal of Applied Physiology*, **64**, 2496–500.

Moriette, G., Van Reempts, P., Moore, M., Cates, D. & Rigatto, H. (1985). The effect of rebreathing CO_2 on ventilation and diaphragmatic electromyography in newborn infants. *Respiration Physiology*, **62**, 387–97.

Mortola, J. P., Milic-Emili, J., Noworaj, A., Smith, B., Fox, G. & Weeks, S. (1984). Muscle pressure and flow during expiration in infants. *American Review of Respiratory Disease*, **129**, 49–53.

Mortola, J. P. & Rezzonico, R. (1988). Metabolic and ventilatory rates in newborn kittens during acute hypoxia. *Respiration Physiology*, **73**, 55–68.

Mortola, J. P., Okubo, S & Carroll, J. L. (1988). The newborn lung. In *Hypoxia: The Tolerable Limits*, ed. J. R. Sutton, C. S. Houston & G. C. Coates. pp. 293–304. Benchmark Press, Indianapolis.

Mortola, J. P., Rezzonico, R. & Lanthier C. (1989). Ventilation and oxygen consumption during acute hypoxia in newborn mammals: a comparative analysis. *Respiration Physiology*, **78**, 31–43.

Mortola, J. P., Frappell, P. B., Dotta, A. et al. (1992). Ventilatory and metabolic responses to acute hyperoxia in newborns. *American Review of Respiratory Disease*, **146**, 11–15.

Mott, J. C. (1963). Oxygen consumption of the newborn. *Federal Proceedings*, **22**, 814–17.

Muller, N., Gulston, G., Cade, D. et al. (1979). Diaphragmatic muscle fatigue in the newborn. *Journal of Applied Physiology,* **46**, 688–95.

Nijhuis, J. G., Prechtl, H. F. R., Martin, C. B. & Bots, R. S. G. (1982). Are there behavioural states in the human fetus? *Early Human Development*, **6**, 177–95.

Nijhuis, J. G., Martin, C. B., Gommers, S., Bouws, P., Bots, R. S. G. M. & Jongsma, H. W. (1983). The rhythmicity of fetal breathing varies with behavioural state in the human fetus. *Early Human Development*, **9**, 1–7.

Parmeggiani, P. L. (1987). Interaction between sleep and thermoregulation: an aspect of the control of behavioral states. *Sleep*, **10**, 426–35.

Parmelee, A. H., Wenner, W. H., Akiyama, Y., Schultz, M. & Stern, E. (1967). Sleep states in premature infants. *Developmental Medicine and Child Neurology*, **9**, 70–7.

Pedraz, C. & Mortola, J. P. (1991). CO_2 production, body temperature, and ventilation in hypoxic newborn cats and dogs before and after body warming. *Pediatric Research*, **30**, 165–9.

Phillipson, E. A., Kozar, L. F., Rebuck, A. S. & Murphy, E. (1977). Ventilatory and waking responses to CO_2 in sleeping dogs. *American Review of Respiratory Disease*, **115**, 251–9.

Prechtl, H. F. R (1974). The behavioural states of the newborn infant (a review). *Brain Research*, **76**, 185–212.

Prechtl, H. F. R., VanEykern, L. A. & O'Brien, M. J. (1977). Respiratory muscle EMG in newborns: a non-intrusive method. *Early Human Development*, **1**, 265–83.

Purves, M. J. (1966). The respiratory response of the newborn lamb to inhaled CO_2 with and without accompagnying hypoxia. *Journal of Physiology*, **185**, 78–94.

Read, D. J. C. (1967). A clinical method for assessing the ventilatory response to carbon dioxide. *Australian Annals of Medicine*, **16**, 20–32.

Reinstorff D. & Fenner, A. (1972). Ventilatory response to hyperoxia in premature and newborn infants during the first three days of life. *Respiration Physiology*, **15**, 159–65.

Remmers, J. E. & Bartlett, Jr., D. (1977). Reflex control of expiratory airflow and duration. *Journal of Applied Physiology,* **42**, 80–7.

Rigatto, H. (1979). A critical analysis of the development of peripheral and central respiratory chemosensitivity during the neonatal period. In *Central Nervous Control Mechanisms in Breathing*, ed. C. von Euler & H. Lagercrantz. pp. 137–148. Pergamon Press, New York.

Rigatto, H. & Brady, P. (1972a). A new nosepiece for measuring ventilation in preterm infants. *Journal of Applied Physiology,* **32**, 423–4.

Rigatto, H. & Brady, J. P. (1972b). Periodic breathing and apnea in preterm infants. I. Evidence for hypoventilation possibly due to central respiratory depression. *Pediatrics*, **50**, 202–18.

Rigatto, H., Brady, J. P., Chir, B. & de la Torre Verduzco, R. (1975a). Chemoreceptor reflexes in preterm infants: I. The effect of gestational and postnatal age on the ventilatory response to inhalation of 100% and 15% oxygen. *Pediatrics*, **55**, 604–13.

Rigatto, H., Brady, J. P. & de la Torre Verduzco, R. (1975b). Chemoreceptor reflexes in preterm infants: II. The effect of gestational and postnatal age on the ventilatory response to inhaled carbon dioxide. *Pediatrics*, **55**, 614–21.

Rigatto, H., de la Torre Verduzco, R. & Cates, D. B. (1975c). Effects of O_2 on the ventilatory response to CO_2 in preterm infants. *Journal of Applied Physiology*, **39**, 896–9.

Rigatto, H., Kalapesi, Z., Leathy, F. N., Durand, M., Maccallum, M. & Cates, D. (1980). Chemical control of respiratory frequency and tidal volume during sleep in preterm infants. *Respiration Physiology*, **41**, 117–25.

Rigatto, H., Kalapesi, Z., Leathy, F. N., Mccallum, M. & Cates, D. (1982). Ventilatory response to 100% and 15% O_2 during wakefulness and sleep in preterm infants. *Early Human Development*, **7**, 1–10.

Rigatto, H., Moore, M. & Cates, D. (1986). Fetal breathing and behavior measured through a double-wall Plexiglas window in sheep. *Journal of Applied Physiology*, **61**, 160–4.

Rigatto, H., Wiebe, C., Rigatto, C., Lee, D. S. & Cates, D. (1988). Ventilatory response to hypoxia in unanesthetized newborn kittens. *Journal of Applied Physiology*, **64**, 2544–51.

Roffwarg, H. P., Muzio, J. N. & Dement, W. C. (1966). Ontogenic development of the human sleep–dream cycle. *Science*, **152**, 604–19.

Ruckebusch, Y. (1972). Development of sleep and wakefulness in the foetal lamb. *Electroencephalography and Clinical Neurophysiology*, **32**, 119–28.

Ruckebusch, Y., Gaujoux, M. & Eghbali, B. (1977). Sleep cycles and kinesis in the foetal lamb. *Electroencephalography and Clinical Neurophysiology*, **42**, 226–37.

Saetta, M. & Mortola, J. P. (1987). Interaction of hypoxic and hypercapnic stimuli on breathing pattern in the newborn rat. *Journal of Applied Physiology*, **62**, 506–12.

Sankaran, K., Wiebe, H., Seshia, M. M. K., Boychuk, R. B., Cates, D. & Rigatto, H. (1979). Immediate and late ventilatory response to high and low O_2 in preterm infants and adult subjects. *Pediatric Research*, **13**, 875–8.

Schwieler, G. H. (1968). Respiratory regulation during postnatal development in cats and rabbits and some of its morphological substrate. *Acta Physiologica Scandinavica Supplement*, **304**, 1–123.

Schramm, C. M. & Grunstein, M. M. (1987). Respiratory influence of peripheral chemoreceptor stimulation in maturing rabbits. *Journal of Applied Physiology*, **63**, 1671–80.

Schulze, K, Kairam, R., Stefanski, M. et al. (1981). Spontaneous variability in minute ventilation oxygen consumption and heart rate of low birth weight infants. *Pediatric Research*, **15**, 1111–16.

Scott, S. C., Inman, J. D. G. & Moss, I. R. (1990). Ontogeny of sleep–wake and cardiorespiratory behavior in unanesthetized piglets. *Respiration Physiology*, **80**, 83–102.

Sidi, D., Kuipers, J. R. G., Heymann, M. A., & Rudolph, A. M. (1983). Effects of ambient temperature on oxygen consumption and the circulation in newborn lambs at rest and during hypoxemia. *Pediatric Research*, **17**, 254–8.

Spiers, D. E. & Adair, E. R. (1986). Ontogeny of homeothermy in the immature rat: metabolic and thermal responses. *Journal of Applied Physiology*, **60**, 1190–7.

Steele, A. M. (1986). Developmental changes in neural control of respiration. In *Developmental Neurobiology of the Autonomic Nervous System*, ed. P. M. Gootman. pp. 327–401. Humana Press, Clifton.

Steinschneider, A. & Weinstein, S. (1983). Sleep respiratory instability in term neonates under hyperthermic conditions: age, sex, type of feeding, and rapid eye movements. *Pediatric Research*, **17**, 35–41.

Stothers, J. K. & Warner, R. M. (1978). Oxygen consumption and neonatal sleep states. *Journal of Physiology*, **278**, 435–40.

Sullivan, C. E., Kozar, L. F. & Phillipson, E. A. (1978). Primary role of respiratory afferents in sustaining breathing rhythm. *Journal of Applied Physiology*, **48**, 11–17.

Thach, B. T., Abroms, I. F., Frantz, I. D., Sotrel, A., Bruce, E. N. & Goldman, M. D. (1980). Intercostal muscle reflexes and sleep breathing patterns in the human infant. *Journal of Applied Physiology*, **48**, 139–46.

Woodrum, D. E., Standaert, T. A., Mayock, D. E. & Guthrie, R. D. (1981). Hypoxic ventilatory response in the newborn monkey. *Pediatric Research*, **15**, 367–70.

Wyszogrodski, I., Thach, B. T. & Milic-Emili, J. (1978). Maturation of respiratory control in unanesthetized newborn rabbits. *Journal of Applied Physiology*, **44**, 304–10.

Pathophysiology

9

Apnoea, sudden infant death and respiratory control

CHRISTIAN F. POETS
and DAVID P. SOUTHALL

Introduction

The sudden infant death syndrome (SIDS) is defined as 'the sudden death of an infant under one year of age which remains unexplained after the performance of a complete postmortem investigation, including an autopsy, an examination of the scene of death and review of the case history' (Zylke, 1989). It is the leading cause of postneonatal mortality in non-third world countries, accounting for about 1500 deaths per year in the UK and 5500 in the United States during the late 1980s (Foundation for the Study of Infant Deaths, 1989; Wegman, 1990). The sudden fatality of this syndrome and the absence of any morphological finding that would explain death have made it, as yet, impossible to identify its pathophysiology.

For many centuries sudden unexpected infant deaths were thought to be caused by the parents accidentally overlying or deliberately suffocating their babies. It was only at the end of the eighteenth century that organic causes started to be considered, namely that an enlarged thymus would interfere with heart or lung function ('thymic death'). This theory persisted, despite good evidence against it, until the first half of this century, and led to the prophylactic irradiation of the thymus (with subsequent carcinomas of the thyroid) in the 1930s. Still (1923) was the first to describe episodes of arrested respiration and to relate such episodes to sudden death in infants. Steinschneider (1972) after observing such episodes in five infants, two of whom later died of SIDS, renewed the hypothesis that prolonged apnoeic pauses are part of the final pathway leading to SIDS. Since then a growing body of evidence suggests that SIDS may not always be as sudden an event as might be implied by its name. Instead, most infants who die of SIDS appear to have experienced a certain degree of hypoxia for some time prior to death (Naeye, 1988; Rognum et al., 1988). Initially this was considered to support the concept that a disturbance in the control of breathing, leading to recurrent and potentially fatal cessations of respiration, is responsible for death (Naeye, 1988). More recently, however, attention has been drawn away from the (central) control of breathing towards a disturbance in the regulation of the matching of ventilation to perfusion in the lungs (Southall, Samuels & Talbert, 1990; Martinez, 1991). This latter approach has introduced new concepts which might help to improve our understanding of the pathophysiology of SIDS. Whether or not they will enable us to prevent SIDS in the future remains, however, still speculative.

This chapter aims (a) to review briefly the characteristic epidemiological and morphological features of SIDS, (b) to highlight some of the recent theories regarding the pathophysiology of SIDS, and (c) to summarize current attempts to prevent SIDS.

Epidemiology

Incidence

There is considerable variability in the rate of SIDS between different countries and between different ethnic groups within a country (Table 9.1). The reasons for these differences are unclear, but both genetic and socioeconomic factors appear to be involved (Black et al., 1986). Recently, an alarming trend towards an increase in SIDS rates was reported from several countries, leading to a doubling of the number of SIDS cases in Norway (Irgens, Skjaerven & Lie, 1989) and an almost threefold increase in The Netherlands over the last 20 years (Engelberts & de Jonge, 1990). This increase could not be sufficiently explained by changes in diagnostic fashions (Mitchell, 1990). It may be due to changes in child care practices (Engelberts & de Jonge, 1990).

Age distribution

One of the most striking epidemiological features of SIDS is its characteristic age distribution. SIDS occurs relatively infrequently during the neonatal period; its frequency then increases rapidly to reach a peak at 2–4 months of age, and decreases gradually thereafter. Hence, 75% of

Table 9.1. *SIDS incidence in various countries and ethnic groups in the world*

Country	Year	Rate (death/1000)	Reference
Cook County, USA	1975–80	2.7	Black et al., 1986
– Blacks		5.1	
– Hispanics		1.2	
– Whites		1.3	
England	1985	2.2	Foundation for the Study of Infant Deaths, 1989
Lübeck, Germany	1980–83	2.2	Dittmann & Pribilla, 1983
Norway	1983–84	2.4	Irgens et al., 1989
Sweden	1984–86	0.9	Wennergren et al., 1987
Hong Kong	1986–87	0.3	Lee et al., 1989
Christchurch, New Zealand	1983	6.3	Mitchell, 1990

deaths occur between 2–4 months of age, and 95% of SIDS victims are younger than 10 months of age (Grether & Schulman, 1989).

Season and time of death

There is a clear preponderance in the cold season, with up to 95% of deaths occurring between October and April in the northern hemisphere (Rajs & Hammarquist, 1988). This seasonal distribution has been related to viral infections, which also occur predominantly during the cold season and are frequently reported to precede death (Guntheroth, 1989a). The outbreak of a viral epidemic in a community may coincide with a clustering of SIDS cases in the same region (Uren et al., 1980).

There is a tendency for SIDS to occur most frequently on Saturdays and Sundays (Kaada & Sivertsen, 1990). This finding has been related to the fact that the infants' daily routine is more likely to be disturbed at weekends (Kaada & Sivertsen, 1990).

SIDS occurs predominantly during the night time, a period when both infants and parents are most likely to be asleep. For example, in a study from Dittmann & Pribilla (1983), 58% of their 155 SIDS cases had died between midnight and 8 am. Kahn et al. (1984) compared the histories of SIDS victims with those of infants who were successfully resuscitated from an apparent life-threatening event (ALTE). They found that most

Table 9.2. *Risk factors for SIDS*

Maternal factors	Infantile factors
Young age	Male gender
Multiparity	Low birthweight
Smoking during pregnancy	Premature birth
Anaemia during pregnancy	Low Apgar scores
Low social class	Prone sleeping position
Short interpregnancy interval	Overheating
Unmarried mother	Previous SIDS in family
Maternal drug abuse	Previous cyanotic episode

Derived from Golding, 1989; Naeye, Ladis & Drage, 1976; Engelberts & De-Jonge, 1990; Hoffman et al., 1988.

SIDS victims had died during the night, while most ALTE were discovered during the afternoon, i.e. at a time when their caretakers were awake and the infants were, therefore, more likely to be under observation. Hence, although the characteristic time distribution may suggest this, there is as yet no conclusive evidence that SIDS is a sleep disorder. In fact, most ALTE seem to occur whilst the infants are awake (Krishna, Wolde-Tsadik & Keens, 1987).

Risk factors

There is a large number of epidemiologically defined risk factors for SIDS (Table 9.2). Based on these risk factors, scoring systems have been developed to identify a group of infants at high risk (Peters & Golding, 1986). Unfortunately, none of these scoring systems has as yet been able to identify a risk-group with a sensitivity and specificity high enough to make them practical tools in an intervention programme aimed at reducing the incidence of SIDS in a community (see below). Nevertheless, a programme of parent education to avoid (1) the prone sleeping position, (2) smoking before and after birth, and (3) over-insulation leading to overheating has been recently implemented in New Zealand and in the UK. Preliminary results are extremely encouraging as they show a 50–70% reduction in SIDS rates, but await confirmation, since it is yet unclear whether this trend will persist over the coming years (Mitchell et al., 1992; Wigfield et al., 1992; Foundation for the Study of Infant Deaths, 1993).

Clinical risk groups

In clinical practice, and only partially in accordance with the risk factors mentioned above, three main risk groups have been identified: (1) infants who have suffered an ALTE, (2) subsequent siblings or surviving twins of SIDS victims, and (3) infants who were born very prematurely (at <32 weeks gestation). Although contributing to less than 10% of all SIDS victims (Hoffman et al., 1988), infants who have suffered an ALTE have a high risk of SIDS, particularly if the events are recurrent. In them the SIDS rate may increase to more than 13% (Oren, Kelly & Shannon, 1986), particularly if the ALTE has been treated by cardiopulmonary resuscitation.

Infants who have lost a previous sibling from SIDS have a risk which is about four to six times that of the total population (Guntheroth, Lohmann & Spiers, 1990). SIDS siblings also have a higher infant mortality from causes other than SIDS. For example, Guntheroth et al. (1990), in the above population-based study involving 251,124 live births, found a SIDS rate of 13.0/1000 and an overall infant mortality rate of 20.8/1000 for subsequent siblings (the corresponding rates for the total population of infants were 2.2 and 5.1/1000, respectively). A 2% risk of losing a baby after already suffering the sudden death of a baby is unacceptably high.

The risk of SIDS in preterm infants increases with decreasing gestational age at birth (Yount et al., 1979), reaching values of up to 24/1000 for those who were born at less than 32 weeks gestation (Wariyar, Richmond & Hey, 1989). Although it has been questioned whether a sudden unexpected death in an infant with bronchopulmonary dysplasia can be classified as SIDS, it is noteworthy that these infants have a particularly high rate of sudden unexpected deaths (up to 11%) (Werthammer et al., 1982).

Pathology

As mentioned above, there are no morphological findings that can explain the death. Nevertheless, there are characteristic findings present in a majority of cases. The most consistent amongst these findings are intrathoracic petechiae, which are present in 52–87% of cases (Valdes-Dapena, 1988; Beckwith, 1988). These are thought to be caused by large intrathoracic pressure swings, possibly in combination with sympathetic stimulation or a respiratory tract infection (Beckwith, 1988; Guntheroth et al., 1980).

Another characteristic finding is the occurrence of blood-stained froth around the nose and mouth, which is found in approximately 60% of SIDS victims (Beckwith, 1973). This phenomenon may be caused by a combination of pulmonary oedema and high transpulmonary pressures (e.g. due to vigorous breathing movements) immediately prior to death (Martinez, 1991).

Finally, as mentioned above, there are a number of morphological changes which have been interpreted as indicative of chronic tissue hypoxia. These so-called 'hypoxic tissue markers' include the retention of periadrenal brown fat, gliosis of the brainstem, hyperplasia of pulmonary neuroendocrine cells, and an increased wall thickness of both pulmonary arteries and airways (Naeye, 1988; Valdes-Dapena, 1988; Gillan et al., 1989; Haque et al., 1991). The interpretation of these markers, however, is difficult, particularly as the latter three observations may not only reflect the presence of chronic hypoxia but may, in turn, indicate an increased reactivity of the pulmonary airways and vessels in these infants (Gillan et al., 1989), thereby pointing to a potential pathophysiology which might have resulted in, or contributed to, the development of potentially fatal hypoxia (see below).

Current theories on mechanisms

The persisting lack of objective data concerning the final pathways leading to SIDS has given rise to a large number of theories concerning the pathogenesis of these tragedies. Only a minute proportion of these proposed theories correlate with the known epidemiological and pathological data on SIDS. A critical review of all these theories would go beyond the scope of this chapter. We therefore concentrate on the four major theories currently under debate.

Cessations of respiratory efforts ('central apnoea')

Following Steinschneider's observation of prolonged apnoeic pauses in two subsequent SIDS victims (Steinschneider, 1972), it soon became widely postulated that this was the major mechanism for SIDS. It was considered to be similar to 'apnoea of prematurity' and related to an immaturity of, or disturbance in, the brainstem centres regulating the control of breathing. This concept was apparently supported by recordings of breathing movements and oxygenation, particularly in preterm infants, which showed that prolonged apnoeic pauses may be one mechanism for severe hypoxaemia. A causal relationship of these apnoeic pauses to SIDS, however, remains unproven. A large, prospective, population-based study, involving 24-hour recordings of breathing movements and ECG in 9856 infants, 29 of whom subsequently died of SIDS (Southall et al., 1983) did not show prolonged apnoeic pauses (≥ 20 s) in any of the SIDS cases. Compared with controls, the SIDS cases in this and a similar, though not population-based study involving 30 future SIDS victims (Kahn et al., 1992) also did not exhibit significantly increased numbers of short apnoeic pauses or a higher proportion of periodic breathing. In fact, in a recent analysis, SIDS infants showed less short apnoeic pauses than controls (Schechtman et al., 1991). Thus, although these prospective studies do not allow conclusions regarding the final pathways for SIDS, they failed to support Steinschneider's original concept that prolonged apnoeic pauses occur repeatedly in infants who subsequently die of SIDS.

Moreover, the few existing studies which obtained physiological recordings during death or 'near-death' events using event recorders at home have found prolonged apnoeic pauses at the onset of these events in only a very small minority of infants (Kelly, Pathak & Meny, 1991; Poets et al., 1992b). Finally, some of the most characteristic morphological findings in SIDS, namely intrathoracic petechiae and the blood-stained froth around the mouth, are difficult to explain if death had been due to a central inhibition of respiration. Instead, both findings point to the presence of large intrathoracic pressure swings immediately prior to death (see above). In conclusion, although prolonged cessations of respiratory efforts may undoubtedly cause severe hypoxaemia, there is as yet no conclusive evidence that this mechanism is of key importance in the majority of SIDS cases.

Cessations of nasal airflow with continued respiratory efforts ('obstructive apnoea')

Guilleminault et al. (1975) described short episodes of arrested airflow, but continued breathing movements, in eight infants who had suffered apparent life-threatening events. This breathing pattern, occurring either alone ('obstructive apnoea') or in combination with a cessation of breathing movements ('mixed apnoea'), has since been identified as the predominant form of apnoea in preterm infants (Barrington & Finer, 1991) (Fig. 9.1). It may also occur in healthy full-term infants. A potential relationship between this breathing pattern and SIDS has been proposed

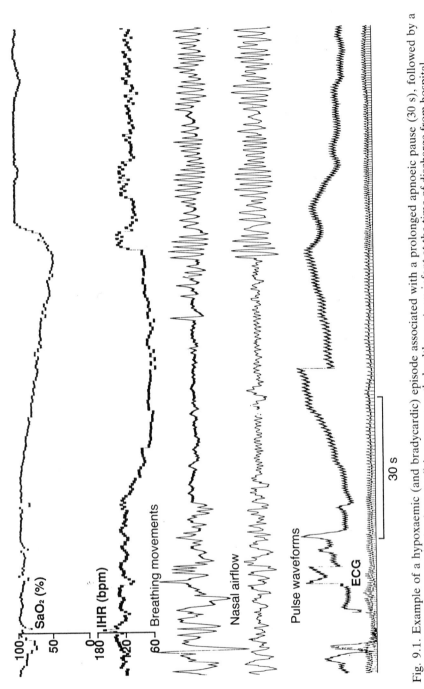

Fig. 9.1. Example of a hypoxaemic (and bradycardic) episode associated with a prolonged apnoeic pause (30 s), followed by a cessation of airflow only ('mixed apnoea') in an apparently healthy preterm infant at the time of discharge from hospital.

by several investigators (Guilleminault et al., 1975), particularly as a terminal episode of airway obstruction might well correlate with some of the morphological findings in SIDS mentioned above. Brief (3–15 s) episodes of interrupted airflow, but continued breathing movements, were also significantly more frequently found in polygraphic sleep recordings from 30 infants who subsequently died of SIDS when compared with matched controls (Kahn et al., 1992).

The pathophysiology resulting in intermittent airway obstruction, and its potential relationship to sudden death remains, however, poorly understood. Even the site of the airway obstruction is unclear. Thus pharyngeal pressure recordings in preterm infants have suggested closure at the pharyngeal level (Mathew, Roberts & Thach, 1982). In contrast, video recordings of the upper airway using an ultrafine fibreoptic bronchoscope showed hypopharyngeal closure (Ruggins, 1991). Moreover, episodes of continued breathing movements and yet absent airflow have also been observed in infants with an endotracheal airway, suggesting that these episodes involve not only obstruction of the upper but possibly also of the lower airways (Poets, Samuels & Southall, 1992c). It may thus be speculated that the site of airway obstruction may either vary between different episodes or infants, or that it involves the simultaneous closure of different parts of the intra- and extrathoracic airways.

Intrapulmonary shunting

Severe hypoxaemia may not only result from a cessation of breathing movements and/or nasal airflow, but may also occur despite continuation of both breathing movements and airflow (Fig. 9.2). This pattern has been found in preterm infants (Poets et al., 1991a), particularly in those presenting with cyanotic episodes of unknown cause (Samuels et al., 1992), in term infants during respiratory tract infections, particularly pertussis and respiratory syncytial virus (Southall, Thomas & Lambert, 1988a; Southall et al., 1988b), and in older infants and young children with cyanotic breath-holding spells (Southall et al., 1990). The pathophysiology of these hypoxaemic episodes has been most rigorously investigated in the latter group. Southall et al. (1990) studied 51 infants and young children with cyanotic breath-holding spells involving loss of consciousness, eight of whom subsequently died suddenly and unexpectedly. Arterial blood gas measurements in eight of these 51 patients obtained during the course of a breath-holding spell showed that PaO_2 fell to 17–32 mmHg within 10–25 seconds of the onset of breath-holding.

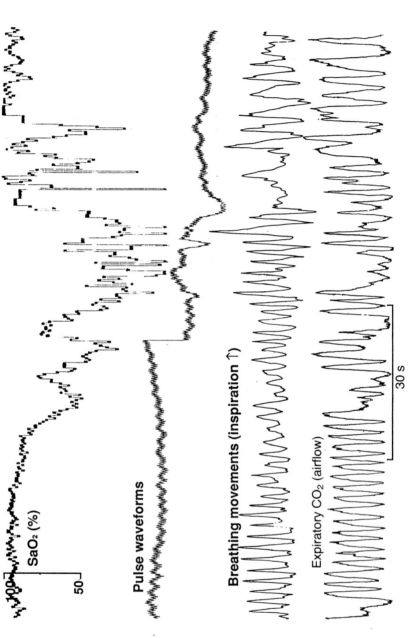

Fig. 9.2. Example of an episode of severe hypoxaemia despite continuation of breathing movements and airflow in a fullterm infant with cyanotic breath-holding spells from (Southall et al., 1990).

Contrast-echocardiography performed during cyanotic attacks in six patients showed no right-to-left intracardiac passage of air bubbles. Moreover, Krypton infusion scans performed in five patients showed an increase in background body counts during cyanotic episodes, suggesting the presence of an intrapulmonary right-to-left shunt. Thus the rapidity of the development of hypoxaemia and the presence of continued ventilation observed at the onset of some of the cyanotic episodes were suggested by these investigations to be due to the sudden development of a shunt of mixed venous deoxygenated blood through to the systemic circulation.

The occurrence of a sudden intrapulmonary shunt leading to severe hypoxaemia could well explain many of the pathological and epidemiological findings in SIDS victims mentioned above. The mechanism(s) by which such a shunt may develop, however, is still unknown (Southall et al., 1990; Martinez, 1991).

Cardiac arrhythmias

Schwartz proposed in 1976 that there might be a transient prolongation of the QT-interval which creates an increased susceptibility to SIDS (Schwartz, 1976). The same author then found a 'markedly prolonged QTc' in six of nine SIDS victims, identified in a prospective population-based study on 8 000 infants (Schwartz, 1987). In contrast, Southall et al. (1983, 1986*b*), in the prospective study mentioned above, and in an additional prospective study involving standard electrocardiograms on 7254 neonates, found no abnormal prolongation of the QT-interval in their 29 and 15, respectively, SIDS victims. Weinstein & Steinschneider (1985) were also unable in a prospective study to identify a prolonged QT-interval in any of their eight SIDS victims. Differences between these studies have been discussed in a recent review by Guntheroth (1989*b*).

Despite the above evidence against a primary cardiac disturbance in SIDS, such a mechanism was recently re-introduced to explain the finding of marked bradycardia without apnoea in recordings of documented infant deaths using event recorders at home (Kelly et al., 1991). These event recordings, however, did not include information about oxygenation. It is thus impossible, on the basis of these recordings, to distinguish between a primary bradycardia and one secondary to hypoxaemia. Therefore, the bradycardias observed in that study may well have been the result of non-apnoeic hypoxaemia (resulting from mechanisms 2 or 3 above) rather than the primary cause of death (Poets et al., 1992*c*).

Intervention strategies

Principal considerations

SIDS is unpredictable and relatively rare. Strategies aiming at reducing the incidence of SIDS in a community are therefore bound to be either non-specific or non-sensitive. A non-specific approach would, for example, be an attempt to modify general child care practices known to be related to SIDS. Such an attempt is currently being undertaken by the British Ministry of Health in their campaign against the prone sleeping position, smoking and overheating. This campaign is based on recent retrospective (and one prospective) studies which showed a relative risk of SIDS for the prone sleeping position of between 2 and 12 (Engelberts & de Jonge, 1990; Dwyer et al., 1991). However, apart from some encouraging preliminary prospective post-intervention data from Avon, New Zealand and The Netherlands (Wigfield et al., 1992; Mitchell et al., 1992; Engelberts & de Jonge, 1990) there is as yet no study that has been able to show a persistent reduction in the incidence of SIDS following such campaigns.

An alternate approach is to identify individual infants at relatively high risk of SIDS and apply to them specific preventive measures. Such an approach was first and most extensively performed in Sheffield, where a predictive risk-score for sudden unexpected infant deaths was developed and infants with high scores regularly seen by a team of health visitors (Carpenter et al., 1983). Although a reduction in overall infant mortality rates was reported, the rate of true SIDS apparently remained unchanged (Alexander & Southall, 1986). Moreover, a randomized controlled trial based on this approach was terminated prematurely. A recent meta-analysis of this and other risk scores showed that 20% of a population would have to be included to identify 40–70% of the SIDS cases in this population (Peters & Golding, 1986). Thus, any intervention programme that aims to reach at least 50% of all future SIDS victims in a community would have to include very large numbers of infants to even come close to this goal.

Clinical management of infants at risk of SIDS

In day-to-day practice, intervention has mostly been limited to the application of preventive measures in the three clinical risk groups mentioned above. These measures are aimed foremost at excluding any treatable disorder potentially resulting in sudden death, particularly in infants presenting with an ALTE. In this latter group, a full medical examination including an ECG, a chest X-ray, a whole blood count, measurements of serum electrolytes and blood glucose, and taking of a specimen for viral and bacteriological analysis should therefore be performed. If clinically indicated, additional investigations such as standard EEG, brainscan, radiography, and pH monitoring of the lower oesophagus might be appropriate.

Only if the above measures have not helped to identify a treatable cause for the ALTE, a sleep study or polysomnography should be performed. This includes the continuous, if necessary long-term, recording of physiological variables such as breathing movements, ECG, nasal airflow, arterial oxygen saturation, transcutaneous PO_2 and PCO_2, electroencephalogram, and electro-oculogram. These recordings have been valuable in the identification of disorders which require specific therapy such as subclinical baseline hypoxaemia (particularly in preterm infants), sleep-related upper airway obstruction, imposed upper airway obstruction, or epileptic seizure-induced cyanotic episodes. However, screening recordings (pneumograms or oxy-pneumograms) have not been shown to have any predictive value with regard to SIDS, and it has been recommended that decisions concerning clinical management should not be based on results of single overnight recordings of breathing movements and ECG (Hunt & Brouillette, 1987; Little et al., 1987).

The next step in the clinical work-up of infants at risk of SIDS is a decision as to whether a child should be commenced on a home monitor. These devices are, at present, the only preventive measure routinely applied in infants considered to be at increased risk of SIDS. Following Steinschneider's hypothesis that a prolonged cessation of respiratory efforts is part of the final pathway in sudden infant death, initially most home monitoring devices monitored only breathing efforts. However, it soon became clear that this type of home monitor would not identify episodes of absent airflow with continuous breathing movements ('obstructive apnoeas'). Based on the assumption that these latter episodes, if severe, would invariably be accompanied by a significant fall in heart rate, many home monitors, particularly in the US, now also include registration of the electrocardiogram.

Recently, however, data obtained during 69 prolonged hypoxaemic episodes (defined as a fall in SaO_2 to $\leq 80\%$ for ≥ 20 s and/or the occurrence of clinically apparent central cyanosis) showed that prolonged apnoeic pauses (≥ 20 s) or bradycardias (HR ≤ 80 bpm) occurred only during 10% and 28%, respectively, of these episodes (Poets et al.,

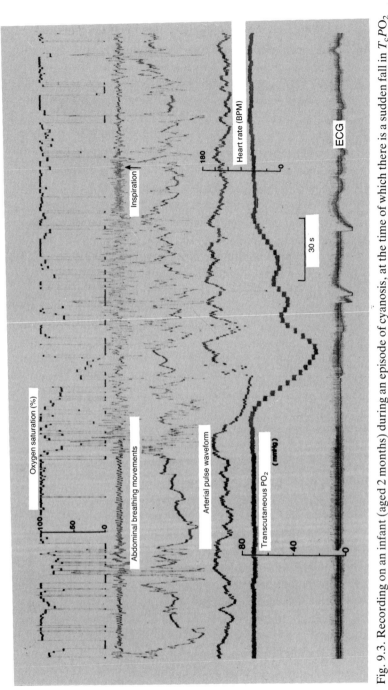

Fig. 9.3. Recording on an infant (aged 2 months) during an episode of cyanosis, at the time of which there is a sudden fall in T_cPO_2 lasting 90 seconds. This is accompanied by continuous breathing movements and a fall in heart rate to 65 beats/minute. The pulse oximeter signal is lost due to movement artefact and might not, therefore, have identified this event (from Poets et al., 1991*b*).

1991*b*). The only recorded variable that would invariably have identified all of these episodes was the transcutaneous PO_2 (the saturation signal from the pulse oximeter was disturbed, due to movement artefact, in 10% of episodes; Fig. 9.3). As a consequence we began to use a modified transcutaneous PO_2 monitor in infants at risk of hypoxaemia and/or sudden death. Experience with this monitor, now in over 600 infants, has shown that it provides a reliable and early detection of sudden changes in PO_2, that it is safe, and that it can be used by parents at home (Poets et al., 1991*b*). However, as with other home monitoring devices, these data are uncontrolled, and there is as yet no proof that home monitoring will reduce the incidence of SIDS.

Conclusions

SIDS is still a mystery. However, there is growing evidence from recent pathological and epidemiological studies and from investigations into hypoxaemic episodes in infancy that the sudden onset of hypoxaemia may play an important role in the pathophysiology leading to these deaths. At the same time, the technical feasibility of recording data during deaths or near-death events in a large number of infants using event-recorders offers the opportunity of gaining direct access to information about the final pathways of SIDS. There are therefore good reasons to hope that the mechanisms leading to SIDS could soon be elucidated.

References

Alexander, J. R. & Southall, D. P. (1986). Cot death and the Sheffield score. *Lancet*, **ii**, 399.

Barrington, K. & Finer, N. (1991). The natural history of the appearance of apnea of prematurity. *Pediatric Research*, **29**, 372–5.

Beckwith, J. B. (1973). The sudden infant death syndrome. *Current Problems in Pediatrics*, **3**, 3–35.

Beckwith, J. B. (1988). Intrathoracic petechial hemorrhages: a clue to the mechanism of death in sudden infant death syndrome? *Annals of the New York Academy of Sciences*, **533**, 37–47.

Black, L., David, R. J., Brouillette, R. T. & Hunt, C. E. (1986). Effects of birth weight and ethnicity on incidence of sudden infant death syndrome. *Journal of Pediatrics*, **108**, 209–14.

Carpenter, R. G., Gardner, A., Jepson, M. et al. (1983). Prevention of unexpected infant death. *Lancet*, **i**, 723–7.

Dittmann, V. & Pribilla, O. (1983). Zur Epidemiologie des plötzlichen Säuglingstodes im Lübecker Raum. *Zeitschrift für Rechtsmedizin (Berlin)*, **90**, 277–92.

Dwyer, T., Ponsonby, A-L. B., Newman, N. M. & Gibbons, L. E. (1991). Prospective cohort study of prone sleeping position and sudden infant death syndrome. *Lancet*, **337**, 1244–7.

Engelberts, A. C. & de Jonge, G. A. (1990). Choice of sleeping position for infants: possible association with cot death. *Archives of Disease in Childhood*, **65**, 462–7.

Foundation for the Study of Infant Deaths (1989). *Newsletter* 35. London.

Foundation for the Study of Infant Deaths (1993). *Newsletter* 44. London.

Gillan, J. E., Curran, C., O'Reilly, E., Cahalane, S. F. & Unwin, A. R. (1989). Abnormal patterns of pulmonary neuroendocrine cells in victims of sudden infant death syndrome. *Pediatrics*, **84**, 828–34.

Golding, J. (1989). The epidemiology and sociology of the sudden infant death syndrome. In *Paediatric Forensic Medicine and Pathology*, ed. J. K. Masons. pp. 141–155. Chapman & Hall, London.

Grether, J. K. & Schulman, J. (1989). Sudden infant death syndrome and birth weight. *Journal of Pediatrics*, **114**, 561–7.

Guilleminault, C., Peraita, R., Souquet, M. & Dement, W. C. (1975). Apneas during sleep in infants: possible relationship with sudden infant death syndrome. *Science*, **190**, 677–9.

Guntheroth, W. G. (1989*a*). *Crib Death: The Sudden Infant Death Syndrome*. Futura Publishing Company, New York.

Guntheroth, W. G. (1989*b*). Theories of cardiovascular causes in sudden infant death syndrome. *Journal of the American College of Cardiology*, **14**, 443–7.

Guntheroth, W. G., Kawabori, I., Breazeale, D. G., Garlinghouse, L. E. & van Hoosier, G. L. (1980). The role of respiratory infection in intrathoracic petechiae. *American Journal of Diseases of Children*, **134**, 364–6.

Guntheroth, W. G., Lohmann, R. & Spiers, P. S. (1990). Risk of sudden infant death syndrome in subsequent siblings. *Journal of Pediatrics*, **116**, 520–4.

Haque, A. K., Mancuso, M. G., Hokanson, J., Nguyen, N. D. & Nichols, M. M. (1991). Bronchiolar wall changes in sudden infant death syndrome: morphometric study of a new observation. *Pediatric Pathology*, **11**, 551–68.

Hoffman, H. J., Damus, K., Hillman, L. & Krongrad, E. (1988). Risk factors for SIDS: Results of the National Institute of Child Health and Human Development Cooperative Epidemiological Study. *Annals of the New York Academy of Sciences*, **533**, 13–20.

Hunt, C. E. & Brouillette, R. T. (1987). Sudden infant death syndrome: 1987 perspective. *Journal of Pediatrics*, **110**, 669–78.

Irgens, L. M., Skjaerven, R. & Lie, R. T. (1989). Secular trends of sudden infant death syndrome and other causes of post perinatal mortality in Norwegian birth cohorts 1967–1984. *Acta Paediatrica Scandinavica*, **78**, 228–32.

Kaada, B. & Sivertsen, E. (1990). Sudden infant death syndrome during weekends and holidays in Norway in 1967–1985. *Scandinavian Journal of the Society of Medicine*, **18**, 17–23.

Kahn, A., Blum, D., Hennart, P. et al. (1984). A critical comparison of the history of sudden-death infants and infants hospitalised for near-miss for SIDS. *European Journal of Pediatrics*, **143**, 103–7.

Kahn, A., Groswasser, J., Rebuffat, E. et al. (1992). Sleep and cardiorespiratory characteristics of infant victims of sudden death: a prospective case-control study. *Sleep*, **15**, 287–92.

Kelly, D. H., Pathak, A. & Meny, R. (1991). Sudden severe bradycardia in infancy. *Pediatric Pulmonology*, **10**, 199–204.

Krishna, V., Wolde-Tsadik, G. & Keens, T. G. (1987). Serious subsequent apneas in infants presenting with ALTE while awake (abstract). *Pediatric Pulmonology*, **3**, 456.

Lee, N. N. Y., Chan, Y. F., Davies, D. P., Lau, E. & Yip, D. C. (1989). Sudden infant death syndrome in Hong Kong: confirmation of low incidence. *British Medical Journal*, **298**, 721.

Little, G. A. & Members of Consensus Development Panel (1987). National Institutes of Health consensus development conference on infantile apnea and home monitoring, Sept 29 to Oct 1, 1986. *Pediatrics,* **79**, 292–9.

Martinez, F. D. (1991). Sudden infant death syndrome and small airway occlusion: facts and a hypothesis. *Pediatrics* **87**, 190–8.

Mathew, O. P., Roberts, J. L. & Thach, B. T. (1982). Pharyngeal airway obstruction in preterm infants during mixed and obstructive apnea. *Journal of Pediatrics*, **100**, 964–8.

Mitchell, E. A. (1990). International trends in postneonatal mortality. *Archives of Disease in Childhood*, **65**, 607–9.

Mitchell, E. A., Ford, R. P. K, Taylor, B. J. et al. (1992). Further evidence supporting a causal relationship between prone sleeping position and SIDS. *Journal of Paediatric Child Health*, **28**, S9-S12.

Naeye, R. L. (1988). Sudden infant death syndrome, is the confusion ending? *Modern Pathology*, **1**, 169–74.

Naeye, R. L., Ladis, B. & Drage, J. S. (1976). Sudden infant death syndrome. A prospective study. *American Journal of Diseases of Children*, **130**, 1207–10.

Oren, J., Kelly, D. & Shannon, D. C. (1986). Identification of a high-risk group for sudden infant death syndrome among infants who were resuscitated for sleep apnea. *Pediatrics*, **77**, 495–9.

Peters, T. J. & Golding, J. (1986). Prediction of sudden infant death syndrome: an independent evaluation of four scoring methods. *Statistics in Medicine*, **5**, 113–26.

Poets, C. F., Stebbens, V. A., Alexander, J. R., Arrowsmith, W. A., Salfield, S. A. W. & Southall, D. P. (1991*a*). Oxygen saturations and breathing patterns in infancy. II preterm infants at discharge from special care. *Archives of Disease in Childhood*, **66**, 574–8.

Poets, C. F., Samuels, M. P., Noyes, J. P., Jones, K. A. & Southall, D. P. (1991*b*). Home monitoring of transcutaneous oxygen tension in the early detection of hypoxaemia in infants and young children. *Archives of Disease in Childhood*, **66**, 676–82.

Poets, C. F., Samuels, M. P. & Southall, M. P. (1992*a*). Sudden severe bradycardia secondary to hypoxaemia (letter). *Pediatric Pulmonology*, **12**, 59.

Poets,C. F., Neuber, K., Noyes, J. P., Samuels, M. P. & Southall, D. P. (1992*b*) Event recordings of oxygenation, breathing movements and ECG in infants and young children with recurrent apparent life-threatening events. *Pediatric Pulmonology*, **14**, 257.

Poets, C. F., Samuels, M. P. & Southall, M. P. (1992*c*) The potential role of intrapulmonary shunting in the genesis of hypoxemic episodes in infants and young children. *Pediatrics*, **90**, 385–92.

Rajs, J., Hammarquist, F. (1988). Sudden infant death in Stockholm. *Acta Paediatrica Scandinavica*, **77**, 812–20.

Rognum, T. O., Saugstad, O. D., Oyasæter, S. & Olaisen, B. (1988). Elevated levels of hypoxanthine in vitreous humour indicate prolonged cerebral hypoxia in victims of sudden infant death syndrome. *Pediatrics*, **82**, 615–18.

Ruggins, N. R. (1991). Pathophysiology of apnoea in preterm infants. *Archives of Disease in Childhood*, **66**, 70–3.

Samuels, M. P., Poets, C. F., Stebbens, V. A., Alexander, J. R. & Southall, D. P. (1992). Oxygen saturation and breathing patterns in preterm infants with cyanotic episodes. *Acta Paediatrica Scandinavica*, **82**, 875–80.

Schechtman, V. L., Harper, R. M., Wilson, A. J. & Southall, D. P. (1991). Sleep apnea in infants who succumb to the sudden infant death syndrome. *Pediatrics*, **87**, 841–6.

Schwartz, P. J. (1976). Cardiac sympathetic innervation and the sudden infant death syndrome. *American Journal of Medicine*, **60**, 167–72.

Schwartz, P. J. (1987). The quest for the mechanisms of the sudden infant death syndrome: doubts and progress. *Circulation*, **75**, 677–83.

Southall, D. P., Richards, J. M., de Swiet, M. et al. (1983). Identification of infants destined to die unexpectedly during infancy: evaluation of predictive importance of prolonged apnoea and disorders of cardiac rhythm or conduction. *British Medical Journal*, **286**, 1092–6.

Southall, D. P., Richards, J. M., Stebbens, V., Wilson, A. J., Taylor, V. & Alexander, J. R. (1986*a*). Cardiorespiratory function in 16 full-term infants with sudden infant death syndrome. *Pediatrics*, **78**, 787–96.

Southall, D. P., Arrowsmith, W. A., Stebbens, V. & Alexander, J. R. (1986*b*). QT interval measurements before sudden infant death syndrome. *Archives of Disease in Childhood*, **61**, 327–33.

Southall, D. P., Thomas, M. G. & Lambert, H. P. (1988*a*). Severe hypoxaemia in pertussis. *Archives of Disease in Childhood*, **63**, 598–605.

Southall, D. P., Thomas, M., Gurney, A. & Lambert, H. P. (1988*b*). Prolonged expiratory apnoea and respiratory tract infections in infancy (abstract). *Early Human Development*, **17**, 91.

Southall, D. P., Samuels, M. P. & Talbert, D. G. (1990). Recurrent cyanotic episodes with severe arterial hypoxaemia and intrapulmonary shunting: a mechanism for sudden death. *Archives of Disease in Childhood* **65**, 953–61.

Steinschneider, A. (1972). Prolonged apnea and the sudden infant death syndrome: clinical and laboratory observations. *Pediatrics*, **50**, 646–54.

Still, G. F. (1923). Attacks of arrested respiration in the new-born. *Lancet*, **i**, 431–2.

Uren, E. C., Williams, A. L., Jack, I. & Rees, J. W. (1980). Association of respiratory virus infections with sudden infant death syndrome. *Medical Journal of Australia*, **1**, 417–19.

Valdes-Dapena, M. (1988). Sudden infant death syndrome: overview of recent research developments from a pediatric pathologist's perspective. *Pediatrician*, **15**, 222–30.

Wariyar, U., Richmond, S. & Hey, E. (1989). Pregnancy outcome at 24–31 weeks'gestation: mortality. *Archives of Disease in Childhood* **64**, 670–7.

Wegman, M. E. (1990). Annual summary of vital statistics – 1989. *Pediatrics*, **86**, 835–47.

Weinstein, S. L. & Steinschneider, A. (1985). QTc and R-R intervals in victims of the sudden infant death syndrome. *American Journal of Diseases of Children*, **139**, 987–90.

Wennergren, G., Milerad, J., Lagercrantz, H. et al. (1987). The epidemiology of sudden infant death syndrome and attacks of lifelessness in Sweden. *Acta Paediatrica Scandinavica*, **76**, 898–906.

Werthammer, J., Brown, E. R., Neff, R. K. & Taeusch, H. W. (1982). Sudden infant death syndrome in infants with bronchopulmonary dysplasia. *Pediatrics*, **69**, 301–4.

Wigfield, R. E., Fleming, P. J., Berry, P. J., Rudd, P. T. & Golding, J. (1992) Can the fall in Avon's sudden death rate be explained by changes in the sleeping position. *British Medical Journal*, **304**, 282–3.

Yount, J. E., Flanagan, W. J., Dingley, E. F. & Lewman, L. V. (1979). Evidence for an exponentially increasing incidence of sudden infant death syndrome with decreasing birth weight (abstract). *Pediatric Research*, **13**, 510 A.

Zylke, J. W. (1989). Sudden infant death syndrome: resurgent research offers hope. *Journal of the American Medical Association*, **262**, 1565–6.

10

Pulmonary hypoplasia, hyaline membrane disease and chronic lung disease

STEPHEN J. GOULD

Pulmonary hypoplasia

Pulmonary hypoplasia is one of the most common problems encountered at the fetal and perinatal autopsy. It has excited considerable interest and study not only because of this high incidence and its attendant morbidity and mortality but because of the insights that it provides into the mechanisms of normal lung growth.

Incidence

The precise incidence of lung hypoplasia is difficult to ascertain. Data are almost inevitably derived from autopsy series, as reliable criteria for its diagnosis in liveborn infants are not available. Even at autopsy, there is evidence that pulmonary hypoplasia may be missed (Rushton, 1991), although the diagnosis is usually only problematic following lengthy neonatal survival when additional pathology may obscure the presence of hypoplasia.

In a study of 756 consecutive autopsies of newborn infants, Page and Stocker (1982) identified pulmonary hypoplasia in approximately 10% (77 cases). A not too dissimilar figure of 14% was reported by Wigglesworth and Desai in the same year (1982) from a series of 235 perinatal necropsies. In a two-year period at the John Radcliffe Hospital, hypoplastic lungs were present in 12.5% of 248 fetuses greater than 20 weeks of gestation, in 16% of neonatal deaths but only 7% of aborted fetuses less than 20 weeks gestation.

Associations and causes

Pulmonary hypoplasia is associated with a wide range of abnormalities and Table 10.1 provides a classification based on current understanding

Table 10.1. *Causes of pulmonary hypoplasia*

Mechanism	Subgroup	Examples
Primary malformation or idiopathic	• Chromosomal abnormality • Familial	Trisomy 21, 18, 13.
Inadequate thoracic volume	• Skeletal • Diaphragmatic hernia • Effusions	Skeletal dysplasia Rhesus disease Fetal hydrops
Impairment of fetal breathing	• Cerebral • Muscular • Diaphragm	Hypoxia/ischaemia Malformation Congenital dystrophy Amyoplasia ? Exomphalos
Oligohydramnios	• Inadequate production • Excessive loss	Renal agenesis Renal cystic dysplasia Urinary tract obstruction Chronic leakage of Liquor amnii

of the main underlying mechanisms. It should be acknowledged, however, that while the major associations are well established, the precise reasons as to why they impair normal lung growth are not. The percentages quoted below are very approximate and are a synthesis of reported autopsy series, with many potential biases.

Primary or idiopathic (5–10%)

A thorough autopsy and adequate clinical history will usually reveal a known cause or association but a proportion of hypoplastic lungs remain unexplained and can be regarded as a primary malformation (Mendelsohn & Hutchins, 1977; Swischuk et al., 1979; George, Handorf & Suttle, 1981; Langer & Kaufmann, 1986). The presence of a chromosomal abnormality such as trisomy 13, 18 or 21 suggests that there is a genetic basis in some instances (Page & Stocker, 1982), a factor also suggested by the very rare examples in twins (Marechal, Gillerot & Chef, 1984), or of familial idiopathic pulmonary hypoplasia (Boylan et al., 1977).

Inadequate thoracic volume (30–40%)

The lungs need adequate space to grow and any reduction of thoracic volume may cause lung hypoplasia. The lethality of many skeletal dysplasias is due to the pulmonary hypoplasia associated with poor rib growth and small thoracic volume, although it might be argued that a genetic component could be contributory.

Due to displaced abdominal organs in the pleural space, a small diaphragmatic hernia may produce a non-lethal unilateral hypoplastic lung but the mediastinal shift associated with large herniation can cause the contralateral lung to be also affected (Fig. 10.1). Pleural effusions from any source are a potent cause of lung hypoplasia.

Impairment of fetal breathing (5–10%)

A number of pathological conditions may be associated with hypoplasia and the common thread appears to be an interference with normal fetal breathing (Wigglesworth, 1987a). This interference may be central in origin owing to congenital or acquired abnormality of the respiratory centres in the brain stem, such as craniorachischisis or hypoxic-ischaemic disease. Inadequate muscular activity, e.g. in some congenital muscular dystrophies, may produce a similar result as well as diaphragmatic abnormalities such as congenital amyoplasia (Wigglesworth, 1987b). Interference with normal diaphragmatic movement may also be the important aspect in some cases of severe exomphalos, the postulated mechanism being a reduction in the normal movement of the diaphragm by traction of displaced organs such as the liver.

Oligohydramnios (30–40%)

Oligohydramnios is probably the single most common cause of pulmonary hypoplasia, although the underlying reasons for the lack of amniotic fluid are varied. It may result from a lack of urine production due to renal or urinary tract anomalies (see Table 10.1) or from chronic leakage of liquor amnii. Of interest, the lung structure in the hypoplastic lungs associated with oligohydramnios appears to be different to that seen in hypoplasia from other causes (see pathology).

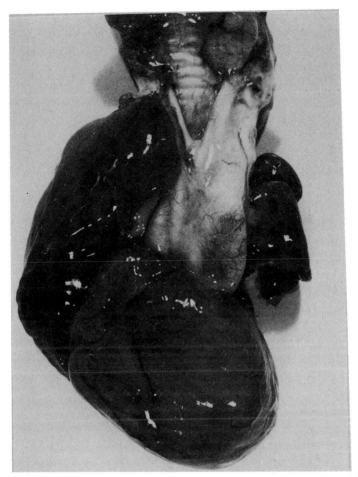

Fig. 10.1. Hypoplastic lungs from an infant born at 37 weeks gestation with left diaphragmatic aplasia and dying at 11 hours of age. The left lung is minute, weighing 2.5 g, and shows the severe compressive effect of liver and bowel in the left thoracic space. The right lung is also small (10 g) following compression due to the mediastinal shift. The diaphragmatic surfaces of both lungs should be at a similar level to the apex of the heart.

Pathology

Macroscopic

At autopsy, diagnosis in stillborn infants and early neonatal deaths is usually straightforward, and lungs are obviously small within the thorax.

A more objective measure is a reduction in the combined lung/body weight ratios; ratios are less than 0.015 in fetuses <28 weeks of gestation, and less than 0.012 in fetuses or infants 28 weeks of gestation or more (Wigglesworth, Desai & Guerrini, 1981).

Microscopy

Morphometry shows reduced radial alveolar counts in hypoplastic lungs from any cause (Emery & Mithal, 1960) but two main patterns of histology are distinguishable. In hypoplasia from any cause other than oligohydramnios, lung growth is reduced but epithelial maturation is normal for the gestation of the infant. In hypoplastic lungs associated with oligohydramnios (OH-lungs), there is not only poor growth but a delay in epithelial maturation and lungs appear immature for gestation. In late third trimester, it is also apparent histologically that elastin does not form properly, being absent from septal crests (Wigglesworth et al., 1981; Haidar, Ryder & Wigglesworth, 1991a; Wigglesworth, Hislop & Desai, 1991). Abnormalities of matrix maturation are also suggested by evidence of disturbed collagen IV development in OH-lungs (Haidar, Wigglesworth & Krausz, 1990).

Detailed morphometry indicates that the epithelial immaturity in OH-lungs is due to lack of differentiation of undifferentiated cells into type I pneumocytes (Haidar, Ryder & Wigglesworth, 1991b). They found that at both 24 and 36 weeks gestation, the percentage of type II pneumocytes is approximately the same in OH-lungs and normal controls. However, the percentage of type I pneumocytes at 36 weeks gestation in hypoplastic OH-lungs is significantly less than those seen in the controls (20% v 46%). Airspace size and proportion of lung occupied by airspace is also considerably reduced in pulmonary hypoplasia.

Biochemistry

Some components of both major subtypes of hypoplastic lungs have been studied and compared with normal (Wigglesworth & Desai, 1981; Wigglesworth, Desai & Aber, 1987; Desai, Wigglesworth & Aber, 1987; Wigglesworth et al., 1991). Not surprisingly, total DNA levels are significantly reduced in both hypoplastic lung subtypes reflecting reduced cell numbers. Disaturated phosphatidylcholine concentration, as a measure of surfactant enzyme system maturation, is lower in OH-lungs than in non-OH hypoplastic lungs. Because detailed morphometry indicates that the proportion of type II cells is similar in OH-lungs compared with normal (Haidar et al., 1991b), the surfactant deficiency suggests there may be a functional impairment of type II cells in OH-lungs not reflected in the simple quantitative measures.

Compared with controls, desmosine, a component of elastic tissue, is reduced in concentration in both subtypes of pulmonary hypoplasia (>30 weeks). This is despite the histologically apparent lack of elastic tissue in septal crests of OH-lung, probably because the septal elastic tissue is a relatively small component of overall lung elastic tissue when the vasculature is taken into account.

Pathogenesis

Although there is a considerable body of evidence to indicate that impaired fetal breathing and oligohydramnios are closely associated with pulmonary hypoplasia, these associations by themselves do not provide an explanation of the poor lung growth. Initial hypotheses suggested that, in oligohydramnios, compression of the fetal thorax was important but experimental studies show that even relatively small losses of amniotic fluid can produce detectable impairment of lung growth (Hislop et al., 1984).

Current concepts suggest that the most important factor in the development of pulmonary hypoplasia, when associated with both oligohydramnios and impairment of fetal breathing, is the production and retention of lung liquid.

Experimental procedures which enhance the loss of lung liquid such as chronic drainage via a tracheal cannula (Alcorn et al., 1977), will produce pulmonary hypoplasia. In contrast, obstruction to lung fluid efflux either surgically or in the natural experiment of laryngeal atresia, produces grossly expanded hyperplastic lungs (Carmel, Friedman & Adams, 1965; Wigglesworth, Desai & Hislop, 1987; Silver, Thurston & Patrick, 1988). In oligohydramnios, Nicolini et al. (1989) hypothesize that there is a reduction in amniotic fluid pressure associated with oligohydramnios and this allows more rapid passage of lung liquid into the amniotic cavity. Harding, Hooper & Dickson (1990; Dickson & Harding, 1991) likewise suggest this pressure gradient exists, but that it results from a relative increase in thoracic and abdominal pressures due to increased spinal curvature and compression.

Besides the clinical associations suggesting the importance of fetal breathing to normal lung growth, evidence of close linkage can be directly obtained in animals following experimentally produced damage to brain stem respiratory centres. In the rabbit, transection of medulla and phrenic nucleus (the latter causing diaphragmatic atrophy) gives rise to severe pulmonary hypoplasia. The link with lung liquid is again suggested by prevention of these effects by simultaneous occlusion of the trachea (Wigglesworth & Desai, 1979). In the fetal lamb, manoeuvres to negate pressure swings within the thorax by the introduction of a silastic window into the chest wall also impair lung growth (Liggins et al., 1981). Despite these observations, it is still not clear how fetal breathing affects lung growth although it does produce an increase in lung volume (Kitterman, 1984) (see also Chapter 4).

Another, but not mutually exclusive, mechanism which might operate in oligohydramnios is suggested by work on hypoplastic lungs associated with renal abnormalities. Hislop, Hey & Reid (1979) reported a reduction in the bronchial branching in some hypoplastic lungs associated with renal agenesis. Further, this abnormality must have occurred early in gestation, before oligohydramnios from lack of fetal urine could have been established. They postulated that there may be an important pulmonary growth factor in fetal urine, such as proline. Peters et al. (1991a,b) have presented further experimental evidence that normal kidneys may be important in early lung growth. To date, however, there is no direct evidence to support a defect in proline metabolism within hypoplastic human fetal lungs and indeed this hypothesis is considered untenable by some (Wigglesworth et al., 1991).

Why should an increase in lung fluid egress lead to hypoplasia? An answer to this question can barely be formulated but one approach is to consider the factors which determine normal pneumocyte differentiation, a fundamental component of OH-lungs being a failure of epithelial maturation. Epithelial differentiation is highly dependent on interaction with the underlying basement membrane and mesenchyme. Thus fibroblasts, under hormonal influence, produce fibroblast-pneumocyte-factor (FPF) which stimulates type II pneumocyte differentiation (Smith & Post, 1989). The basement membrane beneath type I pneumocytes is not the same physically or biochemically as that beneath type II cells; the former shows discontinuities whereas the latter is continuous (Lwebuga-Mukasa, 1991). It is possible that lung liquid retention, via mechanical factors such as stretching, is critical in shaping the matrix with which the overlying epithelium interacts.

Hyaline membrane disease

In any discussion of neonatal lung disease, the terms hyaline membrane disease (HMD) and respiratory distress syndrome (RDS) are often used interchangeably, both being used equally as clinical and pathological diagnoses. To add to the potential for confusion, there is often, *but not invariably*, a distinction made between respiratory distress and RDS. For clarity, therefore, this present discussion will use the term HMD as a *pathological* term, referring to a specific histological picture. Respiratory distress will be used to refer to the clinical picture of a baby with tachypnoea, expiratory grunting, recession and cyanosis. The distinction is worth retaining because, whilst HMD almost invariably causes respiratory distress, only approximately 75–80% of respiratory distress has HMD as the underlying pathology.

The long-term sequelae of neonatal HMD will be discussed together with those of chronic lung disease at the end of this chapter.

Incidence and clinical aspects

The respiratory distress associated with HMD typically presents in the very preterm infant within the first few hours of life (<4 hours). The signs as described above last for at least 24 hours although of course the natural history is often obscured by therapy. In most cases, there is a gradual improvement after the first few days when respiratory support can be discontinued.

In Cambridge, Morley (1986) recorded an incidence of respiratory distress from all causes as 1.9%, rising to 15% of infants <2500 g and 60% <1500 g. Although about a third of very low birthweight infants are recorded as dying from RDS, the recent advent and more widespread use of artificial surfactant has significantly reduced this figure.

By far the most important factor associated with HMD is prematurity and surfactant deficiency. However, HMD has also been recorded in association with birth asphyxia (important in the older infant), some forms of infection and pulmonary haemorrhage. In some cases, more than one factor will be present at the same time.

Pathology

Acute phase

Babies dying in the first few hours of life from HMD have collapsed red/purple lungs with a texture resembling that of liver. Histologically the earliest change, often seen within an hour, is necrosis of bronchial and bronchiolar epithelium which may become dislodged and block some of the more distal airways (de la Monte, Hutchins & Moore, 1986). The

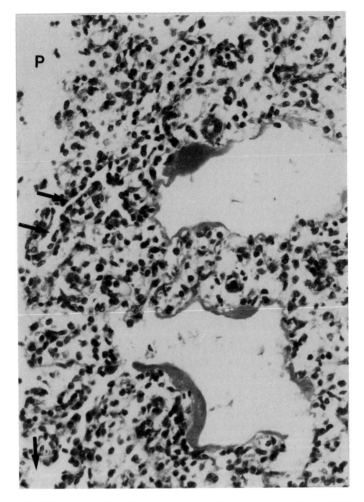

Fig. 10.2. Histology of hyaline membrane disease in an infant of 28 weeks gestation, dying at 12 hours of age. Pleural surface is at the top left (P). The hyaline membranes line the distended terminal airways rather than the more distal terminal sacs which are collapsed (arrowed).

hyaline membranes (HMs) follow rapidly and line distal airways and some parts of the respiratory units but rarely involve the terminal sacs (Fig. 10.2). The eosinophilic, fibrillary membranes are composed primarily of a proteinaceous exudate from plasma including fibrin but also contain a few necrotic epithelial cells. Inflammatory reaction to the membranes comprises macrophages and a few neutrophils but the latter may not be a prominent feature.

Repair phase

Evidence of repair and regeneration can usually be found within 2 or 3 days. Macrophages ingesting membrane are visible in the bronchiolar lumen and wall. Epithelial regeneration is marked by cuboidal type II pneumocytes proliferating beneath membranes and, occasionally, epithelium growing over the surface of membranes, incorporating it into the lung wall. Fibroblastic proliferation beneath the damaged bronchial and bronchiolar walls does occur, but is probably far more limited than the degree seen in the more severely affected lungs coming to autopsy.

Pathogenesis of HMD

Lung function depends on both epithelial and endothelial integrity. It allows gaseous exchange to occur and prevents fluid from both the vasculature and interstitium passing into the airspaces; any insult to this epithelial/endothelial barrier will compromise function. The initiating event in the production of HMD is damage to the epithelium of bronchioli and alveolar ducts resulting in a protein-rich transudation into the airways. Precipitation of protein, a component of which is fibrin, together with necrotic epithelial cells forms the hyaline membranes lining the damaged airways.

Epithelial damage may result from a number of sources including bacterial (Group B *Streptococcus*) and viral infections, pulmonary haemorrhage and asphyxia. At term, there is a subgroup of infants that have a clinical picture and pathology more akin to the adult respiratory distress syndrome than that seen in the typical preterm neonate (Royall & Levin, 1988; Faix et al., 1989). Here, damage may be due to toxic radical production, fibrin microthrombi and leucocyte accumulation in the microvasculature – this latter component amplifying any initial injury. The extent to which factors, important in the more typical neonatal HMD, are significant is not clear, but surfactant depletion may occur as a secondary phenomenon (Royall & Levin, 1988).

In the very preterm neonate, there is a close correlation between the presence of HMD and surfactant deficiency, so it is not unreasonable to assume surfactant is important in the pathogenesis of HMD. However, although there is good evidence that lack of surfactant might compound lung damage and promote the formation of hyaline membrane and respiratory distress, it is still not clear whether the lack of surfactant alone is enough to explain the initial lung injury.

Surfactant is necessary at the air/liquid interface to reduce the pressures needed to expand a small diameter sphere – in this case the terminal sacs. It is probable that the high trans-pulmonary pressures produced by the neonate or ventilator, in an attempt to maintain lung expansion in the face of surfactant deficiency, cause uneven expansion of presaccular airways. The sheer forces generated across these airways leads to epithelial necrosis (Robertson, 1991). It is probable that protein passing into air-spaces further inhibits surfactant so compounding the initial surfactant deficiency (Fuchimukai et al., 1987).

An alternative hypothesis has been suggested by de la Monte et al. (1986) who emphasize that the earliest visible damage, that of epithelial cell necrosis, is critical but that it is not due to surfactant deficiency. This group propose that evidence of pulmonary circulatory disturbances, together with the observation that HMD can be seen (albeit extremely rarely) in stillbirths, suggesting that initial airway damage may be initiated by asphyxia. The initial injury is caused by pulmonary vaso-constriction with secondary reflow injury. They suggest that the early, ischaemically mediated type II pneumocyte necrosis leads to secondary surfactant deficiency. A positive relationship between some cases of intrauterine pneumonia and hyaline membrane disease reported by the same group was considered supporting evidence (Lee, Moore & Hutchins, 1991). A contributory role for ischaemia in preterm HMD is also suggested by a recent study which provides evidence of increased pulmonary intravascular coagulative activity (Schmidt et al., 1992).

Chronic lung disease

Introduction and definition

From the start of neonatal intensive care, it has been recognized that a proportion of infants, usually preterm, become dependent on some form of long-term ventilatory support. In their initial description, Northway, Rosan & Porter (1967) coined the term broncho-pulmonary dysplasia (BPD) with a range of severe clinical and pathological features. One set of criteria is provided by O'Brodovich and Mellins (1985), who considered that an infant with BPD is one requiring assisted ventilation and/ or supplementary oxygen to maintain life at greater than 28 days of life after an initial acute lung injury (usually HMD). In addition, there will be significant clinical (tachypnoea, retractions), radiologic (hyperinflation or pulmonary cystic change) and blood gas abnormalities.

However, there has been a gradual decrease in the use of the term BPD primarily because the clinical criteria as defined above may not be fulfilled entirely (Krauss, Klain & Auld, 1975; Tooley, 1979). In addition, the pathological features are rarely as florid as the initial descriptions, particularly the bronchial changes. As an all-embracing descriptive title, therefore, chronic lung disease is frequently used to describe an infant, usually preterm, who is chronically dependent on some form of respiratory support. Chronic lung disease will often be, in effect, BPD at the less severe end of the spectrum, but it should be recognized that other, but more poorly defined, chronic pulmonary conditions may exist (Wilson & Mikity, 1960; Krauss et al., 1975). Also implicit in the distinction, is that BPD suggests a particular aetiology whereas chronic lung disease does not; chronic lung disease may represent the final common pathway for a variety of initiating or contributing insults.

Incidence

Given the above, it is not surprising that it is difficult to provide consistent data on the incidence of chronic lung disease. In a population-based study reviewing a single year's data – 1984, Kraybill, Bose & D'Ercole (1987) found chronic lung disease in 54% of all very-low-birthweight infants at 30 days of age falling to 5% of survivors at 6 months of age. Importantly, these overall figures hide striking variation due to gestation and major differences in incidence between treatment centres (23–83% at 30 days).

Pathology

The lung has a limited repertoire of responses to injury. Consequently, the pathology of chronic lung disease is broadly similar no matter what the initiating insult.

Most pathological descriptions of chronic lung disease refer to BPD, even though, if the strict clinical definition is adhered to, the term could be argued to be inappropriate. The pathology of BPD has been classified into three phases (Anderson & Engel, 1983; Askin, 1991): early reparative stage, weeks 1–2; subacute fibroproliferative stage, weeks 2–4; chronic fibroproliferative stage, >1 month of age.

The third, chronic fibroproliferative stage can probably be taken to represent the pathology of all forms of chronic lung disease. The first two stages, however, are descriptions of the lung in very severe forms of BPD and, due to improvement in ventilatory techniques, are now more rarely encountered by the pathologist. It is worth noting that the early stages of BPD clearly merge with the repair and regenerative phases of the acute lung injury and it is debatable as to whether a diagnosis of chronic lung disease or BPD can or should be made by histopathological criteria alone early in its evolution. Further, it is not certain whether the descriptions of early, typical BPD can be extrapolated to chronic lung disease of all aetiologies.

The pathology described below is divided into that affecting the airways – bronchi and bronchioles; the respiratory unit distal to bronchioles – primarily alveoli and interstitium; and the vasculature. Each is described in terms of (i) a transitional phase – correlating with stages 1 and 2 and above – indicating a transition from acute to probable established chronic disease, and (ii) established chronic disease.

Airways

Transitional: Severe bronchial or bronchiolar damage is associated with destruction of the respiratory epithelium and excessive fibroblastic proliferation in airway lumen producing an obliterative bronchiolitis. The obliterative process may lead to distal pulmonary collapse. More modest airway injury, a more common situation with modern ventilatory strategies, may be associated with smooth muscle proliferation and lesser degrees of fibrosis without complete airway obliteration (Stocker, 1986; Hislop & Haworth, 1989).

Chronic: In the chronic state, the main airway lesions are continuing smooth muscle hypertrophy and squamous epithelial metaplasia; persistence of the obliterative lesions is distinctly unusual. Glandular hyperplasia and patchy inflammation may be found in 25–50% of cases (Stocker, 1986; Margraf et al., 1991).

Respiratory unit

Transitional: There is good evidence that infants with chronic lung disease have poor development of their alveoli with a reduction in the total numbers and consequent loss of alveolar surface area (Hislop et al., 1987; Margraf et al., 1991). Many of the interstitial changes form a continuum with the repair processes of HMD; this includes interstitial fibrosis, peri-alveolar duct fibrosis with smooth muscle proliferation and type–2 pneumocyte proliferation.

Chronic: The main persistent change is that of interstitial fibrosis but it may be notably patchy with areas of relatively normal alveolar septae alternating with septae up to 10–25 μm in thickness (Fig. 10.3). Emphysematous lung interspersed with foci of fibrosis and collapse may be present in some lungs but, alongside the obliterative bronchiolitis, it is less a feature of modern chronic lung disease.

Vasculature

Transitional: Early changes are often related to hypoxia and persistence of fetal vascular structure. Under normal circumstances, neonatal pulmonary arteries dilate with reduction in the thickness of the media and thinning of the endothelial cells. More muscular arteries are also recruited to the pulmonary circulation to accommodate the increased blood flow but without a parallel increase in vascular resistance. These adaptive changes are fixed over the subsequent weeks by structural changes such as increased connective tissue within the media (Haworth, 1988). In the early stages of chronic lung disease, these vascular adaptations may not occur and vessels remain thick walled and lined by plump endothelium.

Chronic: Abnormalities in the vasculature to some extent depend on the severity of the underlying lung disease and chronic hypoxia. Clearly, the vascular changes in turn may induce further cardiovascular compromise and hypoxia. In some cases, the endothelial cells remain plump and contribute to vascular obstruction (Hislop & Haworth, 1990) but, in general, intimal lesions are not common. The major vascular feature of chronic lung disease is hypertrophy of medial smooth muscle (Fig. 10.3). Adventitial fibrous tissue appears to be increased in thickness (Hislop & Haworth, 1990), although it has been suggested it is reduced in overall area (Gorenflo, Vogel & Obladen, 1991). In severe chronic lung disease there is evidence that a reduction in the peripheral arterial density occurs, a feature that would contribute significantly to increased pulmonary vascular resistance. This may be due to failure of normal recruitment in the early neonatal period.

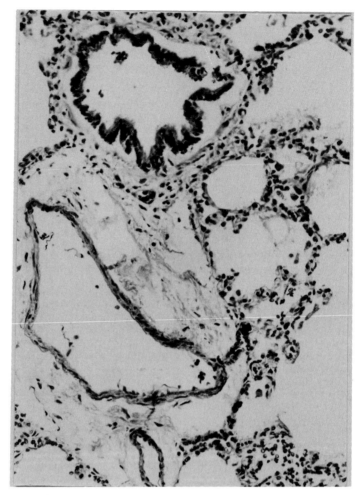

Fig. 10.3. (*a*) Lung from an infant dying from sudden infant death syndrome approximately 8 weeks after being ventilated for hyaline membrane disease. Interalveolar septae remain slightly thickened but artery and terminal bronchiole are normal.

Pathogenesis

By definition, BPD and therefore most chronic lung disease is initiated during a period of acute neonatal lung damage, usually HMD, but its emergence as a disease entity was closely linked to the respiratory support used in treatment, especially the use of increased inspired oxygen concentrations.

Particularly in conditions of hyperoxia a number of highly reactive

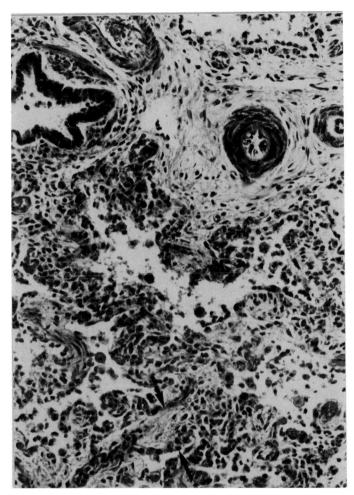

Fig. 10.3. (*b*) Chronic stage bronchopulmonary dysplasia from an infant of similar corrected gestation to (*a*) for comparison. The terminal bronchiole shows increased smooth muscle, although the respiratory epithelium is normal. Arteries demonstrate gross medial hypertrophy with small lumen and interalveolar septae are thickened with fibrous tissue (between arrows).

toxic radicals are produced during normal cellular metabolism, including superoxide and hydroxy radicals, hydrogen peroxide and singlet oxygen. Sources of these toxic species are pulmonary epithelial cells but recruited inflammatory cells may also contribute (Barry & Crapo, 1985; Clement et al., 1988). Toxic effects include membrane lipid peroxidation, enzyme inactivation and base hydroxylation of nucleic acids (Frank & Sosenko,

1987*a,b*). To counteract these toxic by-products, a number of antioxidant enzyme systems have evolved but, similar to those of surfactant, these systems are not usually very active until near term (Frank & Groseclose, 1984; Frank & Sosenko, 1987*a,b*), when, at least in a number of animal species, there is a rapid increase 'in preparation' for birth. Susceptibility to oxygen toxicity may be related partly to low baseline antioxidant enzyme levels, but perhaps more importantly, to the rate at which the enzymes increase in response to hyperoxic conditions (Frank & Sosenko, 1991). The main effect of continuing alveolar and interstitial damage is to produce protein leakage and oedema, which may be a stimulant for fibrosis. In rat lungs, platelet-derived-growth-factor produced by pulmonary interstitium in response to hyperoxia, stimulates early fibroblast hyperplasia (Han et al., 1992). It has also been suggested that there may be damage to surfactant but evidence for this is limited (Nogee & Wispe, 1988).

As well as generation of toxic radicals, inflammatory cells recruited to deal with the acute lung injury may be associated with the release of a number of inflammatory mediators and enzymes including leukotrienes, neutrophil elastase and fibronectin (Ogden et al., 1984; Barry & Crapo, 1985; Gerdes, Harris & Polin, 1988; Mirro, Armstead & Leffler, 1990; Yoder, Chua & Tepper, 1991). The major effects of these mediators is to increase vascular permeability and enzymic damage to the lung parenchyma. Experimentally, plasminogen activators produced after exposure of endothelial monolayers to hyperoxic conditions, are associated with restructuring of matrix proteins (Phillips et al., 1992).

Another aetiological factor implicated in chronic lung disease includes barotrauma associated with ventilator therapy. Indeed in many circumstances it may not be possible to dissociate the effects of barotrauma from that of hyperoxia. High peak inflationary pressures appear to be especially damaging to the airways and the production of the obliterative bronchiolitis (Taghizadeh & Reynolds, 1976). Recently it has been suggested that intralipid might increase the risk of chronic lung disease by augmenting lipid peroxidation, particularly if administered too early in the course of the acute injury (Cooke, 1991).

Infants dying as a direct result of chronic lung disease do so either from chronic respiratory failure or cor pulmonale, although it is difficult to predict those infants who will develop fatal chronic disease from the severity of initial illness (Truog et al., 1985). The main related extra respiratory tract abnormalities in chronic lung disease reflect raised pulmonary vascular resistance (Bush et al., 1990) and include right ventricular hypertrophy and dilatation, and hepatic congestion. It is presumed that the increased pulmonary vascular resistance results from medial hypertrophy of the muscular pulmonary arteries induced by chronic hypoxia.

However, studies have not always shown good correlation between clinical outcome and the pathology visible macro- or microscopically at autopsy. Right ventricular hypertrophy is not necessarily associated with severe airway disease and alveolar fibrosis may not be prominent, despite good evidence of pulmonary hypertension (Hislop & Haworth, 1990; Bush et al., 1990). Gorenflo et al. (1991), however, did find that severe BPD was associated with a fall in peripheral arterial density.

Long-term outcome of neonatal lung disease

In attempting to describe the long-term effects of neonatal lung disease, it needs to be borne in mind that the lungs which become available for study pathologically, may not be representative of those in survivors. Further, it may be impossible to disentangle the various elements, including premature birth and mechanical ventilation, that contribute to a particular outcome.

Clinical studies suggest that respiratory problems attributable to prematurity or respiratory distress alone are minimal (Stahlman et al., 1982) or associated with only a slight increase in airway reactivity (Mansell, Driscoll & James, 1987; Tammela, Linna & Koivisto, 1991). Children who have had chronic lung disease, however, show evidence of increased airway reactivity and are at an increased risk of respiratory infection (Betrand et al., 1986; Gibson et al., 1988).

Pathological studies suggest that premature birth in isolation has no effect on lung growth which continues without interruption (Hislop & Haworth, 1989). However, ventilation for respiratory distress interferes with lung growth, causing impaired alveolar development, reflected in a reduction of alveolar number and surface area (Hislop et al., 1987; Margraf et al., 1991). It is postulated that positive pressure ventilation itself may lead to impaired growth but with effects possibly enhanced by underlying lung disease. There is also evidence of an increase in bronchial smooth muscle and the area of bronchial mucous glands (Hislop & Haworth, 1989). These authors suggest that this may be reflected in the increased airway reactivity and risk of infection shown by some clinical studies on children subject to neonatal intensive care.

References

Alcorn, D., Adamson, T. M., Lambert, T. F., Maloney, J. E., Ritchie, B. C. & Robinson, P. M. (1977). Effects of chronic tracheal ligation and drainage in the fetal lamb lung. *Journal of Anatomy*, **123**, 649–60.

Anderson, W. R. & Engel, R. R. (1983). Cardiopulmonary sequelae of reparative stages of bronchopulmonary dysplasia. *Archives of Pathology and Laboratory Medicine*, **107**, 603–8.

Askin, F. (1991). Respiratory tract disorders in the fetus and neonate. In *Textbook of Fetal and Perinatal Pathology*, ed. J. S. Wigglesworth & D. B. Singer. pp. 643–88. Blackwell Scientific Publications, Oxford.

Barry, B. E. & Crapo, J. D. (1985). Patterns of accumulation of platelets and neutrophils in rat lungs during exposure to 100% and 85% oxygen. *American Review of Respiratory Disease*, **132**, 548–55.

Betrand, J. M., Riley, S. P., Popkin, J. & Coates, A. I. (1986). The longterm pulmonary sequelae of prematurity: the role of familial airway reactivity and the respiratory distress syndrome. *New England Journal of Medicine*, **312**, 742–5.

Boylan, P., Howe, A., Gearty, J. & O'Brien, N. G. (1977). Familial pulmonary hypoplasia. *Irish Journal of Medical Science*, **146(6)**, 179–80.

Bush, A., Busst, C. M., Knight, W. B., Hislop, A. A., Haworth, S. G. & Shinebourne, E. (1990). Changes in pulmonary circulation in severe bronchopulmonary dysplasia. *Archives of Disease in Childhood*, **65**, 739–45.

Carmel, J. A., Friedman, F. & Adams, F. H. (1965). Fetal tracheal ligation and lung development. *American Journal of Diseases in Children*, **109**, 452–6.

Clement, A., Chadelat, K., Sardet, A., Grimfeld, A. & Tournier, G. (1988). Alveolar macrophage status in bronchopulmonary dysplasia. *Pediatric Research*, **23**, 470–3.

Cooke, R. W. I. (1991). Factors associated with chronic lung disease in preterm infants. *Archives of Disease in Childhood*, **66**, 776–9.

de la Monte, S., Hutchins, G. M. & Moore, G. W. (1986). Respiratory epithelial cell necrosis is the earliest lesion of hyaline membrane disease of the newborn. *American Journal of Pathology*, **123**, 155–60.

Desai, R., Wigglesworth, J. S. & Aber, V. (1987). Assessment of elastin maturation by radioimmunoassay of desmosine in the developing human lung. *Early Human Development*, **16**, 61–71.

Dickson, K. A. & Harding, R. (1991). Fetal breathing and pressures in the trachea and amniotic sac during oligohydramnios in sheep. *Journal of Applied Physiology*, **70**, 293–9.

Emery, J. L. & Mithal, A. (1960). The number of alveoli in the terminal respiratory unit of man during late intrauterine life and childhood. *Archives of Disease in Childhood*, **35**, 544–7.

Faix, R. G., Viscardi, R. M., DiPietro, M. A. & Nicks, J. J. (1989). Adult respiratory distress syndrome in full-term newborns. *Pediatrics*, **83**, 971–6.

Frank, L. & Groseclose, E. E. (1984). Preparation for birth into an O_2-rich environment: the antioxidant enzymes in the developing rabbit lung. *Pediatric Research*, **18**, 240.

Frank, L. & Sosenko, I. R. S. (1987*a*). Prenatal development of lung antioxidant enzymes in four species. *Journal of Pediatrics*, **110**, 106–10.

Frank, L. & Sosenko, I. R. S. (1987*b*). Development of lung antioxidant enzyme system in late gestation: Possible implications for the prematurely born infant. *Journal of Pediatrics*, **110**, 9–14.

Frank, L. & Sosenko, I. R. S. (1991). Failure of premature rabbits to increase antioxidant enzymes during hyperoxic exposure: Increased susceptibility to pulmonary oxygen toxicity compared with term rabbits. *Pediatric Research*, **29**, 292–6.

Fuchimukai, T., Fujiwara, T., Takahashi, A. & Enhorning, G. (1987). Artificial surfactant inhibited by proteins. *Journal of Applied Physiology*, **62**, 429–37.

George, P., Handorf, C. R. & Suttle, E. A. (1981). Primary pulmonary hypoplasia. *Southern Medical Journal*, **74**, 884–7.

Gerdes, J. S., Harris, M. C. & Pollin, R. A. (1988). Effects of dexamethasone and indomethacin on elastase α_1-proteinase inhibitor, and fibronectin in bronchoalveolar lavage fluid from neonates. *Journal of Pediatrics*, **113**, 727–31.

Gibson, R. L., Jackson, J. C., Twiggs, G. A., Redding, G. J. & Truog, W. E. (1988). Bronchopulmonary dysplasia. Survival after prolonged mechanical ventilation. *American Journal of Diseases of Children*, **142**, 721–5.

Gorenflo, M., Vogel, M. & Obladen, M. (1991). Pulmonary vascular changes in bronchopulmonary dysplasia: A clinical pathologic correlation in short- and long-term survivors. *Pediatric Pathology*, **11**, 851–66.

Haidar, A., Wigglesworth, J. S. & Krauz, T. (1990). Type IV collagen in developing human lung: A comparison between normal and hypoplastic fetal lungs. *Early Human Development*, **21**, 175–80.

Haidar, A., Ryder, T. A. & Wigglesworth, J. S. (1991*a*). Failure of elastin development in hypoplastic lungs associated with oligohydramnios; an EM study. *Histopathology*, **18**, 471–47.

Haidar, A., Ryder, T. A. & Wigglesworth, J. S. (1991*b*). Epithelial cell morphology and airspace size in hypoplastic human fetal lungs associated with oligohydramnios. *Pediatric Pathology*, **11**, 839–50.

Han, R. N. N., Buch, S., Freeman, B. A., Post, M. & Tanswell, A. K. (1992). Platelet-derived growth factor and growth-related genes in rat lung. II Effect of exposure to 85% O_2. *American Journal of Physiology*, **262**, L140–6.

Harding, R., Hooper, S. B. & Dickson, K. A. (1990). A mechanism leading to reduced lung expansion and lung hypoplasia in fetal sheep during oligohydramnios. *American Journal of Obstetrics and Gynecology*, **163**, 1904–13.

Haworth, S. G. (1988). Pulmonary vascular remodelling in neonatal pulmonary hypertension. State of the Art. *Chest*, **93**, 133–8S.

Hislop, A. A., Fairweather, D. V. I., Blackwell, R. J. & Howard, S. (1984). The effect on amniocentesis and drainage of amniotic fluid on lung development in Macaca fascicularis. *British Journal of Obstetrics and Gynaecology*, **91**, 835–42.

Hislop, A. A. & Haworth, S. G. (1989). Airway size and structure in the normal fetal and infant lung and the effect of premature delivery and artificial ventilation. *American Review of Respiratory Disease*, **140**, 1717–26.

Hislop, A. A. & Haworth, S. G. (1990). Pulmonary vascular damage and the development of cor pulmonale following hyaline membrane disease. *Pediatric Pulmonology*, **9**, 152–6.

Hislop, A. A., Hey, E. & Reid, L. (1979). The lungs in congenital bilateral renal agenesis and dysplasia. *Archives of Disease in Childhood*, **54**, 32–8.

Hislop, A. A., Wigglesworth, J. S., Desai, R. & Aber,V. (1987). The effects of preterm delivery and mechanical ventilation on human lung growth. *Early Human Development*, **15**, 147–64.

Kitterman, J. A. (1984). Fetal lung development. *Journal of Developmental Physiology*, **6**, 67–82.

Krauss, A. N., Klain, D. B. & Auld, P. A. M. (1975). Chronic pulmonary insufficiency of prematurity (CPIP). *Pediatrics*, **55**, 55–8.

Kraybill, E. N., Bose, C. L. & D'Ercole, J. (1987). Chronic lung disease in infants with very low birth weight. A population-based study. *American Journal of Diseases of Children*, **141**, 784–8.

Langer, R. & Kaufmann, H. J. (1986). Primary (isolated) bilateral pulmonary hypoplasia: a comparative study of radiologic findings and autopsy results. *Pediatric Radiology*, **16**, 175–9.

Lee, D. R., Moore, G. W. & Hutchins, G. M. (1991). Lattice theory analysis of the relationship of hyaline membrane disease and fetal pneumonia in 96 perinatal autopsies. *Pediatric Pathology*, **11**, 223–33.

Liggins, G. C., Vilos, G. A., Campos, G. A., Kitterman, J. A. & Lee, C. H. (1981). The effect of bilateral thoracoplasty in lung development in fetal sheep. *Journal of Developmental Physiology*, **3**, 275–82.

Lwebuga-Mukasa, J. S. (1991). Matrix-driven pneumocyte differentiation. *American Review of Respiratory Disease*, **144**, 452–7.

Mansell, A. L., Driscoll, J. M. & James, L. S. (1987). Pulmonary follow-up of moderately low birth weight infants with and without respiratory distress syndrome. *Journal of Pediatrics*, **110**, 111–5.

Marechal, M., Gillerot, Y. & Chef, R. (1984). L'hypoplasie pulmonaire. A propos d'une observation chez des jumeaux. *Journal of Gynecology, Obstetrics and Biology of Reproduction*, **143**, 897–902.

Margraf, L. R., Tomashefski, J. F. Jr, Bruce, M. C. & Dahms, B. B. (1991). Morphometric analysis of the lung in bronchopulmonary dysplasia. *American Review of Respiratory Disease*, **143**, 391–400.

Mendelsohn, G. & Hutchins, G. M. (1977). Primary pulmonary hypoplasia: report of a case with polyhydramnios. *American Journal of Diseases of Children*, **131**, 1220–3.

Mirro, R., Armstead, W. & Leffler, C. (1990). Increased airway leukotriene levels in infants with severe bronchopulmonary dysplasia. *American Journal of Diseases of Children*, **144**, 160–1.

Morley, C. J. (1986). The respiratory distress syndrome. In *Textbook of Neonatology*, ed. N. R. C. Robertson. pp. 274–339. Churchill Livingstone: London.

Nicolini, U., Fisk, N. M., Rodeck, C. H., Talbert, D. G. & Wigglesworth, J. S. (1989). Low amniotic pressure in oligohydramnios – Is this the cause of pulmonary hypoplasia? *American Journal of Obstetrics and Gynecology*, **161**, 1098–101.

Nogee, L. M. & Wispe, J. R. (1988). Effects of pulmonary oxygen injury on airway content of surfactant-associated protein A. *Pediatric Research*, **24**, 568–73.

Northway, W. H., Rosan, R. C. & Porter, D. Y. (1967). Pulmonary disease following respiratory therapy for hyaline membrane disease. *New England Journal of Medicine*, **276**, 357–68.

O'Brodovich, H. M. & Mellins, R. B. (1985). Bronchopulmonary dysplasia. *American Review of Respiratory Disease*, **132**, 694–709.

Ogden, B. E., Murphy, S. A., Saunders, G. C., Pathak, D. & Johnson, J. D. (1984). Neonatal lung neutrophils and elastase/proteinase imbalance. *American Review of Respiratory Disease*, **130**, 817–21.

Page, D. V. & Stocker, J. T. (1982). Anomalies associated with pulmonary hypoplasia. *American Review of Respiratory Disease*, **125**, 216–21.

Peters, C. A., Reid, L. M., Docimo, S., Luetic, T., Carr, M., Retik, A. B. & Mandell, J. (1991*a*). The role of the kidney in lung growth and maturation in the setting of obstructive uropathy and oligohydramnios. *Journal of Urology*, **146**, 597–600.

Peters, C. A, Docimo, S. G., Luetic, T., Reid, L. M., Retik, A. B. & Mandell, J. (1991*b*). Effect of in utero vesicostomy on pulmonary hypoplasia in the fetal lamb with bladder outlet obstruction and oligohydramnios: a morphometric analysis. *Journal of Urology*, **146**, 1178–83.

Phillips, P. G., Birnby, L., Di Bernardo, L. A., Ryan, T. J. & Tsan, M-F. (1992). Hyperoxia increases plasminogen activator activity of cultured endothelial cells. *American Journal of Physiology*, **262**, L21–31.

Robertson, B. (1991). The origin of neonatal lung injury. (Editorial). *Pediatric Pathology*, **11**, iii–vi.

Royall, J. A. & Levin, D. L (1988). Adult respiratory distress syndrome in pediatric patients. 1. Clinical aspects, pathophysiology, pathology and mechanisms of lung injury. *Journal of Pediatrics*, **112**, 169–80.

Rushton, I. (1991). West Midlands perinatal mortality survery, 1987. An audit of 300 perinatal autopsies. *British Journal of Obstetrics and Gynaecology*, **98**, 624–7.

Schmidt, B., Vegh, P., Weitz, J., Johnson, M., Caco, C. & Roberts, R. (1992). Thrombin/Antithrombin III complex formation in the neonatal respiratory distress syndrome. *American Review of Respiratory Disease*, **145**, 767–70.

Silver, M. M., Thurston, W. A. & Patrick, J. E. (1988). Perinatal pulmonary hyperplasia due to laryngeal atresia. *Human Pathology*, **19**, 110–3.

Smith, B. T. & Post, M. (1989). Fibroblast pneumocyte factor. *American Journal of Physiology*, **257**, L174-L178.

Stahlman, M., Hedvall, G., Lindstrom, D. & Snell, J. (1982). Role of hyaline membrane disease in production of later childhood lung abnormalities. *Pediatrics*, **69**, 572–6.

Stocker, J. T. (1986). Pathologic features of long-standing 'healed' bronchopulmonary dysplasia: a study of 28 3- to 40-month-old infants. *Human Pathology*, **17**, 943–61.

Swischuk, L. E., Richardson, C. J., Nichols, M. M. & Ingman, M. J. (1979). Primary pulmonary hypoplasia in the neonate. *Journal of Pediatrics*, **95**, 573–7.

Taghizadeh, A. & Reynolds, E. O. R. (1976). Pathogenesis of bronchopulmonary dysplasia following hyaline membrane disease. *American Journal of Pathology*, **82**, 241–64.

Tammela, O. K. T., Linna, O. V. E. & Koivisto, M. E. (1991). Long-term pulmonary sequelae in low birth weight infants with and without respiratory distress syndrome. *Acta Paediatrica Scandinavica*, **80**, 542–4.

Tooley, W. H. (1979). Epidemiology of bronchopulmonary dysplasia. *Journal of Pediatrics*, **95**, 851–5.

Truog, W. E., Jackson, J. C., Badura, R. J., Sorensen, G. K., Murphy, J. H. & Woodrum, D. E. (1985). Bronchopulmonary dysplasia and pulmonary insufficiency of prematurity. *American Journal of Diseases of Children*, **139**, 351–4.

Wigglesworth, J. S. (1987*a*). Factors affecting fetal lung growth. In *Physiology of the Fetal and Neonatal Lung*, ed. D. V. Walters & F. Geubelle. pp. 25–37. MTP Press Limited, Lancaster.

Wigglesworth, J. S. (1987*b*). Pathology of the lung in the fetus and neonate, with particular reference to problems of growth and maturation. *Histopathology*, **11**, 671–89.

Wigglesworth, J. S. & Desai, R. (1979). Effects on lung growth cervical cord section in the rabbit fetus. *Early Human Development*, **3**, 51–65.

Wigglesworth, J. S. & Desai, R. (1981). Use of DNA estimation for growth assessment in normal and hypoplastic fetal lungs. *Archives of Disease in Childhood*, **56**, 601–5.

Wigglesworth, J. S. & Desai, R. (1982). Is fetal respiratory function a major determinant of perinatal survival? *Lancet*, **i**, 264–7.

Wigglesworth, J. S., Desai, R. & Aber, V. (1987). Quantitative aspects of perinatal lung growth. *Early Human Development*, **15**, 203–12.

Wigglesworth, J. S., Desai, R. & Guerrini, P. (1981). Fetal lung hypoplasia: biochemical and structural variations and their possible significance. *Archives of Disease in Childhood*, **56**, 606–15.

Wigglesworth, J. S., Desai, R. & Hislop, A. A. (1987). Fetal lung growth in congenital laryngeal atresia. *Pediatric Pathology*, **7**, 515–25.

Wigglesworth, J. S., Hislop, A. A. & Desai, R. (1991). Biochemical and morphometric analyses in hypoplastic lungs. *Pediatric Pathology*, **11**, 537–49.

Wilson, M. G. & Mikity, V. G. (1960). A new form of respiratory disease in premature infants. *American Journal of Diseases of Children*, **99**, 489–99.

Yoder, M. C., Chua, R. & Tepper, R. (1991). Effect of dexamethasone on pulmonary inflammation and pulmonary function of ventilator dependent infants with bronchopulmonary dysplasia. *American Review of Respiratory Disease*, **143**, 1044–8.

Clinical applications

11

Physiological measurement of lung function in newborn babies

MICHAEL SILVERMAN

Introduction

Why measure neonatal lung function?

Disturbances of the mechanical function of the respiratory system are central to many perinatal disorders. They may be the direct result of lung disease, for instance in pulmonary hypoplasia or hyaline membrane disease, or result indirectly, from cardiovascular or neuromuscular disorders for example. Whatever the mechanism, measurement of respiratory mechanics has important applications in developmental physiology, epidemiology and clinical practice.

Knowledge of *developmental physiology* and of the adaptive changes which occur in the respiratory system at the time of birth is a prerequisite for clinical measurement and interpretation. In the perinatal period, the establishment of gas filled lungs, an effective pulmonary circulation and pulmonary gas exchange are accompanied by great changes in the mechanical properties of the respiratory system (Chernick & Mellins, 1991; Kafer, 1990). Subsequent bodily growth, with structural changes in the lungs and chest wall, also has mechanical correlates (Wohl, 1991; Mortola, Chapter 7). Great care is needed in the interpretation of age- or growth-related changes in respiratory function. Where changes can be expressed as dimensionless ratios independent of bodily dimensions, direct comparisons are possible between groups of infants or between different stages of development for individual infants. Otherwise relevant population-based reference data, using identical measurement techniques, must be consulted. In many cases, such information is not available. Hence one of the most urgent and important applications of neonatal pulmonary function measurements is to describe the physiology of reference populations of normal infants by means of standardized techniques (Quanjer et al., 1989).

239

Epidemiological studies employing pulmonary function measurements in the newborn period provide important clues to the pathogenesis of pulmonary disease. The effect of maternal smoking during pregnancy on fetal airway growth (Hanrahan et al., 1992) and the relationship between airway function at birth and subsequent recurrent infantile wheeze (Martinez et al., 1988) are recent examples.

In the *clinical* realm, measurements of lung mechanics have had little influence in diagnosis, since with a few exceptions, only simple, non-specific techniques are widely available. They have found wide application as measures of outcome in antenatal and postnatal therapeutic trials and in relation to intervention studies. As prospects for early intervention based on antenatal diagnosis or on gene therapy for specific defects become more widespread, the contribution of measurements of lung mechanics to outcome measurement will increase. Since there are no direct methods of measuring lung growth in live infants, measurements of lung mechanics are sometimes used as a surrogate. Without complete data, false interpretations are likely. For instance, a low lung volume (FRC) may be due to reduced alveolar number (pulmonary hypoplasia), but is far more likely to be the result of abnormal surface forces, lung destruction, interstitial disease or abnormal chest wall or muscle function.

Short-term change in lung function has been used as a measure of response in trials of management procedures and in therapeutic studies. The management of preterm labour, elective neonatal resuscitation for preterm babies, standardization of mechanical ventilation of the newborn and the surgical treatment of PDA have all been investigated using changes in lung mechanics as outcome measures. The response to drugs, whether antenatal (such as corticosteroids or TRH) or postnatal (corticosteroids, surfactant, bronchodilators and diuretics) has been subject to the rigorous rules of therapeutic trials using lung function as an important determinant of outcome.

There is an important role for qualitative lung function measurement for monitoring babies during mechanical ventilation. The advent of miniature flow-measuring devices, such as the hot-wire anemometer or a miniature pneumotachograph which can be incorporated into an endotracheal tube connector (Vallinis, Davis & Coates, 1990), together with stable, low cost, solid-state pressure transducers will allow tracking of respiratory resistance, dynamic compliance and tidal time constant, for early detection of mechanical complications such as pneumothorax or endotracheal tube blockage. In addition, by having to confront the concepts of lung mechanics, nurses and doctors will become more adept at interpreting respiratory signs in terms of changes in respiratory physiology.

Animal studies

In many fields of human biology, research on animals has provided important clues. In neonatal lung disorders, except for basic studies at cellular or molecular level and basic studies of normal mammalian physiology, direct application of the results of animal work to the human newborn has been of limited value and occasionally has been misleading. Much of the early work on neonatal asphyxia and resuscitation falls into this category. There are great differences between mammalian species in the response to preterm delivery, the circulatory effects of mechanical ventilation, the efficacy of surfactant preparations and the toxic effects of high concentrations of inspired oxygen which preclude direct comparisons. Measurement conditions for animal research are often inappropriate for human application. For instance, methods which are suitable for intubated, paralysed, healthy newborn animals may not be accurate in diseased, human, preterm newborns. Recent advances in higher primate biology have, however, largely overcome these objections, allowing experimental work which is likely to be relevant to human disease.

Although experiments, in the form of controlled clinical trials, are certainly possible in human neonates, most data are based on observations of nature's experiments rather than on true randomization.

Scope of this chapter

This chapter represents the practical, clinical applications of neonatal respiratory mechanics, the background mammalian biology of which was described by Mortola (Chapter 7). Essentially, the components of the mechanical impedance of the lower respiratory tract (airflow resistance and dynamic compliance), the elasticity of the respiratory system (static compliance) and the end-expiratory lung volume (FRC) will be discussed. Dynamic properties such as the emptying time constant and the level of intrinsic PEEP ($PEEP_i$) have important consequences during mechanical ventilation. New techniques, such as the 'squeeze' technique for measuring forced expiration, and techniques being newly explored in newborns, such as gas mixing methods, will be discussed. A number of excellent reviews of neonatal lung function measurement techniques have recently been published (McCann, Goldman & Brady, 1987; England, 1988; Working Group Paediatrics SEPCR, 1989; Milner, 1990; Stocks, 1991; Dezateux et al., 1991; ATS/ERS Working Party, 1993) of which two provide a wealth of reference values (Quanjer et al., 1989; Dezateux et al., 1991).

Basic considerations

Subjects

The *selection of subjects* for physiological measurement depends on the purpose of the study. Reference populations of healthy infants may very easily be biased by selection procedures, particularly as parental consent must be obtained. Factors which are known to affect neonatal lung mechanics in term infants include: fetal growth pattern, mode of delivery, duration of membrane rupture and maternal smoking during pregnancy. Subsequent lung function and clinical symptoms in infancy are affected by hereditary factors such as a parental history of asthma and environmental influences such as viral infection and air pollution, especially by cigarette smoke. Ethnic differences in neonatal lung function have been little studied, but one investigation showed that upper airway resistance (and hence total airway resistance) was lower in black than white newborn babies (Stocks & Godfrey, 1978). There are differences between newborn boys and girls in indices which seem to depend on the size of major airways relative to lung compliance. Thus, $\dot{V}_{max,FRC}$ (the maximum expiratory flow rate at FRC from the 'squeeze technique') is generally greater in relation to lung volume in newborn girls than boys (Tepper et al., 1986), although controversy about this exists (Hanrahan et al., 1990).

Selection procedures for sick infants may be even more complex. Confounding factors abound. For instance, among very low birth weight infants, those born by emergency Caesarian section are predominantly the growth retarded products of hypertensive pregnancies, whereas the group of infants delivered vaginally has a predominant history of prolonged rupture of membranes or amnionitis. Endotracheal intubation and mechanical ventilation affect lung function, by imposing a high-resistance tube in series with the lungs and by imposing an arbitrary distending pressure on the respiratory system. The effects of mechanical ventilation limit our ability to detect the effects of therapeutic intervention, as has been amply illustrated with respect to surfactant therapy (England, 1988).

Table 11.1. *The effect of various procedures on neonatal lung function during quiet sleep*

	Sedation	Application of face mask	Increased deadspace
Respiratory frequency	± ↑	↓	↑
Tidal volume	± ↓	↑	↑
FRC	0	?	↑
Gas mixing indices	0	?	?
Reflexes (Hering-Breuer)	0	?	0

? no data available; ± possible change.

Measurement conditions for neonates contrast in several important ways with those for older children. Healthy infants are usually studied asleep, supine and nose-breathing via a face mask in a pulmonary function laboratory. Sleeping term neonates spend up to 50% of the time in active sleep, with sleep cycles of about 20 minutes. Behavioural assessment of sleep state is usually adequate, although full electrophysiological recording may be important for specialised studies (Prechtl, 1974). The measurement of lung mechanics is affected by sleep state, mainly because during active sleep, bodily movement, irregular breathing and asynchrony of chest and abdominal motion render most measurements impossible or too variable (see Chapter 8). For this reason, most measurements of lung mechanics are conducted during quiet sleep. Sedation with chloral hydrate (or triclofos sodium) has remarkably little effect on lung mechanics, but the application of a facemask with its attendant dead space, does cause changes (Table 11.1).

During resuscitation or mechanical ventilation, even when muscle paralysis is used, the mechanical function of the respiratory system can be dominated by the characteristics of the equipment. Endotracheal tubes impose a high, flow-dependent series resistance, while the expiratory valve and circuit of a mechanical ventilator impede expiratory airflow, so that the time constant of tidal expiration is prolonged. The duration of expiration and level of PEEP affect the end-expiratory lung volume (FRC) and therefore intrinsic PEEP, as well as the tidal volume and respiratory compliance. It is possible to obtain false results from studies of therapeutic interventions, if the artefactual effects of the ventilator system, the endotracheal tube resistance and any leakage are not considered.

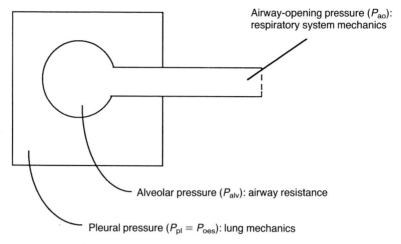

Fig. 11.1. Partitioning of intrathoracic pressures.

Major assumptions

In spite of the sophistication of computer-aided analysis, in practice we tend to view the respiratory system as a single-compartment, linear model (Fig. 11.1). For most clinical purposes, this assumption is adequate. Where it breaks down in disease, for instance in the analysis of gas mixing efficiency or in measurements which depend on a single expiratory time constant (Celluci et al., 1991), either new techniques are needed or accurate measurement must be abandoned.

Equipment

Maintenance and sterilization of equipment are important aspects of lung function measurement. Equally, calibration by appropriate means must incorporate the measurement devices and recording equipment, whether chart recorder or computer. Calibration of pressure, volume, flow and gas composition devices should be performed every time a set of measurements is made. Suitable techniques have been fully reviewed (Working Group Paediatrics SEPCR, 1989; Dezateux et al., 1991).

Sampling rates of 100 s^{-1} for A–D computer cards are acceptable for most purposes during tidal breathing. Where high frequency components are expected, for instance following release of an occluded airway, or during the interrupter technique for measuring R_{rs}, sampling frequencies of $200–1\,000 \text{ s}^{-1}$ may be needed (Richardson, 1989). It is essential that the operator understands the algorithms used in any computer-based lung function system and that data scrutiny for artefact and selection for analysis are permitted by the system.

Techniques

Lung volume

Definition. The volume of gas in the lungs at the end of a tidal breath is the functional residual capacity (FRC). This is the only lung volume which can easily be measured in infants. At equilibrium in a fully relaxed (or paralysed) respiratory system, it represents the volume of the lungs when the inward and outward elastic recoil of the lungs and chest wall respectively, are equal and opposite. In disease, this passive volume may be increased by airway obstruction leading to airway closure and hence incomplete emptying of the lungs ('gas trapping'), or decreased in conditions which lead to reduced lung compliance (increased elastance) such as pulmonary hypoplasia or hyaline membrane disease. The chest wall contributes little to the overall compliance of the respiratory system in infancy (Mortola, 1987). Nevertheless, any severe chest wall disease (neuromuscular disorder, thoracic dystrophy) or disturbance (muscle paralysis) will lead to a reduction in FRC. In newborns, the only condition under which FRC is passively determined is artificial venti-lation with muscle paralysis and a prolonged expiratory time (T_E). Under all other conditions, dynamic factors which determine the expiratory time constant of the respiratory system (T_{rs}) and the duration of expiration, affect the end tidal lung volume. In a freely breathing infant over the first year of life, T_{rs} is actively modified by variable expiratory braking, using the glottis and the diaphragm (Mortola, 1987 & Chapter 7). During artificial ventilation, FRC is additionally affected by externally applied PEEP. The expiratory recoil of the respiratory system produces a pressure which at end-tidal lung volumes above the truly relaxed FRC, is sometimes called 'intrinsic PEEP' ($PEEP_i$). $PEEP_i$ can be measured as the airway opening pressure (P_{ao}) during a brief end-tidal airway occlu-sion, under conditions of muscle relaxation.

Since lung mechanics and gas exchange are affected by changes in lung volume, their measurement is handicapped and the interpretation of results may be impossible if concomitant FRC measurement does not take place (England, 1988).

Techniques. There are three established methods: closed circuit helium dilution, open circuit nitrogen washout and whole body plethysmogra-phy. Gas-based techniques measure the accessible volume of gas in the lungs; plethysmographic methods include all intrathoracic gas (and a small proportion of abdominal gas). The discrepancy between gas equilibration and plethysmographic results increases in the presence of airway disease, and is a measure of 'gas trapping'. The decline in this discrepancy over the first few days of life has been used to chart the establishment of the normal FRC (Boon et al., 1981). No method is ideal for intubated infants, because of potential air leaks (for all methods) or equipment complexity (plethysmography), although both gas based and plethysmographic methods have been attempted during neonatal intensive care.

The helium dilution method is most widely used. In this closed circuit method, the infant either breathes from a bag in a bottle or a spirometer circuit (Working Group Paediatrics SEPCR, 1989; Dezateux et al., 1991; ATS/ERS Working Party, 1993; Tepper et al., 1986; Hanrahan et al., 1990) containing about 10% of the insoluble gas helium, until equilibration is achieved. Knowing the initial apparatus volume, the mask dead space and the initial and final helium concentrations, FRC can be calculated. Changing concentrations of helium preclude pneumotachography during the procedure, but the bag-in-a-bottle technique overcomes this problem. Repeatable results require: stable breathing; estimation of the tidal volume included when rebreathing commences; correction for CO_2 absorbed in the circuit or for deviation of the RQ from unity; absence of leak. Intubated infants can be studied but correction for leakage around the tube introduces unquantifiable inaccuracies.

The *nitrogen washout* technique (Working Group Paediatrics SEPCR, 1989; ATS/ERS Working Party, 1993; Tepper & Adsell, 1992) depends on the fact that nitrogen is very insoluble in body fluids. During oxygen breathing, the quantity of nitrogen exhaled depends on the initial and final concentration in the lungs, and the lung volume. The traditional method relied on 100% oxygen breathing. This is unsuitable for preterm babies and may lead to microatelectasis. The technique is also unsuitable for sick infants who require high ambient oxgyen therapy, since the fractional nitrogen content of the lungs at the start of the washout cannot accurately be determined. Gas mixing indices, based on the efficacy of nitrogen clearance during the washout procedure, can be determined concurrently with FRC. The nitrogen washout technique has become more widely available in commercial equipment. Babies can be studied while intubated (provided there is no leak) but not easily during mechanical ventilation (Sivan, Deakers & Newth, 1990; Edberg et al., 1991).

Plethysmographic techniques depend on the application of Boyle's law to the infant breathing against an occluded airway inside a hermetically sealed (constant mass) or volume displacement (constant pressure) whole-body plethysmograph. Techniques are exacting and apply in practice only to spontaneously breathing infants who can be taken to the infant lung function laboratory. Measurements can only be made during natural or sedated sleep. Values for FRC by plethysmography (often referred to as thoracic gas volume, TGV or V_{tg}) are substantially higher than by the gas dilution or washout methods, even in healthy infants. The difference diminishes with age. It is difficult to impute the difference entirely to 'gas trapping' or airway closure. Suspicion remains that unidentified artefacts may be responsible. With disease, the difference widens. The plethysmographic technique for FRC has been fully reviewed (Working Group Paediatrics SEPCR, 1989). An adaptation of the volume displacement plethysmograph for infant use has been recently described (Marchal et al., 1991), with a re-evaluation of the factors which lead to a discrepancy in V_{tg} based on end-inspiratory compared with end-expiratory occlusions.

Techniques which merit further exploration include radiological lung volume by simple radiology or variants of CT such as echoplanar imaging (Chapman et al., 1990).

Applications. The establishment of FRC in normal infants and its relation to fetal and intrapartum factors has been instructive in evaluating therapeutic interventions such as amniocentesis, mode of delivery and the assessment of fetal lung hypoplasia. The most important applications, however, relate to the use of FRC measurement in the interpretation of data on lung mechanics, which are affected by variation in the lung volume at which measurements are made. In the evaluation of pulmonary hyperinflation and the response to the treatment of airway disease, FRC measurement is vital.

During mechanical ventilation, absolute lung volume measurement is difficult. Here, change in FRC by measurement of $PEEP_i$ and C_{rs} or by body surface techniques such as respiratory inductance plethysmography (RIP), may be used as alternatives, in studying the effects of thera-peutic agents (for instance, surfactant) or techniques (such as levels of PEEP).

In the future, automated equipment for measuring absolute lung volume by nitrogen washout during mechanical ventilation may be expected. Techniques are at present unwieldy (Sivan et al., 1990). This will provide vital information which, together with data on pulmonary perfusion, can only improve techniques of mechanical ventilation.

Other static lung volumes, such as TLC or RV cannot easily be measured at the moment. However, an inflation technique which allows the lungs of spontaneously breathing infants to be inflated at predefined pressures, may eventually permit these lung volumes to be measured (Turner et al., 1992).

Compliance and resistance

Definitions. This section will deal with the elastic and resistive properties of the respiratory system and their product, which by analogy with electrical circuit theory, is the time constant of the respiratory system (T_{rs}).

The basis of the most commmonly used methods is the equation of motion of the respiratory system:

$$P_{dr} = (E . V) + (R . \dot{V}) + (I . \ddot{V}) \tag{1}$$

where P_{dr} is the driving pressure for the system, E is the elastance (the inverse of compliance), V is volume, R is resistance, $\dot{V}$ is flow, I is inertance and $\ddot{V}$ is convective acceleration. The final term is normally ignored, although it may make a significant contribution to pressure losses during rapid breathing, in high frequency mechanical ventilation and relatively speaking, in infants with normal lungs, in whom elastance and resistance are low. For the whole respiratory system, the driving pressure can be determined as the airway opening pressure (P_{ao}) during occlusion or during imposed pressure oscillations or mechanical ventilation; hence the mechanical properties of the whole system can be computed by measuring P_{ao}, flow and its integral, volume. In order to partition C_{rs} and R_{rs} into chest wall and lung components, oesophageal pressure (an approximation to pleural pressure) is measured by an oesophageal air-filled balloon or fluid filled catheter (Coates & Stocks, 1991; Fig. 11.1).

Because the compliance of the newborn chest wall is high in relation to the lung compliance (C_l), especially in infants with lung disease, for most practical purposes C_{rs} gives reasonable estimate of C_l. Under dynamic conditions, convective (flow resistive) pressure losses have to be separated from elastic forces. The difference between static and dynamic compliance measurements depends on a number of physiological factors: chest wall distortion, viscoelastic properties of the lungs and uneven or prolonged time constants within the lungs which determine the validity of airway opening pressure measurements under dynamic conditions. Similarly, the determination of resistance assumes the compliance is constant over the tidal range and that resistance can be expressed by a single value. The latter is clearly incorrect both for intubated babies (since the value of the resistance produced by the endotracheal tube is flow-dependent) and for freely breathing infants in whom glottic braking is common.

Techniques. The variety of techniques available is an indication that none is ideal. Variables such as health or disease, spontaneous breathing or mechanical ventilation, complexity of equipment and availability of computer analysis determine the choice of method. Measurement of airflow (for resistance), tidal volume and airway opening pressure are common to all the methods, with oesophageal pressure for the Mead and Whittenberger technique. Body surface displacement for tidal volume measurement has an occasional role (see section entitled 'Other techniques' below). Techniques have been reviewed in detail (England, 1988; Dezateux et al., 1991; ATS/ERS Working Party, 1993.)

Total respiratory system mechanics

A number of techniques have gained popularity recently because of their simplicity or adaptability to computer automation. All are based on measurements of pressure, flow and volume made at the airway opening (P_{ao}), and hence provide an assessment of the mechanical properties of the whole respiratory system (C_{rs}, the compliance of the respiratory system & R_{rs} the resistance of the respiratory system). There are three main methods: the occlusion/passive flow volume method (R_{rs} & C_{rs}); forced oscillation (R_{rs}); weighted spirometer (C_{rs}). Other techniques, such as the interrupter method for R_{rs}, have yet to be validated in infants (Sly & Bates, 1988).

The best established technique is based on single or multiple, brief, expiratory airway occlusions (Thomson et al., 1985; Stocks, 1991). When flow is interrupted by occluding a pneumotachograph at the airway opening at end-inspiration or during expiration, pressure equilibrates throughout the lungs. P_{ao} is then equal to the elastic recoil pressure of the respiratory system. From the relationship between P_{ao} and the increment of lung volume above FRC at which the occlusion was performed, a value of C_{rs} can be derived. Multiple occlusions enhance the accuracy of determination and provide data over much of the tidal volume range (Fig. 11.2). The intercept on the volume axis is a measure of dynamic elevation of FRC. There are several important assumptions, the most important of which are (i) that the measurement is truly passive i.e. that the Hering–Breuer inflation reflex induced by occlusion leads to total relaxation of

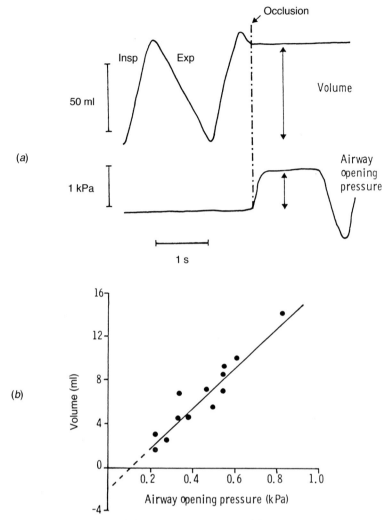

Fig. 11.2. From multiple brief expiratory occlusions (*a*), a plot of airway opening pressure against occluded volume (above FRC) is constructed (*b*). The calculated slope (by linear regression) represents C_{rs} and the y-intercept is the dynamic elevation of FRC. (From Thomson, Beardsmore & Silverman M., 1985.)

the muscles of breathing and (ii) that equilibration has indeed been achieved in the 0.2–0.5 s occlusion which is possible before the next spontaneous breath. In the presence of airway disease, equilibration may take longer. Underestimation of P_{ao} will lead to overestimation of C_{rs}. A further source of error in non-intubated infants is brought about by a shunt of air from lungs to upper airway during occlusion, which will again

(*a*) Passive flow–volume curve

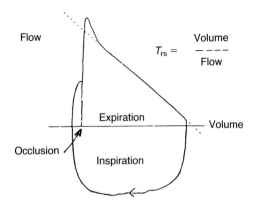

$$T_{rs} = \frac{- - - -}{Flow}$$

Flow

Volume

Expiration

Occlusion

Inspiration

Volume

(*b*) Time-based trace

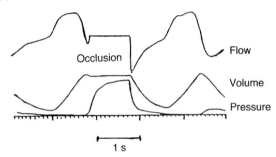

Occlusion

Flow

Volume

Pressure

1 s

Fig. 11.3. The passive flow volume technique. (*a*) the reciprocal slope of the descending expiratory flow volume curve (i.e. volume/flow), during muscle relaxation induced by brief airway occlusion, represents the time constant of the respiratory system (T_{rs}). Simultaneous measurement of elastic recoil pressure developed during occlusion (*b*) enables compliance and resistance of the respiratory system to be assessed. ($T_{rs} = C_{rs} \times R_{rs}$). (From Stocks, 1991.)

lead to a small underestimate of P_{ao}, particularly after end-inspiratory occlusion, when the respiratory recoil pressure is maximal. Two techniques had been described for extending the range of lung volumes over which compliance can be measured, by 'volume clamping' (Grunstein et al., 1987) or by 'pumping' the lungs (Turner, Stick & Le Souef, 1991).

On release of the occlusion, assuming continued muscle relaxation and assuming that the respiratory system behaves as a single compartment, the lungs empty exponentially. The slope of the passive flow-volume curve (Fig. 11.3) represents the time constant of the respiratory system (T_{rs}) (Mortola et al., 1982). From the relationship $T_{rs} = C_{rs} \cdot R_{rs}$, having measured C_{rs}, R_{rs} can be calculated. Again the validity of the assumptions is critical. The main problems encountered in freely breathing infants relate to the upper airways: glottic braking of expiration and flutter from turbulence in the nasopharynx may lead to spurious results, even though the passive flow–volume curve appears linear. In disease and in the presence of a small calibre endotracheal tube (with flow-dependent resistance), the lungs no longer behave as a single compartment; the flow-volume curve is alinear (Prendiville, Thomson & Silverman, 1986) and the technique becomes inaccurate (Celluci et al., 1991).

In the forced oscillation technique (FOT), single or multiple frequency pressure oscillations are applied at the airway opening, usually by means of a loudspeaker attached to a mouthpiece, or in the case of infants, a face mask (Working Group Paediatrics SEPCR, 1989). The input impedance of the respiratory system (Z_{rs}) is then calculated from the induced pressure/flow relationship, after eliminating any effects of tidal breathing. Z_{rs} can be resolved into an in-phase component which represents the flow-resistive properties of the whole respiratory system (R_{rs}), and an out of phase component, the reactance (C_{rs}), a combined function of elastance and inertance. The simplicity of the technique and its ability to provide data on frequency dependence of lung mechanics are attractive. However in infants with a relatively high breathing frequency, accurate measurements of R_{rs} at low frequencies (2–6 Hz) may be impossible without very prolonged measurement runs. Airway obstruction leads to frequency dependence of resistance, the changes being greatest at low frequencies, so that the sensitivity with which a change in resistance can be identified is reduced in young infants. In addition, in nose-breathing infants, R_{rs} may be dominated by upper airway resistance, again reducing the sensitivity of the technique for detecting changes in the lower airways. Another factor which affects accuracy is the compliance of cheeks and pharynx, which leads to a dissipation of pressure and an underestimation of R_{rs}, especially at high frequencies and when there is increased lower airway obstruction. An ingenious solution to this problem has been devised by Peslin and colleagues (Marchal et al., 1991). By applying oscillatory pressure to a head box, the difference in pressure across the cheeks is minimized in mouth-breathing subjects (and probably to a lesser extent in nose-breathing infants), leading to increased accuracy. The FOT has been used very little in infancy (Tepper, Pagtakhan & Taussig, 1984; Desager et al., 1992).

The only other simple method for determining C_{rs} in infants is the weighted spirometer technique (Tepper et al., 1984), in which a change in end-tidal lung volume (FRC) is brought about by adding weights to the bell of a spirometer circuit, thereby inducing CPAP. The method assumes that the infant does not respond to CPAP by altered pattern of breathing or by altered respiratory muscle activity. These assumptions are unlikely to be met, except at the lowest levels of CPAP. The technique gives results for C_{rs} very close to those obtained from multiple occlusions (Merth & Quanjer, 1990).

In addition to the occlusion and passive flow-volume methods, other techniques which may find application in intubated babies include the least squares linear regression (Bhutani et al., 1988) and the constant flow method (Seear, Wensley & Werner, 1991; Storme et al., 1992). These techniques, which are suitable for computer analysis, assume linear relationships of data, single values for compliance and resistance, absence of interference from the ventilator and absence of tube leak.

Qualitative techniques for monitoring lung mechanics during mechanical ventilation are under development. By simply monitoring pressure, flow and volume at the airway opening during mechanical ventilation, trends in respiratory resistance and compliance can be tracked, providing early warning of mechanical or clinical problems. Air leaks around the endotracheal tube limit the accuracy of measurements made in the intensive care unit.

Methods dependent on oesophageal manometry (pulmonary mechanics)

Classical, dynamic pulmonary mechanics was based on the measurement of changes in oesophageal pressure (P_{oes}), a surrogate for pleural pressure (Fig. 11.1), in relation to flow and volume at the airway opening. Several techniques of analysis can be used, all amenable to computer assistance, the commonest being (i) the Mead and Whittenberger method (Mead & Whittenberger, 1953) and (ii) the least squares linear regression technique (Bhutani et al., 1988; Rousselot, Peslin & Duvivier, 1992). Both methods depend on the assumption that the pressure–volume curve of the lungs is linear and hence that a single value can be assigned to lung compliance and resistance, assumptions which are unlikely to be true in the presence of lung disease (Ratjen et al., 1989; Stocks, Thomson & Silverman, 1985a).

The subject of oesophageal manometry has been recently reviewed (Coates & Stocks, 1991). The techniques are deceptively easy, but the two main methods, balloon-catheter and fluid filled catheter, both have major drawbacks. For both, the validity of the assumption that oesophageal pressure is a measure of mean pleural pressure is assessed by the 'occlusion test', in which the magnitude of change in P_{ao} at the occluded airway of a spontaneously breathing infant should be identical to the change in P_{oes}. The ratio may differ from unity because of poor technique (placement of the oesophageal catheter), severe lung disease with non-uniformity of pleural pressure change, oesophageal spasm, upper airway compliance in the presence of a long pulmonary time constant or air leak at the mask or tube.

Whole-body plethysmography (airway resistance)

When an infant breathes within a sealed, 'constant volume' (actually constant mass) whole body plethysmograph (box), changes in box pressure (P_b) occur due to the compression and rarefaction of alveolar gas which is dependent on the resistance of the airways. The relationship between change in P_b and change in P_{ao} (which is equivalent to P_{alv}) during occluded breathing, can be used to convert P_b to P_{alv}. Airway resistance is determined from the relationship between P_{alv} and flow at the airway opening.

The plethysmographic technique is extremely demanding, and cannot be applied to intubated infants or even to infants who require more than minimal oxygen supplementation. Its main advantage is the simultaneous measurement of lung volume and the possibility with computer analysis, of displaying the pressure–flow relationship which provides far more information than a single value for airway resistance (Stocks et al., 1985 *a,b*).

Applications

Qualitative measurements of lung mechanics have contributed to our understanding of the process of adaptation to extrauterine life and to the influence of fetal factors and obstetric interventions. Understanding the nature and severity of neonatal thoracic and pulmonary disease and its management by techniques of mechanical ventilatory support has been aided by lung function measurement. The action on lung mechanics of agents which alter pulmonary compliance, such as surfactant, or airway resistance, such as bronchodilators, can only be fully appreciated if simultaneous measurements are made of changes in lung volume. Without such measurements, the benefits of therapy are likely to be severely underestimated.

Forced expiratory flow

Definition

By far the commonest techniques for measuring lung function in school children and adults rely on forced expiratory manoeuvres. At lung volumes toward the lower end of the tidal range, when flow limitation occurs, expiratory flow rate reaches a maximum value (and is said to be 'effort' independent) and is determined by intrathoracic pulmonary function. According to wave-speed theory (Dawson & Elliott, 1977), under these conditions the following relationship holds true:

$$\dot{V}_{max} = (1/\delta)^{1/2} \cdot (dP_{tm}/dA)^{1/2} \cdot A^{2/3} \tag{2}$$

where $\dot{V}_{max}$ is the maximum expiratory flow rate, δ is gas density and P_{tm} and A are the transmural pressure and airway cross sectional area at the choke point (site of flow limitation). Airway elastance (the middle term) and cross sectional area are the major physiological variables. P_{tm} is affected by both resistive upstream pressure loss and by the elastic recoil of the lungs, both peripheral ('small airway') functions of the lungs. The factors which affect $\dot{V}_{max}$ in growing infants have recently been reviewed (Wohl, 1991).

Forced expiration can be produced passively in infants by means of an inflatable thoraco-abdominal jacket, the squeeze technique (Silverman, Prendiville & Green, 1986), or in intubated infants by applying a negative pressure to the tube, the forced deflation method (Motoyama et al., 1987). The importance of the method is that whereas other forms of resistance measurement are dominated by the upper airway, this technique measures intrathoracic airway function provided that flow-limitation is achieved. This is doubtful in healthy infants (Motoyama, Nakayama & Walczak, 1991), but clearly occurs in infants with airway obstruction (e.g. chronic lung disease of prematurity).

Technique

The squeeze technique is simple. The infant sleeps supine, encased in an inflatable, flexible thoraco-abdominal jacket which is attached to a pressure source by means of a wide bore tube (Fig. 11.4). At end inspiration, the jacket is rapidly inflated, causing a passive, partial, forced expiration. Flow and volume are measured by face mask and pneumotachograph. During successive squeezes, jacket pressure is increased until $\dot{V}_{max}$ is produced (or the maximum pressure, usually 8–10 kPa) is reached. The reference point for determination of $\dot{V}_{max}$ is FRC, since

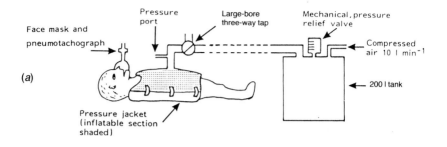

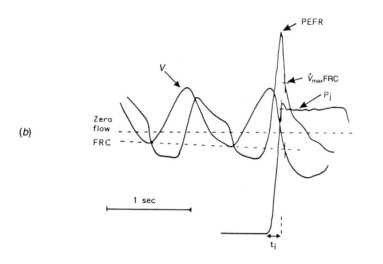

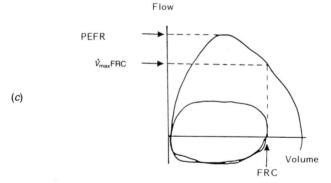

Fig. 11.4. (*a*) Equipment for measuring partial expiratory flow-volume curves in infancy. (*b*) Measurement of maximal flow at FRC from time-based data (note: flow signal inverted). PEFR: peak expiratory flow rate; $\dot{V}_{max}FRC$: maximum flow at FRC; P_j: jacket inflation pressure. (*c*) Partial expiratory flow-volume curve and the preceding tidal breath in a normal infant.

TLC and vital capacity cannot be defined in the sleeping, passive infant (Fig. 11.4). Both in shape and in numerical value, flow volume curves differ in lung disease and in health.

The use of the 'floating' reference point FRC is problematic. Disease, therapy, breathing pattern and even measurement conditions (Table 11.1) may cause shifts in the level of FRC. Ideally, lung volume should be measured at each stage. The assumption that infants remain passive is often untrue, reflex glottic braking and early onset of inspiration are two responses which can disrupt expiratory flows.

The forced deflation method for intubated infants has been used mainly during anaesthesia or intensive care (Motoyama et al., 1987). Flow rates by this technique are greater than by the squeeze in healthy infants, raising doubts about the assumption that flow limitation can be achieved by the squeeze method.

Applications

The squeeze technique has been used to study lung growth, in epidemiological studies (for instance to determine the effects on fetal lung development of maternal smoking), for clinical assessment, to measure the response to therapy and in the assessment of bronchial responsiveness in newborns. Future developments include measuring expiratory flow over the full vital capacity range after passive inflation (Turner et al., 1991) and refinements of the application of the squeeze to minimize reflex responses.

The distribution of ventilation
Definition

Tests which determine how evenly inspired gas is distributed throughout the lung have proved to be extremely sensitive in detecting minor degrees of lung dysfunction, for instance in demonstrating a difference between asymptomatic smokers and nonsmokers. Gas distribution can be adversely affected by any focal or generalized disorder of the lungs. Little use has been made of these techniques in studying infant lung function.

Techniques

Most tests are based on an assessment of the efficiency with which a tracer gas can be removed from or equilibrated with the lungs (Working Group Paediatrics SEPCR, 1989). Nitrogen clearance during oxygen breathing is the usual basis, providing indices of efficiency such as pulmonary clearance delay, gas distribution index or distribution of moments (Edberg et al., 1991; Wall, Misley & Brown, 1988). Techniques which can be applied to oxygen-dependent infants (Edberg et al., 1991) and which treat the lungs as a multi-compartmental system have recently been described.

The multiple inert gas methods, requiring mass spectrometry, which have provided a wealth of data on ventilation/perfusion relationships in adult lung disease await adaptation to the newborn field. Other potentially useful techniques are based on the use of small amounts of radioactive tracers, such as $^{81}Kr^m$ (Working Group Paediatrics SEPCR, 1989).

Applications

The simpler tests of nitrogen clearance may be valuable in epidemiological studies, as sensitive indices of mild disease. At the other extreme, the multiple inert gas technique (Rodriguez-Roisen & Wagner, 1990) should find application in the neonatal intensive care unit, as a means of evaluating mechanical or pharmacological therapy. Ethical factors limit the use of radionuclides to the identification of focal lung disease.

Other techniques

The analysis of *tidal breathing* has received little attention until recently. As suggested by Mortola (Chapter 7), much physiological information can be prised from differences between active/dynamic and passive/dynamic patterns of flow and volume. The frequency of breathing (surely the most often recorded but least useful measure of lung function), the duty cycle (Haddad et al., 1979; Gaultier et al., 1985) and the shape of the flow/time curve (Martinez et al., 1988; Stocks, 1991) provide information which warrants further physiological explanation and clinical exploration. The recent observation that the likelihood of subsequent wheezing can be predicted from flow/time patterns soon after birth in groups of infants, provides a glimpse of further exciting developments in this area (Martinez et al., 1988). The advantage of tidal breathing techniques is that they are amenable to measurement at the body surface, obviating the need for devices at the airway opening.

Body surface measurements can be made using the principles of inductance, impedance or magnetometery, to study patterns of thoraco-abdominal motion during breathing or, by summing thoracic and abdominal signals, tidal volume. In order to calibrate the signals to allow quantitation, simultaneous measurement of flow at the airway opening must be recorded. Changes in breathing pattern, sleep state or posture usually lead to a change in calibration factors and therefore inaccuracy (Wilkes et al., 1987). Thus these techniques provide short-term quantitative data. They are most valuable as long-term monitoring devices, or for tracking physiological functions which do not need quantitation, such as breathing pattern. Body surface measurements have contributed to a number of clinical or physiological studies in infancy (Colin et al., 1989; Maxwell et al., 1988).

Disorders of the *respiratory pump*, including the muscles of breathing and the other structures which make up the chest wall, are relatively common in neonatal clinical practice, encompassing both primary abnormalities and functional disorders such as muscle fatigue. The electrophysiology of muscle fatigue has been studied in detail in newborns (Nichols, 1991), and the mechanical aspects of the muscles of breathing to a lesser extent (Gaultier et al., 1985, Mortola et al., 1984).

Reference values

The issue of reference values and their application in clinical situations is complex (Quanjer et al., 1989). Reference values are needed for several reasons, one of the most important being their value as standards of comparison between different laboratories. Deviation from normality and determination of pathophysiology are based on reference data. While the response to treatment can be determined by internal reference, the completeness of recovery requires data from a reference population. Longitudinal reference data are important in the evaluation of the growth of lung function and for epidemiological studies. Poor specificity and sensitivity of most tests of pulmonary physiology limit their use in diagnosis.

Four phases are involved in obtaining and using reference values: selection of an appropriate population, measurement by means of standardized techniques, expression of results and application to infants.

The choice of a reference population is not simple, and depends on the purpose to which the data are to be put. Measuring deviation from normality presumes reference data derived from an ideal population (full-term, healthy infants without familial respiratory disease). On the other hand, a study of the pulmonary effects of prematurity would be relevant only in comparison with an unselected term population in which other factors (smoking, family history of asthma, etc) were equally represented. Bias can be best avoided by choosing a large enough population base, and by recording all of the important variables for subsequent statistical manipulation.

Standardization of measurement techniques, including length and body weight as well as physiological techniques, is critical. This is the subject of much recent work (Working Group Paediatrics SEPCR, 1989). Reference data should be expressed either graphically or as regression equations, relating physiological values to body size or to each other. In applying reference data, regression formulae rather than ratios should be the basis for assessing normality, since with few exceptions, simple ratios are not age (or size) independent. Degree of abnormality cannot usefully be expressed as '% predicted' where scatter (for instance the residual standard deviation) is not proportional to the mean. Standardized residuals ('Z' units or standard deviation units) or centiles are appropriate. Compilations of reference data have recently been published (Quanjer et al., 1989; Dezateux et al., 1991).

Prospects

The advent of molecular biology has temporarily eclipsed clinical physiology. As the fruits of the new biology are applied to clinical problems, physiological outcome variables will assume renewed importance.

Computer technology has lead to user-friendly commercial equipment, with applications during intensive care and subsequently. Servocontrol of respiratory support equipment can be expected soon, based on miniature sensors and automatic calibration techniques. These advances will widen the scope and availability of lung function measurements in infants.

References

ATS/ERS (American Thoracic Society/European Respiratory Society) Working Party. (1993). Respiratory mechanics in infants; physiologic evaluation in health and disease. *American Review of Respiratory Disease*, **147**, 474–96.

Bhutani, V. K., Sivieri, E. M., Abbasi, S. & Shaffer, T. H. (1988). Evaluation of neonatal pulmonary mechanics and energetics: a two factor least squares analysis. *Pediatric Pulmonology*, **4**, 150–8.

Boon, A. W., Ward-McQuaid J. M. C., Milner, A. D. & Hopkin, I. E. (1981). Thoracic gas volume, helium functional residual capacity and air trapping in the first six hours of life: the effect of oxygen administration. *Early Human Development*, **5**, 157–66.

Celluci, G. L., Brunet, P., Dallava-Santucci, J., Dhainaut, J. F., Paccals, D., Armaganidis, A., Milic Emili, J. & Lockhart, A. (1991). A single compartment model cannot describe passive expiration in intubated, paralysed humans. *The European Respiratory Journal*, **4**, 458–64.

Chapman, B., O'Callaghan, C., Coxon, R., Glover, P., Jaroszkiewicz, G., Howseman, A., Mansfield, P., Small, P., Milner, A. D. & Coupland, R. E. (1990). Estimation of lung volume in infants by echo planar imaging and total body plethysmography. *Archives of Disease in Childhood*, **65**, 168–70.

Chernick, V. & Mellins, R. B. (1991). *Basic Mechanisms of Pediatric Respiratory Disease: Cellular and Integrative*. B. C. Decker, Inc., Philadelphia.

Coates, A. L. & Stocks, J. (1991). Esophageal pressure manometry in human infants. *Pediatric Pulmonology*, **11**, 350–60.

Colin, A. A., Wohl, M. E. B., Mead, J., Ratjen, F. A., Glass, G. & Stark A. R. (1989). Transition from dynamically maintained to related end-expiratory volume in human infants. *Journal of Applied Physiology*, **67**, 2107–11.

Dawson, S. V. & Elliott, E. A. (1977). Wave-speed limitation on expiratory flow – a unifying concept. *Journal of Applied Physiology*, **43**, 498–515.

Desager, K. N., van Bever, H. P., Boven, K., de Backer, W. & Vermeire, P. A. (1992). Respiratory system resistance and functional residual capacity in intermittently wheezing infants treated with nebulised fenoterol. *European Respiratory Journal*, **5**, 275s.

Dezateux, C. A., Fletcher, M. E., Rabbette, P. S., Stanger, L. J. & Stocks, J. (1991). *A Manual of Infant Lung Function Testing*. Institute of Child Health, London.

Edberg, K. E., Sandberg, K., Silberberg, A., Ekstrom-Jodal, B. & Hjalmarson, O. (1991). Lung volume, gas mixing and mechanics of breathing in mechanically ventilated very low birth weight infants with idiopathic respiratory distress syndrome. *Pediatric Research*, **30**, 496–500.

England, S. J. (1988). Current techniques for assessing pulmonary function in the newborn and infant: advantages and limitations. *Pediatric Pulmonology*, **4**, 48–53.

Gaultier, C., Boulé, B., Tournier, G. & Girard, F. (1985). Inspiratory force reserve of the respiratory muscles in children with chronic obstructive pulmonary disease. *American Review of Respiratory Disease*, **131**, 811–5.

Grunstein, M. M., Springer, C., Godfrey, S., Bar-Yishay, E., Vilozni, D., Inscore, S. C. & Schramm C. M. (1987). Expiratory volume clamping: a new method to assess respiratory mechanics in sedated infants. *Journal of Applied Physiology*, **62**, 2107–14.

Haddad, G. G., Epstein, R. A., Epstein, M. A. F., Leistner, H. L., Marino, P. A. & Mellins, R. B. (1979). Maturation of ventilation and ventilatory pattern in normal sleeping infants. *Journal of Applied Physiology*, **46**, 998–1002.

Hanrahan, J. P., Tager, I. B., Castile, R. G., Segai, M. R., Weiss, S. T. & Speizer, F. E. (1990). Pulmonary function measurements in healthy infants. Variability and size correction. *American Review of Respiratory Disease*, **141**, 1135–7.

Hanrahan, J. P., Tager, I. B., Segal, M. R. et al. (1992). The effect of maternal smoking during pregnancy on early infant lung function. *American Review of Respiratory Disease*, **145**, 1129–35.

Kafer, E. R. (1990). Neonatal gas exchange and oxygen transport. In *Fetal and Neonatal Cardiology*, ed W. A. Long. pp. 97–117. W B Saunders, Philadelphia.

McCann, E. M., Goldman, S. L. & Brady, J. P. (1987). Pulmonary function in the sick newborn infant. *Pediatric Research*, **21**, 313–25.

Marchal, F., Duvivier, C., Peslin, R. & Haouzi, P. (1991). Thoracic gas volume at functional residual capacity measured with an integrated-flow plethysmograph in infants and young children. *European Journal of Respiratory Disease*, **4**, 180–7.

Martinez, F. D., Morgan, W. J., Wright, A. L., Holberg, C. J. & Taussig, L. M. (1988). Diminished lung function as a predisposing factor for wheezing respiratory illness in infants. *New England Journal of Medicine*, **319**, 1112–17.

Maxwell, D. L., Prendiville, A., Rose, A. & Silverman, M. (1988). Lung volume changes during histamine induced bronchoconstriction in recurrently wheezy infants. *Pediatric Pulmonology*, **5**, 145–51.

Mead, J. & Whittenberger, J. L. (1953). Physical properties of human lungs measured during spontaneous respiration. *Journal of Applied Physiology*, **5**, 779–96.

Merth, I. & Quanjer, P. H. (1990). Respiratory system compliance assessed by the multiple occlusion and weighted spirometer method in non-intubated healthy newborns. *Pediatric Pulmonology*, **8**, 273–9.

Milner, A. D. (1990). Lung function testing in infancy. *Archives of Disease in Childhood*, **65**, 548–52.

Mortola, J. P. (1987). Dynamics of breathing in newborn mammals. *Physiological Reviews*, **67**, 187–243.

Mortola, J. P., Fisher, J. T., Smith, B., Fox, G. & Weeks, S. (1982). Dynamics of breathing in infants. *Journal of Applied Physiology*, **52**, 1209–15.

Mortola, J. P., Milic-Emili, J., Noworaj, A., Smith, B., Fox, G. & Weeks, S. (1984). Muscle pressure and flow during expiration in infants. *American Review of Respiratory Disease*, **129**, 49–53.

Motoyama, E. K., Fort, M. D., Klesh, K. W., Mutich, R. L. & Guthrie, R. D. (1987). Early onset of airway reactivity in premature infants with bronchopulmonary dysplasia. *American Review of Respiratory Disease*, **136**, 50–7.

Motoyama, E. K., Nakayama, D. & Walczak, S. A. (1991). Absence of flow limitation in partial flow-volume curves by thoracoabdominal compression in healthy infants: a comparison with deflation flow-volume curves. *American Review of Respiratory Disease*, **143**, A809.

Nichols, D. G. (1991). Respiratory muscle performance in infants and children. *Journal of Pediatrics*, **118**, 493–502.

Prechtl, H. F. R. (1974). The behavioural states of the newborn infant. *Brain Research*, **76**, 185–212.

Prendiville, A., Thomson, A. & Silverman, M. (1986). Effect of tracheobronchial suction on respiratory resistance in intubated preterm babies. *Archives of Disease in Childhood*, **61**, 1178–83.

Quanjer, Ph. H., Stocks, J., Polgar G., Wise M., Karlberg, J. & Borsboom G. (1989) Compilation of reference values for lung function measurements in children. *The European Respiratory Journal*, **2** (Suppl. 4), 184s–261s.

Ratjen, F., Zinman, R., Stark, A. R., Leszcyznski, L. E. & Wohl, M. E. B. (1989). Effect of changes in lung volume on respiratory system compliance in newborn infants. *Journal of Applied Physiology*, **67**, 1192–7.

Richardson, P. (1989). Lung mechanics: a discussion of methods for measurements in newborn infants. ARKOS, Dec, 15–21.

Rodriguez-Roisin, R. & Wagner, P. D. (1990). Clinical relevance of ventilation–perfusion inequality determined by inert gas elimination. *European Respiratory Journal*, **3**, 469–82.

Rousselot, J. M., Peslin, R. & Duvivier, C. (1992). Evaluation of the multiple linear regression method to monitor respiratory mechanics in ventilated neonates and young children. *Pediatric Pulmonology*, **13**, 161–8.

Silverman, M., Prendiville, A. & Green, S. (1986). Partial expiratory flow-volume curves in infancy: technical aspects. *Bulletin Européen Physiopathologie Respiratoire*, **22**, 257–62.

Seear, M., Wensley, D. & Werner, H. (1991). Comparison of three methods for measuring respiratory mechanics in ventilated children. *Pediatric Pulmonology*, **10**, 291–5.

Sivan, Y., Deakers, T. W. & Newth, C. J. (1990). An automated bedside method for measuring functional residual capacity by N_2 washout in mechanically ventilated children. *Pediatric Research*, **28**, 446–50.

Sly, P. D. & Bates, J. H. T. (1988). Computer analysis of physical factors affecting the use of the interrupter technique in infants. *Pediatric Pulmonology*, **4**, 215–24.

Stocks, J. (1991). Recent advances in the assessment of lung function in infants. *Pneumologie*, **45**, 881–6.

Stocks, J. & Godfrey, S. (1978). Nasal resistance during infancy. *Respiration Physiology*, **34**, 233–46.

Stocks, J., Thomson, A. & Silverman, M. (1985*a*) The numerical analysis of pressure flow curves in infancy. *Pediatric Pulmonology*, **1**, 19–26.

Stocks, J., Thomson. A., Wong, C. & Silverman, M. (1985*b*). Pressure-flow curves in infancy. *Pediatric Pulmonology*, **1**, 33–40.

Storme, L., Leclerc, F., Kacet, N., Dubos, J. P., Grouillet, C., Tousseau, U. & Lequien, P. (1992). Respiratory mechanics in mechanically ventilated newborns: a comparison between passive inflation and occlusion methods. *Pediatric Pulmonology*, **12**, 203–12.

Tepper, R. S. & Adsell, S. (1992). Comparison of helium dilution and nitrogen washout measurements of functional residual capacity in infants and very young children. *Pediatric Pulmonology*, **13**, 250–4.

Tepper, R. S., Pagtakhan, R. D. & Taussig, L. M. (1984). Noninvasive determination of total respiratory system compliance in infants by the weighted-spirometer method. *American Review of Respiratory Disease*, **130**, 461–6.

Tepper, R. S., Morgan, W. J., Cota, K. & Taussig, L. M. (1986). Physiologic growth and development of the lung during the first year of life. *American Review of Respiratory Disease*, **134**, 513–19.

Thomson, A. H., Beardsmore, C. S. & Silverman, M. (1985). *Bulletin Européen Physiopathologie Respiratoire*, **21**, 411–16.

Turner, D. J., Stick, S. M. & Le Souef, P. N. (1991). Assessment of respiratory function in infants pumped to higher lung volumes. *American Review of Respiratory Disease*, **143**, A126.

Turner, D. T., Stick, S. M., Sly, P. D. & Le Souef, P. N. (1992). Respiratory function from raised lung volumes in normal and wheezy infants. *American Review of Respiratory Disease*, **145**, A248.

Vallinis, P., Davis, G. M. & Coates, A. L. (1990). A very low deadspace pneumotachograph for ventilatory measurements in newborns. *Journal of Applied Physiology*, **69**, 1542–5.

Wall, M. A., Misley, M. C. & Brown, A. (1988). Changes in ventilation homogeneity from preschool through young adulthood as determined by movement analysis of nitrogen washout. *Pediatric Research*, **23**, 68–71.

Wilkes, D. L., Revow, M., Bryan, M. H. & England, S. J. (1987). Evaluation of respiratory inductance plethysmography in infants weighing less than 1500 grams. *American Review of Respiratory Disease*, **136**, 416–19.

Wohl, M. E. B. (1991). Lung mechanics in the developing human infant. In *Basic Mechanisms of Pediatric Respiratory Disease: Cellular and Integrative*, ed V. Chernick & R. B. Mellins. pp. 89–99. B C Decker, Inc, Philadelphia.

Working Group Paediatrics SEPCR (1989). Standardization of lung function tests in paediatrics. *The European Respiratory Journal*, **2** (Suppl. 4).

12

Surfactant replacement

HENRY L. HALLIDAY and BENGT ROBERTSON

Introduction

The idea that a deficiency of pulmonary surfactant might be compensated by 'replacing' the missing (or some equivalent) material via the airways must have occurred to many of the pioneers in surfactant research. For example, Gruenwald in 1947 suggested that 'the addition of surface active substances to the air or oxygen which is being spontaneously breathed in or introduced by a respirator might aid in relieving the initial atelectasis of newborn infants'. However, some erroneous concepts, once shared by many investigators, delayed the transformation of a basically sound idea into principles applicable to clinical practice.

For example, although dipalmitoylphosphatidylcholine (DPPC) is the main component of pulmonary surfactant, it cannot serve alone as a surfactant substitute. Clinical trials in which DPPC was aerosolized into the airways of babies with surfactant deficiency were thus unsuccessful (Robillard et al., 1964; Chu et al., 1967) – at least in comparison with the results of recent studies involving the use of more complex, and complete, surfactant substitutes. Another misconception was the belief that physiologically active chloroform extracts of natural surfactant are protein-free (Metcalfe, Enhörning & Possmayer, 1980) and its correlate that the therapeutic potential of a surfactant substitute would depend solely on its lipid components. We now know that the surfactant system contains at least four specific proteins (Possmayer, 1988; Kuroki, 1992) and that these proteins regulate a number of important mechanisms including surfactant secretion, transformation of secreted lamellar bodies into tubular myelin, adsorption of the surface film, and uptake and recycling of waste surfactant material by the alveolar epithelium. The hydrophilic surfactant-associated proteins, SP-A and SP-D, also stimulate phagocytosis of bacteria and viruses by alveolar macrophages and may thus play an important role in the pulmonary defence system (van Iwaarden et al., 1990, 1991; Kuroki, 1992). Hydrophobic proteins (SP-B,

SP-C), accelerating surface adsorption, are present in all modified natural surfactants prepared by extraction of lung tissue or lung lavage fluid using organic solvents.

Yet another postulate that fortunately turned out to be wrong was the claim that, in order to be effective in a baby with surfactant deficiency, the exogenous substitute would have to be given very soon after birth, preferably before the first breath (Enhörning & Robertson, 1972). Although the distribution of exogenous surfactant is indeed more uniform in immature animals treated at birth than in those treated after a period of ventilation (Jobe et al., 1981), recent clinical trials have shown that the timing of therapy is not critical, and that good results can be obtained by prophylactic administration of surfactant to babies at risk after the onset of breathing. It is now generally accepted that a physiologically active surfactant substitute must contain both DPPC and agents that facilitate adsorption and spreading of the lipid at the air–liquid interfaces of the lung, that hydrophobic proteins are essential components of natural surfactants for replacement therapy (Notter, 1984) and that the time window for surfactant treatment in the neonatal period is surprisingly wide, up to several hours or even days after birth.

With these concepts as a foundation, surfactant treatment of respiratory distress syndrome (RDS) has become part of the clinical routine in many neonatal intensive care units. In this chapter, we will review possible clinical targets for surfactant replacement therapy with emphasis on the neonatal period, methods for quality control of exogenous surfactants, and experience from a large number of clinical trials that confirms efficacy of surfactant replacement for prevention and treatment of RDS, but we will also indicate some limitations of this new therapeutic approach.

Possible targets for surfactant replacement therapy

The most obvious candidate for surfactant replacement therapy is an immature newborn infant with anticipated, or established, respiratory problems due to surfactant deficiency. In babies who develop 'idiopathic' RDS the average pool size of surfactant lipids is about 10 mg/kg body weight (Hallman et al., 1986). This is not much different from the normal adult mammalian pool size (11–14 mg/kg) (Jobe & Ikegami, 1987). It is significantly larger than the amount required to form a complete monolayer at the alveolar air–liquid interfaces (about 3 mg/kg) (Marks et al., 1983), but nevertheless only about one-tenth of the corresponding figure for a full-term neonatal lung (Jobe & Ikegami, 1987).

The purpose of replacement therapy in a baby with immature lungs is to upgrade the intra-alveolar pool of surfactant to a level allowing normal neonatal respiratory function. This dose is not clearly defined, but apparently a large reservoir (including a safety margin) must be present in the fetal lung liquid to ensure rapid adsorption of the surfactant lipids to the expanding air–liquid interfaces at birth, and to provide material for subsequent continuous replenishment of the surface film. Kobayashi et al. (1990) estimated from experiments on immature newborn rabbits treated with modified natural surfactant (prepared by extraction with organic solvents) that the 'critical concentration' of surfactant in fetal lung liquid, needed for adequate neonatal lung function, is about 3 mg/ml. This is close to the concentration required with the same surfactant for rapid adsorption and optimal dynamic surface properties during rapid area oscillation in a pulsating bubble system. The average pool size of a baby with RDS (see above), suspended in a normal volume of fetal lung liquid before onset of respiration (about 30 ml/kg) yields a concentration that is about one-tenth of this critical concentration (Kobayashi et al., 1990), whereas the pool size of a normal full-term neonate matches it fairly well. Although data from animal experiments involving the use of surfactant extracted with organic solvents cannot be directly extrapolated to describe the kinetics of endogenous surfactant in the newborn baby, they help explain why a comparatively large dose of exogenous surfactant (> 50 mg/kg) is required to prevent RDS in an immature newborn lamb (Ikegami et al., 1980) or human baby (Enhorning et al., 1985; Kwong et al., 1985; Shapiro et al., 1985; Merritt et al., 1986; Morley et al., 1988; Gortner et al., 1990a; Corbet et al., 1991). For the reasons explained below, even larger doses (>100 mg/kg) are required to treat babies with established RDS.

Some babies with clinical signs of RDS have a mature phospholipid profile in the airways and therefore probably do not suffer from primary surfactant deficiency. It has been postulated that these babies instead have a disease similar to the adult respiratory distress syndrome (ARDS) (Royall & Levin, 1988; Faix et al., 1989) with increased lung permeability to macromolecules and excessive accumulation of surfactant-inhibitory serum proteins in the airspaces. Although the effect of exogenous surfactant is less striking in these babies than in those with 'classical' RDS, and relapse is common (Segerer et al., 1991), they should be listed among potential candidates for replacement therapy.

Another neonatal lung disease which may reflect mild surfactant dysfunction is transient tachypnoea of the newborn (also known as wet lung syndrome, type II RDS, or pulmonary maladaptation) (Egan,

1989). The resorption of fetal lung liquid at birth is mainly mediated by sodium channels on the luminal side and sodium–potassium pumps on the other side of the lung epithelium (Olver, 1983; Olver et al., 1986), but may be facilitated by low surface tension at the alveolar air–liquid interfaces (Guyton, Moffat & Adair, 1984). However, in our experience, administration of surfactant to immature newborn rabbits (gestational age, 27 days) does not accelerate lung liquid absorption to any significant degree, in spite of considerable improvement in lung compliance (Song et al., 1992). On the other hand, blocking of the sodium channels with topical administration of amiloride in a near-term animal does not influence lung compliance during artificial ventilation (Song et al., 1992), although lung liquid absorption is delayed and signs of respiratory distress develop during spontaneous ventilation (O'Brodovich, Weity & Possmayer, 1990). Treatment with surfactant may be particularly rewarding in babies with moderately severe RDS (Bevilacqua et al., 1992), but so far there is no evidence that this effect is mediated by enhanced reabsorption of fetal lung liquid.

The pathophysiology of meconium aspiration syndrome is usually attributed to a combination of conducting airway obstruction and chemical injury to the lung parenchyma (Tyler, Murphy & Chaney, 1978). However, meconium contains several components that may interfere with surfactant function including free fatty acids, cholesterol, proteins, and bilirubin (Holm, 1992). Surfactant mixed with either the chloroform-soluble or the water-soluble fraction of meconium shows delayed surface adsorption and elevated minimum surface tension during cyclic film compression, but the specific inhibitory activity of the chloroform-soluble fraction is stronger (Sun, Curstedt & Robertson, 1992a). Tracheal instillation of filtered meconium (containing only small particles, not blocking the major airways) in near-term newborn rabbits induces respiratory failure with reduced compliance and alveolar collapse (Sun et al., 1992a). Treatment with a large dose of exogenous surfactant leads to a significant improvement of gas exchange and compliance in these experimental animals, but does not restore normal lung function completely (Sun et al., 1992b). Promising results have also been reported from a pilot study of surfactant treatment in term babies with meconium aspiration (Auten et al., 1991) (see below).

Certain forms of bacterial and viral pneumonia may be associated with surfactant dysfunction and respond, at least in experimental models, favourably to surfactant replacement therapy (Eijking et al., 1991; van Daal et al., 1991, 1992). On the other hand, instillation of large doses of surfactant into an infected lung may influence bacterial growth in different ways depending on the composition of the exogenous surfactant and probably also on the type of micro-organism involved. In experiments on newborn rabbits infected with Group B streptococci (GBS), neither natural nor modified natural surfactant (with or without SP-A) had any influence on bacterial growth, whereas bacterial proliferation was depressed after treatment with a synthetic surfactant (Sherman et al., 1990).

These observations are probably clinically relevant since neonatal pneumonia, especially when caused by infection with GBS, may have clinical signs similar to RDS, and some babies with primary surfactant deficiency may have unrecognized concomitant infection of the lungs. Both these categories of babies are likely to be treated with surfactant on the assumption that they have classical RDS. So far, there is no clinical evidence that administration of surfactant to babies with infection has any adverse effects. On the contrary, Auten et al. (1991) recently reported a beneficial effect of treatment with modified natural surfactant (lacking SP-A) in seven term babies with pneumonia; the therapeutic response was similar to that seen in term infants with meconium aspiration.

Data from the studies summarized above indicate that both meconium aspiration syndrome and neonatal pneumonia should be considered as potential clinical targets for surfactant replacement. Additional experimental and clinical studies are required before strict recommendations can be made.

Surfactants used in clinical practice

Exogenous surfactant preparations, used to treat or prevent neonatal respiratory distress syndrome may be divided into two main groups: synthetic (or protein-free) and naturally sourced (containing apoproteins) (Table 12.1).

Synthetic surfactants

Two protein-free synthetic surfactants are currently used in clinical practice:

(a) *Colfosceril palmitate* (Exosurf[R] Neonatal[TM], Burroughs Wellcome) consists of DPPC, hexadecanol (cetyl alcohol) and tyloxapol mixed in proportion by weight 13.5:1.5:1 (Durand et al., 1985; Dechant & Faulds, 1991). Hexadecanol and tyloxapol are added to facilitate

Table 12.1. *Surfactant preparations in clinical use*

Name	Composition concentration	Dose (mg/kg)	Number of doses	Prophylaxis or treatment	Dose volume (ml/kg)
Synthetic					
ALEC (Pumactant[R]) Britannia	DPPC: PG 7:3 50 mg/ml	100	4	P	2
Colfosceril palmitate Exosurf[R] Burroughs Wellcome	DPPC 13.5 Hexadecanol 1.5 Tyloxapol 1.0 13.5 mg/ml	67.5	2–4	P, T	5
Natural					
Surfactant TA (Surfacten[R]) Tokyo Tanabe	Bovine mince plus DPPC, tripalmitin palmitic acid 30 mg/ml	120	3	P, T	4
Beractant (Survanta[R]) Abbott	Bovine mince plus DPPC, tripalmitin palmitic acid 25 mg/ml	100	4	P, T	4
Bovactant (Alveofact[R]) Boehringer-Ingelheim	Bovine lavage 41.7 mg/ml	50	4	P	1.2
Calf lung Surfactant Extract (CLSE, Infasurf[R]) ONY	Calf lung lavage 25–30 mg/ml	90–100	3	P, T	3–4
Porcine lung surfactant extract (Curosurf[R]) Chiesi	Porcine mince 80 mg/ml	100–200	3	T	1.25–2.5

surface adsorption and spreading of DPPC. Exosurf[R] is a sterile, lyophilized powder which when reconstituted in 0.1 M sodium chloride has a lipid concentration of 13.5 mg/ml. It is given in a dose of 67.5 mg/kg (dose volume 5 ml/kg) intratracheally over 4 to 30 min using an endotracheal tube adaptor with a side-port. Exosurf^R is recommended for babies whose birthweight is 700 g or greater who are being mechanically ventilated. Up to two doses, given at 12 hourly intervals, are currently recommended.

(b) *Pumactant* (ALEC or artificial lung expanding compound, Britannia Pharmaceuticals) contains only DPPC and phosphatidylglycerol (PG) in a ratio of 7:3 (w/w). It is also a sterile, lyophilized powder which was initially used in its dry form (Morley et al., 1981; Wilkinson, Jenkins & Jeffrey, 1985) but is now reconstituted in 1.25 ml of cold, sterile saline with a concentration of 100 mg phospholipids/ml (Morley et al., 1988). ALEC is recommended to be given to all babies of less than 30 weeks' gestation who are at risk of RDS. The first dose is given as near the first breath as possible. It can be deposited into the pharynx before intubation with subsequent doses administered down an endotracheal tube if the baby remains intubated. Up to four doses are recommended.

(c) *Other synthetic surfactants* A surfactant composed of DPPC and high density lipoprotein in a w/w ratio of 10:1 was used in a prophylaxis trial of 100 babies in Belfast (Halliday et al., 1984) but is no longer in clinical practice.

Synthetic surfactants based upon DPPC and apoproteins produced by recombinant DNA technology have not been used in clinical trials and are still in the developmental stage.

Naturally sourced surfactants

These surfactants are derived from animal lungs or human amniotic fluid and contain varying amounts of apoproteins. Four bovine, two porcine and one human amniotic fluid surfactant have been studied clinically, although not all have been developed commercially. The animal lung surfactants are extracted with organic solvents (Folch, Lees & Sloane-Stanley, 1957) which remove water-soluble proteins such as SP-A and SP-D but allow hydrophobic proteins like SP-B and SP-C to remain. SP-B and SP-C are functionally important constituents of an effective exogenous surfactant facilitating surface adsorption and spreading of lipids (Whitsett et al., 1986).

Bovine surfactants

(a) *Surfactant TA* (Surfacten^R, Tokyo Tanabe) This is a saline extract of minced bovine lung isolated by differential centrifugation and flotation at a density of 1.2 g/ml. Cholesterol is removed by mixing with ethyl acetate followed by chloroform–methanol extraction. Synthetic DPPC, palmitic acid and tripalmitin (triacylglycerol) are then added so that the final product contains 84% phospholipids, 7% tripalmitin, 8% palmitic acid and about 1% hydrophobic proteins (SP-B, SP-C). The mixture is dissolved in chloroform and sterilized using a high pressure filter system. Surfactant TA is stored as a freeze-dried, white powder which is suspended in normal saline at a concentration of 30 mg/ml. It is administered intratracheally in a dose of 100 mg of phospholipids/kg (4 ml/kg) for prophylaxis or treatment of neonatal RDS. Repeated doses may be indicated.

(b) *Beractant* (Survanta[R], Abbott) This is a modification of Surfactant TA which is suspended in saline at a concentration of 25 mg/ml, autoclaved for sterilization and stored frozen. It is also given in a dose of 100 mg phospholipids/kg divided into four quarter doses administered with the infant in different positions. Repeat doses of 100 mg/kg may be given no sooner than 6 h after the preceding dose if the baby remains intubated and needs at least 30% inspired oxygen.

(c) *Calf lung surfactant extract* (CLSE, *Infasurf*[R], ONY) CLSE is an organic solvent extract of surfactant isolated from calf lung lavage by differential centrifugation. It contains 97% phospholipids, of which 63% is saturated phosphatidylcholine (PC) and 4% cholesterol and cholesterol esters, and 1% hydrophobic proteins (SP-B, SP-C). CLSE is suspended by vortexing in saline at a concentration of 30 mg/ml, sterilized by flash autoclaving and stored at 4 °C (Shapiro et al., 1985). Infasurf[R], which has a similar lipid and protein composition is suspended in 0.1 M saline and 0.5 mm calcium chloride at a concentration of 25 mg/ml (Enhorning et al., 1985).

This surfactant is given in a dose of 90–100 mg/kg for either prophylaxis or treatment of RDS and multiple doses are recommended for babies who relapse.

(d) *Bovactant* (Alveofact[R], SF-RI1, Boehringer-Ingelheim) This product is an organic solvent extract of a fraction isolated from cow lung lavage by differential centrifugation. It contains 88% phospholipids, 4% cholesterol, 8% other lipids and 1% hydrophobic proteins (SP-B, SP-C). Alveofact[R] is suspended in saline at a concentration of 45 mg/ml. It is recommended for use as prophylaxis in a dose of 50 mg phospholipids/kg (1.2 ml/kg) given within 1 h after birth. Depending on the need for ventilation, a further three doses may be given but the total dose should not exceed 200 mg/kg in the first 5 days of life.

Porcine surfactants

Only one porcine surfactant, Curosurf[R], has been commercially produced although an earlier preparation, Surfactant CK isolated from pig
lung lavage fluid by centrifugation, chloroform-methanol extraction, and
acetone precipitation was used to treat some babies in Japan in the early
1980s with promising results (Kobayashi et al., 1981; Nohara, Matsu-
mura & Oda, 1983).

Porcine lung surfactant extract (Curosurf[R], Chiesi Farmaceutici) is
prepared from minced pig lungs by a combination of washing, centrifugation, extraction with chloroform-methanol, and liquid-gel chromatography. The isolated polar lipid fraction is dissolved in chloroform and
sterilized by a high pressure filter system. Curosurf[R] contains 41–48%
saturated PC, 51–58% other phospholipids and about 1% hydrophobic
proteins (SP-B, SP-C) (Curstedt et al., 1988). It is suspended by gentle
sonication in normal saline at a concentration of 80 mg/ml.

Curosurf[R] is recommended to treat RDS and is used in an initial dose
of 200 mg phospholipids/kg (2.5 ml/kg) followed by up to two further
doses of 100 mg/kg if the baby remains ventilator-dependent and in
oxygen 12 and 24 h later (Speer et al., 1992).

Surfactant from human amniotic fluid

Human surfactant has been obtained from amniotic fluid collected at
elective Caesarean section carried out at term. This surfactant is isolated
by sucrose density gradient centrifugation and filtration (Hallman, Merritt & Schneider, 1983). It contains about 34% saturated PC, 51% other
phospholipids, 19% neutral lipids (mainly cholesterol & free fatty acids),
and 6% protein (including SP-A, SP-D and non-surfactant proteins). It is
lyophilized and suspended by vortexing in 0.6% saline at a phospholipid
concentration of 20 mg/ml.

Initial trials showed that this surfactant was effective when used for
prophylaxis and treatment in a dose of 60 mg/kg, with repeated doses for
babies who relapse (Hallman et al., 1985; Merritt et al., 1986). Recently,
however, because of the risks of viral contamination human surfactant
has been withdrawn from clinical trials.

Experimental evaluation of surfactants for clinical use

In vitro systems

In vitro properties of surfactant preparations are usually evaluated with
reference to surface adsorption, surface spreading and respreading, film

compressibility, and changes in surface tension during cyclic film compression (for review, see Keough, 1992). We believe a surfactant for clinical use should adsorb very rapidly from an aqueous hypophase to the air–liquid interface, generating a film with equilibrium surface tension about 25 mN/m. This rapid spreading is probably essential for the therapeutic effect since it allows the exogenous surfactant to reach its 'site of action' in the terminal airspaces with a minimum of delay, after instillation into the central airways. Other important properties of a surfactant film are low minimum surface tension (less than 10 mN/m) during cyclic compression in a Wilhelmy balance or pulsating-bubble system, and effective respreading after compression beyond film collapse (Notter, 1984). All these physical properties are temperature and concentration dependent, and maximum and minimum surface tension during cyclic film compression also depend on the cycling speed and the degree of area oscillation. Optimal values can therefore only be defined for standardized experimental conditions.

Although most of the surfactants currently used in clinical practice have probably been examined with respect to the in vitro surface properties outlined above, only part of that information is available in current literature. Surfactant TA and Curosurf[R] exhibit rapid spreading with an equilibrium surface tension of 24–27 mN/m when applied in droplet form on to the air–saline interface of a Wilhelmy balance, and minimum surface tension below 5 mN/m during 50% cyclic film compression (Fujiwara & Robertson, 1992). Films of Surfactant TA also have a very low compressibility (less than 0.02 m/mN) at surface tension 10 mN/m (Fujiwara, 1984), reflecting the high proportion of saturated fatty acid chains in the monolayer. Low surface compressibility is probably important for alveolar stability since low minimum surface tension can then be attained with only minimal dimensional changes (King & Clements, 1972). Films of human amniotic fluid surfactant have a higher mean compressibility (0.04 m/mN) and require, in a Wilhelmy balance system, 90% compression to reduce surface tension to 3 mN/m (Hallman et al., 1983). Films of CLSE require only 20% compression to reduce surface tension <5 mN/m and have a respreadability superior to that of DPPC plus unsaturated PG (7:3) (Egan et al., 1983). Minimum surface tension of films of Exosurf[R] is 0 mN/m during a first 90% compression cycle in the Wilhelmy balance, but >8 mN/m during subsequent cycles indicating incomplete replenishment (Tooley et al., 1987). This is similar to the value of 8.5 mN/m reported for films of DPPC and high density lipoprotein at 80% surface compression (Meban, 1981; Halliday et al., 1984). Films of DPPC plus unsaturated PG (7:3) spread from dry particles have a minimum surface tension <5 mN/m at 50% surface compression (Morley et al., 1981).

When examined with the pulsating bubble technique developed by Enhorning (1977), most modified natural surfactants have acceptable surface properties at hypophase concentration > 5 mg/ml, with rapid adsorption and low minimum surface tension. However, at lower hypophase concentrations some potentially important differences between various surfactants can be recognized. Surfactant TA, a preparation enriched with synthetic lipids including DPPC (see above), thus requires a hypophase concentration of only 1 mg/ml to generate a rapidly adsorbing film with minimum surface tension <5 mN/m (Sasaki, 1990). With Curosurf^R this 'critical concentration' is significantly higher (Robertson et al., 1990). In the original description of the product, Exosurf^R at a hypophase concentration of 10 mg/ml was reported to have a minimum surface tension close to zero during 40% surface compression (Tooley et al., 1987), but values for maximum and equilibrium surface tension (56 & 45 mN/m, respectively) were clearly higher than those obtained with natural surfactants. In a more recent study, Hall et al. (1992) found that Exosurf^R at 10 mg/ml had a minimum surface tension of 29 mN/m during 50% surface compression in a pulsating bubble system, whereas corresponding values for CLSE and Survanta^R at 2.5 mg/ml were < 1 and 2 mN/m, respectively.

Animal models for quality control of surfactant substitutes

Unfortunately, simple in vitro tests as described above do not predict the therapeutic effects of exogenous surfactants in animals (Nohara et al., 1986) or patients with surfactant dysfunction. For example, some protein-free synthetic surfactants with seemingly satisfactory surface properties in the pulsating bubble system are ineffective when instilled into the airways of a surfactant-depleted lung, probably because the artificial material becomes easily inactivated by leaking serum proteins (Holm et al., 1990). In general, the resistance to such inhibition depends on the presence of surfactant-specific protein, especially SP-A (Cockshutt, Weitz & Possmayer, 1990; Holm et al., 1990). Although for any particular exogenous surfactant this resistance can be estimated in vitro by measurements of dynamic surface tension (Cockshutt et al., 1990; Holm et al., 1990) or microbubble stability (Berggren et al.,

1992*a*) after exposure to inhibitory proteins under standardized conditions, final pre-clinical evaluation of the product requires animal experiments.

Surfactant-deficient immature newborn rabbits, delivered at a gestational age of 26–27 days, are commonly used for quality control of surfactant substitutes. These animals have a very small pool of endogenous surfactant (Kikkawa, Motoyama & Gluck, 1968), cannot establish functional residual capacity at birth (Lachmann et al., 1979; Robertson, 1992) and require artificial ventilation to survive. The exogenous surfactant to be tested is instilled into the airways via a tracheal cannula, and its effect evaluated from static pulmonary pressure–volume recordings and/ or dynamic physiological measurements under in vivo conditions (Robertson & Lachmann, 1988). Static lung volumes >40 ml/kg at 5 cm H_2O deflation pressure indicate a satisfactory therapeutic response. Such volumes are obtained with, for example, Surfactant TA (Maeta et al., 1983), human surfactant (Schneider et al., 1982), and Curosurf[R] (Fujiwara & Robertson, 1992), but not with synthetic surfactants such as DPPC plus unsaturated PG (Maeta et al., 1983) or Exosurf[R] (Tooley et al., 1987).

Since a disturbance of lung mechanics secondary to moderately delayed adsorption of surfactant may remain unrecognized under static conditions (Nitta et al., 1989), quality control of a surfactant substitute should include studies on ventilated surfactant-deficient animals. Convenient methods have recently been introduced by which multiple animals connected to the same respiratory system can be ventilated with standardized tidal volume by individual adjustment of insufflation pressure (Ikegami et al., 1987*a*; Sun et al., 1991). With this type of equipment, it can be shown that treatment of immature newborn rabbits (gestational age, 27 days) with an adequate surfactant substitute improves lung–thorax compliance and carbon dioxide tension in heart blood to nearly mature levels, reduces the bidirectional leakage of protein in the lungs (Robertson et al., 1985), and increases end-expiratory lung gas volume (Robertson, 1992). Lungs of surfactant-treated immature animals also have significantly improved alveolar volume density (Sun et al., 1991) and well-preserved airway mucosa in contrast to the widespread bronchiolar epithelial necrosis seen in non-treated littermate controls (Grossmann, Nilsson & Robertson, 1986). Treatment with ALEC improved lung–thorax compliance in immature newborn rabbits but did not prevent disruption of airway epithelium, probably because the lungs were not properly stabilized by the artificial surfactant (Morley et al., 1980). Similar observations have been reported after treatment of immature newborn rabbits with Exosurf^R (Berggren et al., 1992*b*) and DPPC plus high density lipoprotein (Halliday et al., 1987).

Pre-term lambs have been used by several workers for evaluation of various natural and synthetic exogenous surfactants. Significant and sustained improvements of oxygenation, carbon dioxide elimination, and lung compliance were observed after administration of comparatively low doses of CLSE (15–30 mg/kg) (Egan et al., 1983) and Alveofact^R (35 mg/kg) (Gortner et al., 1990*b*) to ventilated immature newborn lambs with a gestational age of 124–130 days (term, 145 days) whereas dry DPPC plus unsaturated PG (7:3) had no influence on gas exchange and lung compliance (Egan et al., 1983).

Ikegami et al. (1987*b*) compared the therapeutic effects of four different exogenous surfactants (Surfactant TA, human surfactant, natural rabbit surfactant, and natural sheep surfactant) in very immature lambs (gestational age 120–122 days). All animals received the same dose of surfactant (50 mg/kg), corresponding to the amount of natural surfactant that according to previous observations (Ikegami et al., 1980) was required for an optimal therapeutic effect, and were ventilated for 4 h. In this model, the response to Surfactant TA was inferior to that obtained with natural sheep or rabbit surfactant. Animals receiving human surfactant showed a satisfactory initial improvement of gas exchange, but the effect faded more rapidly than in the other treatment groups. The leak of serum albumin into the air-spaces was larger in animals receiving Surfactant TA than in animals receiving sheep or rabbit surfactant, but on the other hand Surfactant TA was less sensitive to inhibition by alveolar wash protein than the other surfactants. Surfactant TA and human surfactant were lost more quickly from the airspaces than natural sheep or rabbit surfactant. This may be one of several possible reasons why the very immature lambs responded most favourably to treatment with natural surfactant and only transiently to treatment with human surfactant.

In a more recent study, Cummings et al., (1992) compared efficacy of Exosurf^R, Infasurf^R, Survanta^R and natural sheep surfactant in immature lambs delivered at a mean gestational age of 126 days. The commercially available surfactants were administered at the dose recommended by the manufacturer, natural sheep surfactant at a dose of 100 mg/kg. Arterial oxygenation, survival and pulmonary pressure–volume characteristics were significantly improved after treatment with the natural, or modified natural surfactants, but a sustained therapeutic response was seen only in animals receiving Infasurf^R. Lambs treated with Exosurf^R did not differ from untreated controls. These data seem to contradict earlier observations in fetal lambs treated with Exosurf^R (67.5 mg/kg) at a gestational age of 131–133 days; these slightly more mature animals responded to treatment with Exosurf[R] with improved gas exchange and lung compliance, and the effects were reported to be similar to those obtained with natural surfactant (Durand et al., 1985). These seemingly conflicting data can be reconciled if the therapeutic effect of Exosurf[R] depends on some endogenous surfactant component which is absent in very immature lambs, or if Exosurf[R] becomes inactivated more easily than the other surfactants in the airways of very immature lambs. If so, these experimental observations suggest some serious limitations as to the use of Exosurf[R] in clinical practice. Indeed, babies who responded well to treatment with Exosurf[R] in clinical 'rescue' trials (Long et al., 1991a,b; Phibbs et al., 1991) were generally less ill than babies treated successfully with, for example, Curosurf[R] (Collaborative European Multicentre Study Group, 1988) or Surfactant TA (Fujiwara et al., 1990) in large multicentre studies (see below). Recently, Exosurf[R] has been shown to have no effect in reducing mortality of babies who weighed between 500 and 699 g at birth (Stevenson et al., 1992).

The only preparation so far evaluated systematically in a primate model of neonatal RDS is Surfactant TA (Vidyasagar et al., 1985). These studies have confirmed efficacy of surfactant replacement under experimental conditions very similar to a neonatal intensive care unit. Premature newborn baboons with a gestational age of 141 days (corresponding to 77% gestation) with clinical and radiological evidence of RDS were treated, at the age of 2 h, with Surfactant TA at a dose of 100 mg phospholipids/kg. Treated animals showed a significant improvement of gas exchange and lung compliance, sustained for the whole period of observation (14 h) and lung expansion in histological sections was much better than in non-treated controls. In another study using the same model, Maeta et al. (1988), compared the effect of Surfactant TA (100 mg/kg) given within 10 min of birth with that of treatment at the age of 2 h. As in immature newborn lambs (Jobe et al., 1981), the clinical response was superior in animals receiving early treatment, suggesting that prophylactic treatment of infants at risk might be better than therapy for established RDS. Conflicting results have been obtained in randomized clinical trials addressing this important issue (see below).

Results of clinical trials of surfactant treatment for RDS

The first published successful clinical trial of surfactant replacement in RDS was by Fujiwara et al. (1980). In the next 5 years there were a number of uncontrolled or small randomized controlled trials showing promising results with a variety of different surfactant preparations used both for prophylaxis (Morley et al., 1981; Kwong et al., 1985) and for treatment (Hallman et al., 1983; Smyth et al., 1983; Gitlin et al., 1987; Noack et al., 1987; Raju et al., 1987) of RDS.

These preliminary trials were followed by a series of larger, well controlled studies which examined prophylaxis with synthetic surfactant (Halliday et al., 1984; Ten Centre Study Group, 1987; Morley et al., 1988; Bose et al., 1990; Corbet et al., 1991; Phibbs et al., 1991), prophylaxis with natural surfactant (Enhorning et al., 1985; Merritt et al., 1986; Kendig et al., 1988; Gortner et al., 1990*a*; Soll et al., 1990; Ferrara et al., 1991; Hoekstra et al., 1991), treatment with synthetic surfactant (Long et al., 1991 *a,b*; Phibbs et al., 1991) and treatment with natural surfactant (Hallman et al., 1985; Collaborative European Multicenter Study Group, 1988; Horbar et al., 1989, 1990; Lang et al., 1990; Liechty et al., 1991). These trials have been subjected to overviews using meta-analysis (Soll, 1992*a,b,c,d,e*) (Table 12.2). Thirty-two randomized controlled trials enrolling 6240 babies have been used to develop these overviews. There is remarkable consistency throughout the trials demonstrating the effectiveness of both synthetic and natural surfactants in reducing neonatal mortality and pulmonary air leaks (pneumothorax and pulmonary interstitial emphysema). For neonatal mortality the odds ratios (OR) are about 0.55 for prophylaxis and about 0.60 for treatment of established RDS. This means that surfactant therapy reduces the odds of death by between 40 and 45%. The OR for pneumothorax are lower for natural surfactants (0.31–0.34) than for synthetic surfactants (0.52–0.64) but this should not be used to infer that natural surfactants are superior. There have been no fully reported clinical trials comparing synthetic and natural surfactants (see below).

The overviews (Table 12.2) also demonstrate that the incidence of patent ductus arteriosus (PDA) may be increased by prophylactic administration of surfactant (OR synthetic 1.27 and natural 1.16) but not by surfactant treatment of established RDS (OR 0.73 and 0.96, respectively). Surfactant replacement does not influence the incidence of intraventricular haemorrhage or bronchopulmonary dysplasia. A number of questions remaining to be resolved (Halliday, 1991) will be discussed below.

Synthetic or natural surfactant

No published studies have directly compared synthetic and natural surfactants although some are in progress or have recently been completed. As natural surfactants have clear acute effects in improving lung

Table 12.2. *Typical odds ratios (OR) and 95% confidence intervals (CI) for the effects of surfactant in prophylaxis and treatment trials*

	Synthetic surfactant				Natural surfactant			
	Number of trials	Number of babies	OR	95% CI	Number of trials	Number of babies	OR	95% CI
Prophylaxis								
Neonatal death	7	1475	0.56	0.43–0.74	7	930	0.55	0.38–0.80
Pneumothorax	5	1218	0.64	0.45–0.89	8	988	0.31	0.22–0.44
Intraventricular haemorrhage (IVH)	4	1146	0.94	0.73–1.20	8	965	0.95	0.73–1.24
Severe IVH (III/IV)	0	–	–	–	7	940	1.25	0.89–1.50
Patent ductus arteriosus	6	1526	1.27	1.03–1.57	8	988	1.16	0.67–1.15
Bronchopulmonary dysplasia (BPD)	5	1095	1.01	0.75–1.37	7	930	0.88	0.067–1.15
Death or BPD	3	971	0.77	0.58–1.02	7	930	0.64	0.49–0.84
Treatment								
Neonatal death	5	2126	0.61	0.47–0.81	9	1451	0.60	0.43–0.84
Pneumothorax	4	2102	0.52	0.42–0.65	12	1600	0.34	0.27–0.44
IVH	2	1656	0.77	0.62–0.97	10	1473	0.94	0.76–1.15
Severe IVH (III/IV)	0	–	–	–	10	1502	0.91	0.76–1.14
Patent ductus arteriosus	3	1760	0.73	0.60–0.88	12	1597	0.96	0.79–1.18
BPD	3	1680	0.68	0.46–0.99	10	1390	1.01	0.81–1.27
Death or BPD	3	1988	0.56	0.45–0.71	10	1443	0.66	0.53–0.82

From Soll (1992*a–d*) *Oxford Database of Perinatal Trials.*

Table 12.3. *Effect of prophylactic surfactant vs treatment with surfactant on mortality and complications (typical odds ratio and 95% CI)*

	Number of trials	Number of babies	OR	95% CI
Neonatal mortality	1	122	1.10	0.40–3.06
Pneumothorax	2	601	0.55	0.32–0.97
Intraventricular haemorrhage (IVH)	1	112	1.65	0.80–3.42
Severe IVH	1	112	2.90	0.88–9.50
Patent ductus arteriosus	1	112	1.62	0.79–3.33
Bronchopulmonary dysplasia (BPD)	3	804	1.19	0.87–1.63
Mortality prior to discharge	3	804	0.82	0.57–1.17
Death or BPD	3	804	1.08	0.81–1.43

From Soll (1992*f*) *Oxford Database of Perinatal Trials*.

function they might have a major role in therapy of RDS whereas synthetic surfactants with their more gradual effects might be more useful for prophylaxis. Economic aspects of surfactant replacement may also be important in determining which type of surfactant is used in different circumstances.

Prophylaxis or rescue treatment

Three completed trials have compared prophylactic and rescue treatment with natural surfactants (Dunn et al., 1991; Kendig et al., 1991; Merritt et al., 1991). Meta-analysis of these trials suggests a slight benefit of prophylactic administration in reducing the incidence of pneumothorax but there is no difference in neonatal mortality between prophylactic and late treatment groups (Soll, 1992*e*) (Table 12.3). Very recently three trials in progress with Curosurf[R] have reported interim analyses (Egberts et al., 1993). For neonatal mortality there appears to be a definite benefit from prophylactic therapy for babies of less than 31 weeks' gestation compared to rescue treatment (Table 12.4). The odds of neonatal death are reduced by almost 50% and when taken together with the first three comparative trials in Soll's overview give solid evidence supporting prophylaxis for the more immature babies.

A large multicentre trial of Exosurf[R] (the OSIRIS Collaborative Group, 1992) which has recruited more than 7000 babies demonstrated the benefits of early treatment in immature babies.

Table 12.4. *Effect of prophylaxis vs treatment with Curosurf^R of babies
<31 weeks' gestation on neonatal mortality (interim analyses)*

Study	Prophylaxis	Treatment	OR	95% CI
Italian (Bevilacqua et al.)	16/79	27/74	0.44	0.20–0.97
French (Walti et al.)	12/101	19/95	0.54	0.20–1.26
Dutch/Swedish (Egberts et al.)	10/75	15/72	0.58	0.22–1.52
	Typical odds ratio		0.51	0.31–0.82

From Egberts et al., 1993.

Single or multiple doses

Two studies have demonstrated that multiple doses are superior to single doses (Dunn, Shennan & Possmayer, 1990; Speer et al., 1992). Multiple dose treatment with Curosurf^R reduces both mortality and the incidence of pneumothorax (Speer et al., 1992). This study used retreatment criteria of continued need for mechanical ventilation and any oxygen supplementation 12 h and 24 h after the initial treatment dose. About two-thirds of babies needed retreatment (100 mg/kg) but it is possible that second and third doses of surfactant should be reserved for babies needing at least 30–40% oxygen after relapse. Multiple dose treatment is now recommended for Survanta^R, Exosurf^R, Pumactant^R, and Infasurf^R (Table 12.2). The Osiris study (the OSIRIS Collaborative Group, 1992) also compared two and four doses of Exosurf^R, and showed no benefits of the extra doses. A large multicentre trial which enrolled more than 2000 babies (Halliday et al., 1993) compared three doses of 100 mg/kg (maximum total dose 300 mg/kg) with up to five doses (maximum total dose 600 mg/kg) of Curosurf^R, and although there were short-term benefits from the higher dose there were no long-term advantages.

Dose and administration

The doses of surfactant used in clinical trials over the past 12 years have varied from 25 to 200 mg of phospholipids/kg body weight (Halliday, 1989; Morley, 1991; Fujiwara & Robertson, 1992). As mentioned above, these doses are all much larger by at least tenfold than the amount of lipids required to form a monolayer on the interior surface of the lungs

(Marks et al., 1983). For licensed surfactant preparations the doses vary from 50 to 200 mg/kg (dose volumes 1.2 to 5 ml/kg) (Table 12.1). In two recent trials, larger doses have been shown to be superior to smaller ones (Konishi et al., 1988; Gortner et al., 1990). Konishi et al. (1988) showed that treatment of RDS with 120 mg/kg (100 mg phospholipid/kg) of Surfactant TA improved oxygenation and reduced the incidence of BPD compared to 60 mg/kg. Gortner et al. (1990c) compared 100 mg/kg with 50 mg/kg of Alveofact^R and also showed improved oxygenation with the higher dose. For Curosurf^R, 200 mg/kg gives better early physiological changes compared to 100 mg/kg, but there is no difference in 28 day clinical outcome (Halliday et al., 1993; Herting et al., 1993). The dose of surfactant needed for optimal effects is not known but is probably at least 100 mg phospholipid/kg which is close to the 100–250 mg/kg estimated to form the total pulmonary surfactant pool in a full-term neonate (Jobe & Ikegami, 1987; Hallman, 1989).

In some clinical rescue trials, surfactant has been administered as a bolus into each main bronchus or as a single bolus into the lower trachea (Hallman et al., 1985; Collaborative European Multicentre Study Group, 1988). In other trials surfactant has been given as divided doses directed into each lung lobe by positioning the baby (Gitlin et al., 1987; Raju et al., 1987; Konishi et al., 1988; Horbar et al., 1989, 1990; Fujiwara et al., 1990; Liechty et al., 1991). After instillation the baby is either manually ventilated for a short time or reconnected to the ventilator to distribute the surfactant. A sterile feeding tube is often used to deliver the surfactant through the endotracheal tube. With Exosurf^R an endotracheal adaptor with a side-port is used to instil the surfactant very slowly over 5 to 30 min without disconnecting the baby from the ventilator (Phibbs et al., 1991; Long et al., 1991a). It is not clear whether slow instillation has any advantages over rapid bolus dosing, and no randomized trials have examined this issue. Studies comparing methods of administration are needed since acute responses and potentially adverse haemodynamic effects may vary with the duration of instillation.

Pumactant^R (Morley et al., 1981) and a bovine equivalent to Curosurf^R (Victorin et al., 1990) have been administered to babies breathing spontaneously. Pumactant^R (ALEC) was administered by pharyngeal deposition but it is not clear how well this synthetic surfactant performs when used in this way. Victorin et al. (1990) used the bovine preparation in a neonatal unit in Kuwait without facilities for assisted ventilation. Fourteen babies weighing more than 1500 g with moderately severe RDS were intubated only for the instillation of surfactant and then were extubated. Twelve babies showed the expected acute responses and 13 babies survived without sequelae. If surfactant administration could serve as an alternative to mechanical ventilation, or at least reduce the number of babies subsequently needing assisted ventilation this would be a major advance. This hypothesis is currently being tested in a large randomized multicentre trial (Verder et al., 1992).

Response patterns following surfactant treatment

The response pattern following treatment with Exosurf[R] is characterized by slow improvement in oxygenation and mean airway pressure which is different from that seen after treatment with the natural surfactants (Fig. 12.1). The difference in response between synthetic and natural surfactants is likely to be due to differences in the physico-chemical properties favouring the protein-containing preparations but may also be influenced by the slower infusion of Exosurf[R] compared to the more rapid instillation of the natural surfactants.

Not all babies respond optimally to surfactant treatment despite apparently adequate distribution within the lungs (Charon et al., 1989). Some reasons for treatment failure include alternative diagnoses such as congenital infection, persistent fetal circulation, pulmonary hypoplasia and perinatal asphyxia, and the presence of surfactant inhibitors in the airways. Multiple regression analysis has shown that in addition to asphyxia and severity of RDS the outcome after surfactant treatment also varies between neonatal intensive care units, perhaps reflecting variations in admission policies, transportation and other aspects of neonatal care (Collaborative European Multicenter Study Group, 1991).

Follow-up studies

There are now 18 studies that have examined long-term outcome of babies treated with surfactant (Table 12.5); ten with natural surfactants (Dunn et al., 1988; Vaucher et al., 1988; Jain, Vidyasagar & Raju, 1989; Msall et al., 1989; Ferrara et al., 1991; Merritt et al., 1991; Ware et al., 1990; Robertson et al., 1992) and eight with synthetic surfactants (Wilkinson et al., 1985; Halliday, McClure & Reid, 1986; Morley & Morley, 1990; Long, 1991; Corbet, 1992). Some authors have reported more than one study, for example, prophylaxis and treatment in a single paper (Wilkinson et al., 1985; Vaucher et al., 1988; Merritt et al., 1991; Long, 1991). About 6 000 babies have been included in these follow-up studies, the majority in synthetic surfactant trials. They show no significant influence on the odds of disability except perhaps for synthetic rescue

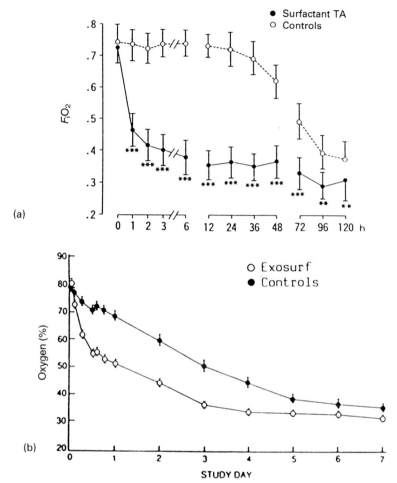

Fig. 12.1. Response patterns, shown as inspired oxygen fraction (F_iO_2) or concentration (%) in babies treated with a natural or a synthetic surfactant compared to controls. (*a*) The response of babies treated with Surfactant TA (100 mg/kg). Data are mean values and 95% confidence intervals. *** $P < 0.001$, ** $P < 0.01$ compared with controls (from Fujiwara et al., 1990 with permission). (*b*) Response of babies treated with Exosurf (67.5 mg/kg). A second dose of Exosurf was given at 12 h to babies who remained on the ventilator. Data are mean and SEM. The differences between the groups are significant ($P < 0.001$) during the first week of life (from Long et al., 1991*a* with permission).

trials where a reduction in disability has been found (Table 12.5). In general between 70% and 90% of surviving babies who had been treated with surfactant at or soon after birth show normal development at age 1–2 years (Halliday, 1991, 1992). Disability or handicap rates are generally lower for babies in prophylactic trials compared to rescue trials as up to

Table 12.5. *Effect of surfactant on the odds of disability in survivors to age at least one year*

	Number of studies	Number of babies	OR	95% CI
Synthetic prophy-laxis	4	2453	0.88	0.68–1.15
Natural prophylaxis	5	164	1.22	0.61–2.47
Synthetic rescue	4	3057	0.83	0.71–0.97
Natural rescue	5	194	0.78	0.38–1.60
All prophylaxis	9	2617	0.91	0.71–1.16
All rescue	9	3251	0.82	0.71–0.96

Table 12.6. *Outcome at 1 year of babies treated with human surfactant: prophylaxis versus rescue*

	Prophylaxis ($N = 33$)	Rescue ($N = 35$)
Major handicap	9 (27%)	3 (9%)
Minor handicap	3 (9%)	1 (3%)
Normal outcome	21 (64%)	32 (88%)[*]
Bayley MDI	73	98[**]
Bayley PDI	67	91[**]

[*] $P < 0.02$. [**] $P < 0.005$.
From Vaucher et al. (1990).

half of the treated babies would not develop RDS and thus would be expected to have an improved outcome compared to babies treated after developing RDS.

One study has compared outcome of babies from a randomized controlled trial of rescue versus prophylactic treatment with human surfactant (Vaucher, Merritt & Hallman, 1990). This small study of 68 babies suggests that the outcome is better for babies treated by rescue rather than prophylactic therapy (Table 12.6). In one follow-up study with Curosurf[R] the risk of retinopathy of prematurity was not increased in surviving treated babies (Tubman et al., 1992).

Other potential targets for surfactant therapy

Recently seven full-term babies with congenital pneumonia and seven with meconium aspiration syndrome have been treated with CLSE (Auten et al., 1991). These results, taken together with in vivo and in vitro studies suggesting that surfactant inhibition occurs in meconium aspiration (Moses et al., 1990; Sun et al., 1993*a*), and that this inhibition can, at least in part, be overcome in newborn experimental animals by treatment with a large dose of exogenous surfactant (Sun et al., 1993*b*) are promising. Multicentre controlled trials of surfactant replacement therapy for meconium aspiration syndrome are beginning in the USA.

Secondary surfactant deficiency has also been implicated in the adult respiratory distress syndrome (ARDS) and some recent reports suggest that natural surfactant replacement may improve the outcome (Lachmann, 1989; Richman et al., 1989; Nosaka et al., 1990). Multicentre randomized controlled clinical trials of surfactants in ARDS are being coordinated in the USA, but results have not yet been published.

Deficiency of pulmonary surfactant has been found in babies dying of sudden infant death syndrome (James, Berry & Fleming, 1990) but it is unclear whether such deficiency is primary or secondary and whether surfactant replacement could have a role in prevention of this disorder.

Other potential targets for surfactant therapy include persistent fetal circulation, congenital diaphragmatic hernia, bronchopulmonary dysplasia and pulmonary hypoplasia as each of these disorders may have surfactant dysfunction, but clinical trials are limited to anecdotal case reports (Bos et al., 1991; Glick et al., 1992).

Problems

Adverse effects of surfactant have been reported relatively infrequently.

Haemodynamic effects

The overviews suggest an increase in the incidence of PDA which is more apparent following use of prophylactic synthetic surfactants (Table 12.2). It has been suggested that PDA causes most of the relapses that occur after surfactant administration (Fujiwara et al., 1987). However, PDA is usually easy to detect using Doppler ultrasound, and intravenous indomethacin is an effective treatment (Halliday, 1988). Sometimes babies with a large left to right shunt develop a low diastolic blood pressure and there has been an association with pulmonary haemorrhage particularly in those babies of less than 27 weeks' gestation treated with Exosurf[R] (Long et al., 1991a; van Houten et al., 1992; Stevenson et al., 1992). Careful management of PDA in these very immature babies should reduce the risk of pulmonary haemorrhage.

PDA has also been suggested as a cause of haemodynamic instability found occasionally after treatment with natural surfactants. These haemodynamic effects are variable, with some studies showing no change in blood pressure and cerebral blood flow velocities (McCord et al., 1989; Jorch et al., 1989), and some showing reductions (van Bel et al., 1992; Cowan et al., 1991). With Exosurf[R] cerebral blood flow velocities tend to increase (van de Bor, Ma & Walther, 1991). Near infrared spectroscopy (Edwards et al., 1992; Skov, Bell & Greisen, 1992a; Skov et al., 1992a,b) and stable isotope studies (Skov et al., 1992a) demonstrate no significant alteration in cerebral blood flow after surfactant administration but an overall increase in cerebral oxygenation. This makes the finding of transient depression of cerebral activity in the EEG (Hellstrom-Westas et al., 1992) difficult to explain. Similar depression of the EEG occurs after suctioning of the airways in babies on ventilators (Skov et al., 1992c), and there is no evidence of long-term harmful effects. One study has looked specifically for evidence of cerebral ischaemia after surfactant treatment (Amato et al., 1991). There were no changes in creatine kinase isoenzyme (CK-BB) levels nor did antibodies to brain antigens develop. This is in keeping with the normal long-term development in surviving babies which has been reported in a number of studies (Halliday, 1992).

Immunological and toxicological problems

Surfactant apoproteins (SP-A, SP-B & SP-C) are potentially immunogenic (Strayer et al., 1989). A transient increase in circulating anti-surfactant antibodies and surfactant-anti-surfactant immune complexes has been found in babies with RDS irrespective of whether they were treated with human surfactant or not (Strayer et al., 1986). These circulating antibodies, detected by a sensitive ELISA technique probably represent an auto-immune response to endogenous surfactant proteins that have leaked into the circulation in both surfactant-treated and non-treated babies with RDS. Harmful effects have not been reported (Strayer & Robertson, 1992). Others, using Western blot analysis, failed to detect circulating antibodies in babies treated with a bovine surfactant (Whitsett, Hull & Luse, 1991). Using a similar modified bovine surfactant, Chida et al. (1991) showed that SP-A did leak into the circulation but that this leak and subsequent antibody formation was reduced by surfactant treatment. This latter observation is in agreement with data from animal experiments showing reduced leakage of albumin in preterm lungs treated with surfactant (Jobe et al., 1983; Robertson et al., 1985). We speculate that endogenous SP-A could serve as a marker of lung permeability and the determination of serum levels of this protein might be used for early diagnosis of lung protein leakage in ARDS and other forms of pulmonary disease.

Conclusions and perspectives for the future

Synthetic, natural and modified natural surfactant preparations reduce neonatal mortality and pulmonary air leaks in preterm babies with RDS or at risk of developing it. In the USA there is now evidence of a significant decline in neonatal mortality on a national basis as a result of the widespread introduction of surfactant therapy. Recently, it has been shown that exogenous surfactant may be effective also in respiratory failure caused by inactivation of surfactant by leaking serum proteins or meconium aspiration. Large doses of surfactant may be required to overcome the inhibitory effects in some of these clinical situations, and the exogenous material should first of all be designed to resist inhibition. There is also anecdotal evidence that exogenous surfactant may have a beneficial effect in neonatal pneumonia. If so, the exogenous surfactant should be tailored to assist, as much as possible, the antimicrobial defence system of the lung. As mentioned above, this may require the presence of SP-A. Various potential new targets for replacement therapy may thus call for a spectrum of exogenous surfactants, adapted to combat different pathophysiological processes operating in the lungs. Surfactant treatment also improves lung function in congenital diaphragmatic hernia and accelerates lung recovery in infants treated with extracorporeal membrane oxygenation (ECMO) (Lotze et al., 1993). Currently, randomized trials in the USA and elsewhere are evaluating surfactant therapy in term infants with severe respiratory failure regardless of aetiology.

Trials of Exosurf[R] and Survanta[R] in ARDS are being undertaken but because of the heterogeneous nature of ARDS it is expected that the outcomes will be less consistent than those of babies with RDS.

It is not clear if nebulization or instillation of surfactant is the better method of administration and further trials are needed. In ARDS large quantities of surfactant will be needed and the cost of treatment may be prohibitive unless prices are reduced on a weight for weight basis by the pharmaceutical companies.

'Third generation', genetically engineered surfactants are undergoing evaluation in animal models. These are composed of synthetic surfactant lipids, reconstitued with recombinant proteins or peptides. These artificial surfactants do not completely match the in vivo physiological properties of natural surfactants but do have clear beneficial effects in animals with surfactant deficiency. SP-B and possibly SP-C may be critical for optimal biophysical function of surfactant. Antibodies against SP-B destroy surfactant function (Kobayashi et al., 1991) but less is known about the specific roles of SP-C. SP-B and SP-C, and SP-C alone with added phospholipids mimic the biological effects of natural surfactant, whereas SP-A alone is less effective in this respect. It has also been reported that partial sequence peptides of SP-B (Waring et al., 1989) or other peptides that mimic SP-B function (Cochrane & Revak, 1991) may serve as critical components of an artificial surfactant. SP-C added to phospholipids does not reduce surface tension as well as SP-B, and SP-C combined with SP-A does not organize phospholipids into tubular myelin (Williams, Hawgood & Hamilton, 1991). Thus, recombinant protein expression of SP-B together with phospholipids appears the likely goal of drug development as third generation surfactants (Yao et al., 1990). Clinical trials comparing these third generation surfactants with the currently used preparations in the treatment of neonatal and adult respiratory failure will soon be undertaken.

Acknowledgements

This work was supported by The Swedish Medical Research Council (Project No. 3351), Oscar II Jubileumsfond, The General Maternity Hospital Foundation, Axel Tielman's Minnesfond, and the Northern Ireland Mother and Baby Appeal.

References

Amato, M., Hüppi, P., Markus, D. & Herschowitz, N. (1991). Neurological function of immature babies after surfactant replacement therapy. *Neuropediatrics*, **22**, 43–33.

Auten, R. L., Notter, R. H., Kendig, J. W., Davis, J. M. & Shapiro, D. L. (1991). Surfactant treatment of full-term newborns with respiratory failure. *Pediatrics*, **87**, 101–7.

Berggren, P., Eklind, J., Linderholm, B. & Robertson, B. (1992*a*). Bubbles and computer-aided image analysis for evaluation of surfactant inhibition. *Biology of the Neonate*, **61** (Suppl 1), 15–20.

Berggren, P., Corcoran, D., Curstedt, T. & Robertson, B. (1992*b*). Exosurf versus Curosurf: comparison of surface properties, resistance to inhibition, and physiological effects in preterm rabbits. European Society for Pediatric Research Annual Meeting, Uppsala.

Bevilacqua, G., Halliday, H. L., Parmigiani, S., Robertson, B. on behalf of the Collaborative European Multicentre Study Group (1992). Randomized multicentre trial of treatment with porcine natural surfactant for moderately severe neonatal respiratory distress syndrome. *Journal of Perinatal Medicine* (in press).

Bos, A. P., Tibboel, D., Hazelrock, F. W., Malenaar, J. C.,Lachmann, B. & Gommes, D. (1991). Surfactant replacement therapy in high-risk congenital diaphragmatic hernia. *Lancet*, **338**, 1279.

Bose, C., Corbet, A., Bose, G., Garcia-Prats, J., Lombardy, L., Wold, D., Donlon, D. & Long, W. (1990). Improved outcome at 28 days of age for very low birth weight infants treated with a single dose of synthetic surfactant. *Journal of Pediatrics*, **117**, 947–53.

Charon, A., Taeusch, H. W., Fitzgibbon, C., Smith, G. B., Treves, S. T. & Phelps, D. S. (1989). Factors associated with surfactant treatment response in infants with severe respiratory distress syndrome. *Pediatrics*, **83**, 348–54.

Chida, S., Phelps, D. S., Soll, R. F. & Taeusch, H. W. (1991). Surfactant proteins and anti-surfactant antibodies in sera from infants with respiratory distress syndrome with and without surfactant treatment. *Pediatrics,* **88**, 84–9.

Chu, J., Clements, J. A., Cotton, E. K., Klaus, M. H., Sweet, A. Y. & Tooley, W. H. (1967). Neonatal pulmonary ischemia. Part I: Clinical and physiologic studies. *Pediatrics*, **40**, 709–82.

Cochrane, C. G. & Revak, S. D. (1991). Pulmonary surfactant protein B (SP-B): structure–function relationship. *Science*, **254**, 566–8.

Cockshutt, A., Weitz, J. & Possmayer, F. (1990). Pulmonary surfactant-associated protein A enhances the surface activity of lipid extract surfactant and reverses inhibition by blood proteins in vitro. *Biochemistry*, **29**, 8424–9.

Collaborative European Multicenter Study Group (1988). Surfactant replacement therapy for severe respiratory distress syndrome: an international randomized clinical trial. *Pediatrics*, **82**, 683–91.

Collaborative European Multicentre Study Group (1991). Factors influencing the clinical response to surfactant replacement therapy in babies with severe respiratory distress syndrome. *European Journal of Pediatrics*, **150**, 433–9.

Corbet, A. J. (1992). Double-blind, one-year follow-up in 2134 infants randomized to synthetic surfactant or air. Satellite Symposium European Congress of Perinatal Medicine, Amsterdam, Surfactant in Practice – Long-term Issues and Consequences, pp. 10–11.

Corbet, A., Bucciarelli, R., Goldman, S., Mammel, M., Wold, D., Long, W. & the American Exosurf Pediatric Study Group (1991). Decreased mortality rate among small premature infants treated at birth with a single dose of synthetic surfactant: a multicenter controlled trial. *Journal of Pediatrics*, **118**, 277–84.

Cowan, F., Whitelaw, A., Wertheim, D. & Silverman, M. (1991). Cerebral blood flow velocity changes after rapid administration of surfactant. *Archives of Disease in Childhood*, **66**, 1105–9.

Cummings, J. J., Holm, B. A., Hudak, M. L., Hudak, B. B., Ferguson, W. H. & Egan, E. A. (1992). A controlled clinical comparison of four different surfactant preparations in surfactant-deficient preterm lambs. *American Review of Respiratory Disease*, **145**, 999–1004.

Curstedt, T., Jörnvall, H., Berggren, P. & Robertson, B. (1988). Artificial surfactants based on different hydrophobic low-molecular-weight proteins. In *Surfactant Replacement Therapy in Neonatal and Adult Respiratory Distress Syndrome*, ed. B. Lachmann. pp. 332–7. Springer, Berlin.

Dechant, K. L. & Faulds, D. (1991). Colfosceril palmitate. A review of the therapeutic efficacy and clinical tolerability of a synthetic surfactant preparation (Exosurf[R] Neonatal [TM]) in neonatal respiratory distress syndrome. *Drugs*, **82**, 877–94.

Dunn, M. S., Shennan, A. T., Hoskins, E. M., Lennox, K. & Enhorning, G. (1988). Two year follow-up of infants enrolled in a randomized trial of surfactant therapy for prevention of neonatal respiratory distress syndrome. *Pediatrics*, **82**, 543–7.

Dunn, M. S., Shennan, A. T. & Possmayer, F. (1990). Single versus multiple-dose surfactant replacement therapy in neonates of 30 to 36 weeks' gestation with respiratory distress syndrome. *Pediatrics*, **86**, 567–71.

Dunn, M. S., Shennan, A. T., Zayack, D. & Possmayer, F. (1991). Bovine surfactant replacement therapy in neonates of less than 30 weeks' gestation: a randomized controlled trial of prophylaxis vs treatment. *Pediatrics*, **87**, 377–86.

Durand, D. J., Clyman, R. I., Heymann, M. A., Clements, J. A., Mauray, F., Kitterman, J. & Ballard, P. (1985). Effects of a protein-free, synthetic surfactant on survival and pulmonary function in preterm lambs. *Journal of Pediatrics*, **107**, 775–80.

Edwards, A. D., McCormick, D. C., Roth, S. C. et al. (1992). Cerebral haemodynamic effects of treatment with modified natural surfactant investigated by near infrared spectroscopy. *Pediatric Research*, **32**, 532–6.

Egan, E. A. (1989). Surfactant and fetal lung liquid absorption at birth. In *Surfactant Replacement Therapy*. ed. D. L. Shapiro & R. H. Notter. pp. 91–8. Alan R Liss, New York.

Egan, E., Notter, R. H., Kwong, M. S. & Shapiro, D. L. (1983). Natural and artificial lung surfactant replacement therapy in premature lambs. *Journal of Applied Physiology*, **55**, 875–83.

Egberts, J., Walte, H., Berilacqua, G. & the Dutch, Swedish and Italian Multicenter Collaborators (1993). Meta analysis of three 'prophylaxis versus rescue' trials with Curosurf. In Proceedings of the 8th International Workshop on Surfactant Replacement, ed. O. D. Sangstad, Oslo, p. 19.

Eijking, E. P., van Daal, G. J., Tenbrinck, R., Luijendijk, A., Slviters, J. F., Hannappel, E. & Lachmann, B. (1991). Effect of surfactant replacement on pneumocystis carinii pneumonia in rats. *Intensive Care Medicine*, **17**, 475–8.

Enhorning, G. (1977). Pulsating bubble technique for evaluating pulmonary surfactant. *Journal of Applied Physiology*, **43**, 198–203.

Enhorning, G. & Robertson, B. (1972). Lung expansion in the premature rabbit fetus after tracheal deposition of surfactant. *Pediatrics*, **56**, 58–66.

Enhorning, G., Shennan, A. T., Possmayer, F., Dunn, M. S., Chen, C. P. & Milligan, J. (1985). Prevention of neonatal respiratory distress syndrome by tracheal instillation of surfactant: a randomized clinical trial. *Pediatrics*, **76**, 145–53.

Faix, R. G., Viscardi, R. M., Di Pietro, M. A. & Nicks, J. J. (1989). Adult respiratory distress syndrome in full-term newborns. *Pediatrics*, **83**, 971–6.

Ferrara, T. B., Hoekstra, R. E., Couser, R. J., Jackson, J. C., Anderson, C. L., Myers, T. F. & Raye, J. R. (1991). Effects of surfactant therapy on outcome of infants with birth weights of 600 grams to 750 grams. *Journal of Pediatrics*, **119**, 455–7.

Folch, J., Lees, M. B. & Sloane-Stanley, G. H. (1957). A simple method for the isolation and purification of total lipids from animal tissue. *Journal of Biology and Chemistry*, **226**, 497–509.

Fujiwara, T. (1984). Surfactant replacement in neonatal RDS. In *Pulmonary Surfactant*. ed. B. Robertson, L. M. G. van Golde & J. J. Batenburg. pp 479–503. Elsevier, Amsterdam.

Fujiwara, T., Konishi, M., Chida, S. & Maeta, H. (1987). Factors affecting response to a single postnatal dose of exogenous surfactant. Surfactant treatment of lung disease: *Report of the 96th Ross Conference on Pediatric Research*, pp. 128–39. Ross Laboratories, Columbus, Ohio.

Fujiwara, T., Konishi, M., Chida, S. et al. (1990). Surfactant replacement therapy with a single post-ventilatory dose of a reconstituted bovine surfactant in preterm neonates with respiratory distress syndrome: final analysis of a multicentre, double-blind, randomized trial and comparison with similar trials. *Pediatrics*, **86**, 753–64.

Fujiwara, T., Maeta, H., Chida, S., Morita, T., Watabe, Y. & Abe, T. (1980). Artificial surfactant therapy in hyaline-membrane disease. *Lancet*, **i**, 55–9.

Fujiwara, T. & Robertson, B. (1992). Pharmacology of exogenous surfactant. In *Pulmonary Surfactant: From Molecular Biology to Clinical Practice*, ed. B. Robertson, L. M. G. van Golde & J. J. Batenburg. pp. 561–92. Elsevier, Amsterdam.

Gitlin, J. D., Soll, R. F., Parad, R. B., Horbar, J. D., Feldman, H. A., Lucey, J. F. & Taeusch, H. W. (1987). Randomized controlled trial of exogenous surfactant for the treatment of hyaline membrane disease. *Pediatrics*, **79**, 31–7.

Glick, P. L., Lerch, C. L., Besner, G. E., et al. (1992). Pathophysiology of congenital diaphragmatic hernia III. Exogenous surfactant therapy for the high-risk neonate with congenital diaphragmatic hernia. *Journal of Pediatric Surgery*, **27**, 866–9.

Gortner, L., Bernsau, U., Hellwege, H. H., Hieronimi, G., Jorch, G. & Reiter, H. L. (1990a). A multicenter randomized controlled clinical trial of bovine surfactant for prevention of respiratory distress syndrome. *Lung*, **168** (Suppl.), 864–9.

Gortner, L., Pohlandt, F. & Weller, E. (1990b). Effects of bovine surfactant in premature lambs after intratracheal application. *European Journal of Pediatrics*, **149**, 280–3.

Gortner, L., Bernsau, U., Hellwege, H. H. et al. (1990c). Surfactant treatment in very premature infants: a multicenter controlled sequential clinical trial of high-dose versus standard-dose of bovine surfactant. In *Hot Topics '90 in Neonatology*, ed. J. F. Lucey. pp. 266–73. Ross Laboratories, Columbus, Ohio.

Grossmann, G., Nilsson, R. & Robertson, B. (1986) Scanning electron microscopy of epithelial lesions induced by artificial ventilation of the immature neonatal lung; the prophylactic effect of surfactant replacement. *European Journal of Pediatrics*, **145**, 361–7.

Gruenwald, P. (1947). Surface tension as a factor in the resistance of neonatal lungs to aeration. *American Journal of Obstetrics and Gynecology*, **53**, 996–1007.

Guyton, A. C., Moffatt, D. S. & Adair, T. H. (1984). Role of alveolar surface tension in transepithelial movement of fluid. In *Pulmonary Surfactant*. ed. B. Robertson, L. M. G. Van Golde & J. J. Batenburg, pp. 171–85. Elsevier, Amsterdam.

Hall, S. B., Venkitaraman, A. R., Whitsett, J. A., Holm, B. A. & Notter, R. H. (1992). Importance of hydrophobic apoproteins as constituents of clinical exogenous surfactants. *American Review of Respiratory Disease*, **145**, 24–30.

Halliday, H. L. (1988). Neonatal patent ductus arteriosus. *Pediatric Review and Communications*, **3**, 1–17.

Halliday, H. L. (1989). Clinical experience with exogenous natural surfactant. *Developmental Pharmacology and Therapeutics*, **13**, 173–81.

Halliday, H. L. (1991). Surfactant replacement. In *Year Book of Neonatal and Perinatal Medicine 1990*, ed. M. H. Klaus & A. A. Fanaroff. pp. XIII-XXI. Year Book Medical Publishers, New York.

Halliday, H. L. (1992). Follow-up data from babies treated with surfactant. In *Surfactant in Clinical Practice*, ed. G. Bevilacqua, S. Parmigiani, S. & B. Robertson. pp. 149–56, Harwood, Chur.

Halliday, H. L., Tarnow-Modi, W. O., Corcoran, J. D. & Patterson, C. C., on behalf of the European Collaborative Multicenter Study Group (1993). Multicenter randomized trial comparing high and low dose surfactant regimes for the treatment of respiratory distress syndrome (the Curosurf 4 trial). *Archives of Disease in Childhood*, **69**, 276–80.

Halliday, H. L., McClure, G. & McReid, M. (1986). Growth and development two years after artificial surfactant replacement at birth. *Early Human Development*, **13**, 323–7.

Halliday, H. L., McClure, G., McReid, M., Lappin, T. R. J., Meban, C. & Thomas, P. S. (1984). Controlled trial of artificial surfactant to prevent respiratory distress syndrome. *Lancet*, **i**, 476–8.

Halliday, H. L., Robertson, B., Nilsson, R., Rigaut, J-P. & Grossman, G. (1987). Automated image analysis of alveolar expansion patterns in immature newborn rabbits treated with natural or artificial surfactant. *British Journal of Experimental Pathology*, **68**, 727–32.

Hallman, M., Merritt, T. A., Jarvenpaa, A. L. et al. (1985). Exogenous human surfactant for treatment of severe respiratory distress syndrome: a randomized prospective clinical trial. *Journal of Pediatrics*, **106**, 963–9.

Hallman, M., Merritt, T. A., Schneider, H. (1983). Isolation of human surfactant from amniotic fluid and a pilot study of its efficacy in respiratory distress syndrome. *Pediatrics*, **71**, 473–82.

Hallman, M., Merritt, T. A., Pohjavuoari, M. & Gluck, L. (1986). Effect of surfactant substitution on lung effluent phospholipids in respiratory distress syndrome: evaluation of surfactant phospholipid turnover, pool size, and the relationship to severity of respiratory failure. *Pediatric Research*, **20**, 1228–35.

Hallman, M. (1989). Recycling of surfactant: a review of human amniotic fluid as a source of surfactant for treatment of respiratory distress syndrome. *Reviews in Perinatal Medicine*, **6**, 197–226.

Hellstrom-Westas, L., Bell, A. H., Skov, L., Greisen, G. & Svenning-sen, N. W. (1992). Cerebro-electrical depression following surfactant treatment in preterm neonates. *Pediatrics*, **89**, 643–7.

Herting, E., Tubman, R., Halliday, H. L. et al. (1993) Einfluß von 2 unterschiedlichen Dosierungen eines porcinen Surfactants auf den pulmonalen Gasaustausch Frühgeborener mit schwerem Atemnotsyndrom. *Monatsschr Kinderheilkd.*, **141**, 721–7.

Hoekstra, R. E., Jackson, J. C., Myers, T. F. et al. (1991). Improved neonatal survival following multiple doses of bovine surfactant in very premature neonates at risk for respiratory distress syndrome. *Pediatrics*, **88**, 10–18.

Holm, B. A. (1992) Surfactant inactivation in adult respiratory distress syndrome. In *Pulmonary surfactant, from Molecular Biology to Clinical Practice*, ed. B. Robertson, L. M. G. van Golde & J. J. Batenburg. pp. 665–84. Elsevier, Amsterdam.

Holm, B. A., Venkitaraman, A. R., Enhorning, G. & Notter, R. H. (1990). Biophysical inhibition of synthetic lung surfactant. *Chemistry and Physics of Lipids*, **52**, 243–50.

Horbar, J. D., Soll, R. F., Sutherland, J. M. et al. (1989). A multicenter randomized, placebo-controlled trial of surfactant therapy for respiratory distress syndrome. *New England Journal of Medicine*, **320**, 956–9.

Horbar, J. D., Soll, R. F., Schachinger, H. et al. (1990). A European multicenter randomized trial of single dose surfactant therapy for idiopathic respiratory distress syndrome. *European Journal of Pediatrics*, **149**, 416–23.

Ikegami, M., Berry, D., Elkady, T., Pettenazzo, A., Seidner, S. & Jobe, A. (1987a). Corticosteroids and surfactant change lung function and protein leaks in the lung of ventilated premature infants. *Journal of Clinical Investigation*, **79**, 1371–8.

Ikegami, M., Agata, Y., Elkady, T., Hallman, M., Berry, D. & Jobe, A. (1987b). Comparison of four surfactants: in vitro surface properties and responses of preterm lambs to treatment at birth. *Pediatrics*, **79**, 38–46.

Ikegami, M., Adams, F. H., Towers, B. & Osher, A. B. (1980). The quantity of natural surfactant necessary to prevent the respiratory distress syndrome in premature lambs. *Pediatric Research*, **14**, 1082–5.

Jain, L., Vidyasagar, D. & Raju, T. N. K. (1989). Developmental outcome of infants from surfactant trials. *Pediatric Research*, **25**, A1512 (abstract).

James, D., Berry, P. J. & Fleming, P. (1990). Surfactant abnormality and the sudden infant death syndrome: a primary or secondary phenomenon? *Archives of Disease in Childhood*, **65**, 774–8.

Jobe, A., Ikegami, M., Glatz, T., Yoshida, Y., Diakomanolis, E. & Padbury, J. (1981). Duration and characteristics of treatment of premature lambs with natural surfactant. *Journal of Clinical Investigation*, **67**, 370–5.

Jobe, A. & Ikegami, M. (1987). Surfactant for treatment of respiratory distress syndrome. *American Reviews of Respiratory Disease*, **136**, 1256–75.

Jobe, A., Ikegami, M., Jacobs, H. et al. (1983). Permeability of premature lamb lungs to protein and the effect of surfactant on that permeability. *Journal of Applied Physiology*, **55**, 169–76.

Jorch, G., Rabe, H., Garbe, M., Michel, E. & Gortner, L. (1989). Acute and protracted effects of intratracheal surfactant application on internal carotid blood flow velocity, blood pressure and carbon dioxide tension in very low birth weight infants. *European Journal of Pediatrics*, **148**, 770–3.

Kendig, J. W., Notter, R. H., Cox, C. et al. (1988). Surfactant replacement therapy at birth: final analysis of a clinical trial and comparison with similar trials. *Pediatrics*, **82**, 756–62.

Kendig, J. W., Notter, R. H., Cox, C. et al. (1991). A comparison of surfactant as immediate prophylaxis and as rescue therapy in newborns of less than 30 weeks' gestation. *New England Journal of Medicine*, **324**, 865–71.

Keough, K. M. W. (1992). Physical chemistry of pulmonary surfactant in the terminal airspaces. In *Pulmonary Surfactant: From Molecular Biology to Clinical Practice*, ed. B. Robertson, L. M. G. van Golde & J. J. Batenburg. pp. 109–164. Elsevier, Amsterdam.

Kikkawa, Y., Motoyama, E. K. & Gluck, L. (1968). Study of the lungs of fetal and newborn rabbits: morphologic, biochemical, and surface physical development. *American Journal of Pathology*, **52**, 177–92.

King, R. J. & Clements, J. A. (1972). Surface active material from dog lung. II. Composition and physiological correlations. *American Journal of Physiology*, **223**, 715–26.

Kobayashi, T., Kataoka, H., Murakami, S. & Haruki, S. (1981). A case of idiopathic respiratory distress syndrome treated with newly developed surfactant (Surfactant CK). *Journal of Japanese Medical Society of Biology Interface*, **12**, 1–6.

Kobayashi, T., Nitta, K., Takahashi, R. et al. (1991). Activity of pulmonary surfactant after blocking the associated proteins SP-A and SP-B. *Journal of Applied Physiology*, **71**, 530–6.

Kobayashi, T., Shido, A., Nitta, K., Inui, S., Ganzuka, M. & Robertson, B. (1990). The critical concentration of surfactant in fetal lung liquid at birth. *Respiration Physiology*, **80**, 181–92.

Konishi, M., Fujiwara, T., Naito, T. et al. (1988). Surfactant replacement therapy in neonatal respiratory distress syndrome. A multicentre randomized clinical trial: comparison of high versus low-dose of Surfactant TA. *European Journal of Pediatrics*, **147**, 20–5.

Kuroki, Y. (1992). Surfactant protein SP-D. In *Pulmonary Surfactant: from Molecular Biology to Clinical Practice*. ed. B. Robertson, L. M. G. van Golde & J. J. Batenburg. pp. 77–85. Elsevier, Amsterdam.

Kwong, M. S., Egan, E. A., Notter, R. H. & Shapiro, D. L. (1985). Double-blind clinical trial of calf lung surfactant extract for the prevention of hyaline membrane disease in extremely premature infants. *Pediatrics*, **76**, 585–92.

Lachmann, B. (1989). Animal models and clinical pilot studies of surfactant replacement in adult respiratory distress syndrome. *European Respiratory Journal*, **2** (Suppl 3), 98s–103s.

Lachmann, B., Grossmann, G., Nilsson, R. & Robertson, B. (1979). Lung mechanics during spontaneous ventilation in premature and full term rabbit neonates. *Respiratory Physiology*, **38**, 283–302.

Lang, M. J., Hall, R. T., Reddy, N. S., Kurth, C. G. & Merritt, T. A. (1990). A controlled trial of human surfactant replacement therapy for severe respiratory distress syndrome in very low birth weight infants. *Journal of Pediatrics*, **116**, 295–300.

Liechty, E. A., Donovan, E., Purohit, D. et al. (1991). Reduction of neonatal mortality after multiple doses of bovine surfactant in low birth weight neonates with respiratory distress syndrome. *Pediatrics*, **88**, 19–28.

Long, W. A. (1991). Follow-up of babies treated with synthetic surfactant. In Satellite Symposium. European Society for Pediatric Research, Zurich. The Value of Surfactant Therapy, pp. 8–10.

Long, W., Thompson, T., Sundell, H. et al. (1991a). Effects of two rescue doses of a synthetic surfactant on mortality rate and survival without bronchopulmonary dysplasia in 700 to 1350-gram infants with respiratory distress syndrome. *Journal of Pediatrics*, **118**, 595–605.

Long, W., Corbet, A., Cotton, R. et al. (1991*b*). A controlled trial of synthetic surfactant in infants weighing 1250 g or more with respiratory distress syndrome. *New England Journal of Medicine*, **325**, 1696–703.

Lotze, A., Knight, G. R., Martin et al. (1993). Improved pulmonary outcome after exogenous surfactant therapy for respiratory failure in term infants requiring extracorporeal membrane oxygenation. *Journal of Pediatrics*, **122**, 261–8.

Maeta, H., Asakura, K., Konishi, M. & Fujiwara, T. (1983). Effect of Surfactant-TA on alveolar stability of premature rabbit fetus: Comparison with term rabbit fetus and dry surfactant (70% DPPC & 30% PG). *Acta Neonatology of Japan*, **48**, 600.

Maeta, H., Vidyasagar, D., Raju, T. N. K., Bhat, R. & Matsuda, H. (1988). Early and late surfactant treatments in baboon model of hyaline membrane disease. *Pediatrics*, **81**, 277–83.

Marks, L. B., Notter, R. H., Oberdoster, G. & McBride, J. T. (1983). Ultrasonic and jet aerosolization of phospholipids and the effects on surface activity. *Pediatric Research*, **17**, 742–7.

McCord, B., Halliday, H. L., McClure, G. & McReid, C. (1989). Changes in pulmonary and cerebral blood flow after surfactant treatment for severe respiratory distress syndrome. In *Surfactant Replacement Therapy in Neonatal and Adult Respiratory Distress Syndrome*, ed. B. Lachmann. pp. 195–200. Berlin, Springer-Verlag.

Meban, C. (1981). Effect of lipids and other substances on the adsorption of dipalmitoylphosphatidylcholine. *Pediatric Research*, **15**, 1029–31.

Merritt, T. A., Hallman, M., Berry, C. et al. (1991). Randomized, placebo-controlled trials of human surfactant given at birth versus rescue administration in very low birth weight infants with lung immaturity. *Journal of Pediatrics*, **118**, 581–94.

Merritt, T. A., Hallman, M., Bloom, B. T. et al. (1986). Prophylactic treatment of very premature infants with human surfactant. *New England Journal of Medicine*, **315**, 785–90.

Metcalfe, I. L., Enhörning, G. & Possmayer, F. (1980). Surfactant-associated proteins: their role in the expression of surface activity. *Journal of Applied Physiology*, **49**, 34–41.

Morley, C. J. (1991). Surfactant treatment for premature babies: a review of clinical trials. *Archives of Disease in Childhood*, **66**, 445–50.

Morley, C. J. & Morley, R. (1990). Follow-up of premature babies treated with artificial surfactant (ALEC). *Archives of Disease in Childhood*, **65**, 667–9.

Morley, C., Robertson, B., Lachmann, B. et al. (1980). Artificial surfactant and natural surfactant. Comparative study of the effects on premature rabbit lungs. *Archives of Disease in Childhood*, **55**, 758–65.

Morley, C. J., Bangham, A. D., Miller, N. & Davis, J. A. (1981). Dry artificial lung surfactant and its effect on very premature babies. *Lancet*, **i**, 64–8.

Morley, C. J., Greenough, A., Miller, N. G. et al. (1988). Randomized trial of artificial surfactant (ALEC) given at birth to babies from 23 to 34 weeks' gestation. *Early Human Development*, **17**, 41–54.

Moses, D., Holm, B. A., Spitale, P., Liu, M. & Enhorning, G. (1990). Inhibition of pulmonary surfactant function by meconium. *American Journal of Obstetrics and Gynecology*, **164**, 477–81.

Msall, M. E., Rogers, B. T., Catanyaro, N., Kwong, M. & Buck, G. (1989). Five year neurodevelopmental outcome of infants less than 28 weeks' gestational age enrolled in a surfactant randomized clinical trial. *Pediatric Research*, **25**, 258, A1532 (abstract).

Nitta, K., Inui, S., Kobayashi, T., Shido, A., Ganzuka, M. & Murakami, S. (1989). Evaluation of pulmonary surfactants by the use of immature animals. *Hokuriku Journal of Anesthesiology (Hokurikumasuishi)*, **23**, 13–17.

Noack, G., Berggren, P., Curstedt, T. et al. (1987). Severe neonatal respiratory distress syndrome treated with the isolated phospholipid fraction of natural surfactant. *Acta Paediatrica Scandinavica*, **76**, 697–705.

Nohara, K., Matusumura, K. & Oda, T. (1983). Six cases of RDS treated with Surfactant CK. *Journal of Japanese Medical Society of Biology Interface*, **14**, 173–8.

Nohara, K., Berggren, P., Curstedt, T., Grossmann, G., Nilsson, R. & Robertson, B. (1986). Correlations between physical and physiological properties of various preparations of lung surfactant. *European Journal of Respiratory Disease*, **69**, 321–35.

Nosaka, S., Sakai, T., Yonekura, M. & Yoshikawa, K. (1990). Surfactant for adults with respiratory failure. *Lancet*, **336**, 947–8.

Notter, R. H. (1984). Surface chemistry of pulmonary surfactant: the role of individual components. In *Pulmonary Surfactant*, ed. B. Robertson, L. M. G. van Golde, & J. J. Batenburg. pp. 17–65. Elsevier, Amsterdam.

O'Brodovich, H. M., Weity, J. I. & Possmayer, F. (1990). Effect of fibrinogen degradation products and lung ground substance on surfactant function. *Biology of the Neonate*, **57**, 325–33.

Olver, R. E. (1983). Fluid balance across the fetal alveolar epithelium. *American Review of Respiratory Diseases*, **127**, 33–6.

Olver, R. E., Ramsden, C. A., Strang, L. B. & Walters, D. V. (1986). The role of amiloride blockable sodium transport in adrenaline induced lung liquid reabsorption in the fetal lamb. *Journal of Physiology*, **376**, 321–40.

Phibbs, R. H., Ballard, R. A., Clements, J. A. et al. (1991). Initial clinical trial of Exosurf, a protein-free synthetic surfactant, for the prophylaxis and early treatment of hyaline membrane disease. *Pediatrics*, **88**, 1–9.

Possmayer, F. A. (1988). A proposed nomenclature for pulmonary surfactant-associated proteins. *American Reviews of Respiratory Diseases*, **138**, 990–8.

Raju, T. N. K., Vidyasagar, D., Bhat, R. et al. (1987). Double-blind controlled trial of single-dose treatment with bovine surfactant in severe hyaline membrane disease. *Lancet*, **i**, 651–6.

Richman, R. S., Spragg, R. G., Robertson, B., Merritt, T. A. & Curstedt, T. (1989). The adult respiratory distress syndrome: first trials with surfactant replacement. *European Respiratory Journal*, **2**, (Suppl 3), 109s–111s.

Robertson, B. (1992). Animal models of neonatal surfactant dysfunction. In *Pulmonary Surfactant. From Molecular Biology to Clinical Practice*, ed. B. Robertson, L. M. G. van Golde & J. J. Batenburg. pp. 459–84. Elsevier, Amsterdam.

Robertson, B. & Lachmann, B. (1988). Experimental evaluation of surfactants for replacement therapy. *Experimental Lung Research*, **14**, 279–310.

Robertson, B., Berry, D., Curstedt, T. et al. (1985). Leakage of protein in the immature rabbit lung: effect of surfactant replacement. *Respiration Physiology*, **127**, 265–76.

Robertson, B., Curstedt, T., Johansson, J., Jörnvall, H. & Kobayashi, T. (1990). Structural and functional characterization of porcine surfactant isolated by liquid-gel chromatography. In *Basic Research on Lung Surfactant. Progress in Respiration Research*, ed. P. von Wichert & B. Müller Vol. 25. pp. 237–46. Karger, Basel.

Robertson, B., Curstedt, T., Tubman, R. et al. (1992). A two year follow up of babies enrolled in a European multicentre trial of porcine surfactant replacement for severe neonatal respiratory distress syndrome. *European Journal of Pediatrics*, **151**, 373–6.

Robillard, E., Alarie, Y., Dagenais-Perusse, P., Baril, E. & Guilbeault, A. (1964). Microaerosol administration of synthetic dipalmitoyl lecithin in the respiratory distress syndrome: a preliminary report. *Canadian Medical Association Journal*, **90**, 55–7.

Royall, J. A. & Levin, D. L. (1988). Adult respiratory distress syndrome in pediatric patients. 1. Clinical aspects, pathophysiology, pathology, and mechanisms of lung injury. *Journal of Pediatrics*, **112**, 169–80.

Sasaki, M. (1990). Comparison of five pulmonary surfactants: in vitro surface properties and ultrastructures. *Journal of Iwate Medical Association*, **42**, 883–96.

Schneider, H. A., Hallman, M., Benirschke, K. & Gluck, L. (1982). Human surfactant: A therapeutic trial in premature rabbits. *Journal of Pediatrics*, **100**, 619–22.

Segerer, H., Stevens, P., Schadow, B. et al. (1991). Surfactant substitution in ventilated very low birthweight infants: factors related to response types. *Pediatric Research*, **30**, 591–6.

Shapiro, D. L., Notter, R. M., Morin, F. C. III et al. (1985). Double-blind randomized trial of a calf lung surfactant extract administered at birth to very premature infants for prevention of respiratory distress syndrome. *Pediatrics*, **76**, 593–9.

Sherman, M. P., Campbell, C. A., Merritt, T. A., Shapiro, D. L., Long, W. A. & Gunkel, J. H. (1990). The infected preterm rabbit lung. A model to test the effect of surfactant replacement on lung host defenses. In *Basic Research on Lung Surfactant. Progress in Respiration Research*, ed. P. von Wichert & B. Müller. vol 25 pp. 204–8, Karger, Basel.

Skov, L., Bell, A. & Greisen, G. (1992*a*). Surfactant administration and the cerebral circulation. *Biology of the Neonate* **61** (Suppl. 1), 31–6.

Skov, L., Hellström-Westas, L., Jacobsen, T., Greisen, G., & Svenning-sen, N. W. (1992*b*). Acute changes in cerebral oxygenation and cerebral blood volume in preterm infants during surfactant treatment. *Neuropediatrics*, **23**, 126–30.

Skov, L., Ryding, J., Pryds, O. & Greisen, G. (1992*c*). Changes in cerebral oxygenation and cerebral blood volume during endotracheal suctioning in ventilated neonates. *Acta Paediatrica*, **81**, 389–93.

Smyth, J. A., Metcalfe, I. L., Duffty, P., Possmayer, F., Bryan, M. H. & Enhorning, G. (1983). Hyaline membrane disease treated with bovine surfactant. *Pediatrics*, **71**, 913–7.

Soll, R. F. (1992*a*). Natural surfactant extract treatment of RDS. In *Oxford Database of Perinatal Trials*, ed. I. Chalmers. Version 1. 3, Disk Issue 7, Record 5206.

Soll, R. F. (1992*b*). Prophylactic administration of natural surfactant extract. In *Oxford Database of Perinatal Trials*, ed. I. Chalmers. 5207 Version 1. 3, Disk Issue 7, Record 5207.

Soll, R. F. (1992*c*). Synthetic surfactant treatment of RDS. In *Oxford Database of Perinatal Trials*, ed. I. Chalmers. Version 1. 3, Disk Issue 7, Record 5252.

Soll, R. F. (1992*d*). Prophylactic administration of synthetic surfactant. In *Oxford Database of Perinatal Trials*, ed. I. Chalmers. Version 1. 3, Disk Issue 7. Record 5253.

Soll, R. F. (1992*e*). Prophylactic administration of any surfactant. In *Oxford Database of Perinatal Trials*, ed. I. Chalmers. Version 1. 3, Disk Issue 7, Record 5664.

Soll, R. F. (1992*f*). Prophylactic surfactant vs treatment with surfactant. In *Oxford Database of Perinatal Trials*, ed. I. Chalmers. Version 1. 3, Disk Issue 7, Record 5675.

Soll, R. F., Hoekstra, R. E., Fangman, J. J. et al. (1990). Multicentre trial of single-dose modified bovine surfactant extract (Survanta) for prevention of respiratory distress syndrome. *Pediatrics*, **85**, 1092–102.

Song, G. W., Sun, B., Curstedt, T., Grossmann, G. & Robertson, B. (1992). Effect of amiloride and surfactant on lung liquid clearance in mechanically ventilated newborn rabbits. *Respiration Physiology*, **88**, 233–46.

Speer, C. P., Robertson, B., Curstedt, T. et al. (1992). Randomized European multicenter trial of surfactant replacement therapy for severe neonatal respiratory distress syndrome: single versus multiple doses of Curosurf. *Pediatrics*, **89**, 13–20.

Stevenson, D., Walther, F., Long, W. et al. (1992). Controlled trial of a single dose of synthetic surfactant at birth in premature infants weighing 500 to 699 grams. *Journal of Pediatrics*, **120**, S3-S12.

Strayer, D. S. & Robertson, B. (1992). Surfactant as an immunogen: implications for therapy of respiratory distress syndrome. *Acta Paediatrica*, **81**, 446–7.

Strayer, D. S., Merritt, T. A., Lwebuga-Mukasa, J. & Hallman, M. (1986). Surfactant – anti-surfactant immune complexes in infants with respiratory distress syndrome. *American Journal of Pathology*, **122**, 353–62.

Strayer, D. S., Merritt, T. A., Makunike, C. & Hallman, M. (1989). Antigenicity of low molecular weight surfactant species. *American Journal of Pathology*, **134**, 723–32.

Sun, B., Kobayashi, T., Curstedt, T., Grossmann, G. & Robertson, B. (1991). Application of a new ventilator – multi-plethysmograph system for testing efficacy of surfactant replacement in newborn rabbits. *European Respiratory Journal*, **4**, 364–70.

Sun, B., Curstedt, T. & Robertson, B. (1993*a*). Surfactant inhibition in experimental meconium aspiration. *Acta Paediatrica*, **82**, 182–9.

Sun, B., Curstedt, T., Song, G-W. & Robertson, B. (1993*b*). Surfactant improves lung function and nephrology in newborn rabbits with meconium aspiration. *Biology of the Neonate*, **63**, 96–104.

Ten Centre Study Group (1987). Ten centre trial of artificial surfactant (artificial lung expanding compound) in very premature babies. *British Medical Journal*, **294**, 991–6.

The OSIRIS Collaborative Group (1992). Early versus delayed neonatal administration of a synthetic surfactant – the judgement of OSIRIS. *Lancet*, **340**, 1363–9.

Tooley, W. H., Clements, J. A., Muramatsu, K., Brown, C. L. & Schleuter, M. A. (1987). Lung function of prematurely delivered rabbits treated with a synthetic surfactant. *American Review of Respiratory Disease*, **136**, 347–51.

Tubman, T. R. J., Rankin, S. J., Halliday, H. L. & Johnston, S. S. (1992). Surfactant replacement therapy and the prevalance of acute retinopathy of prematurity. *Biology of the Neonate*, **61** (Suppl. 1): 54–8.

Tyler, D. C., Murphy, J. & Chaney, F. W. (1978). Mechanical and chemical damage to lung tissue caused by meconium aspiration. *Pediatrics*, **62**, 454–9.

van Bel, F., de Winter, P. J., Wijnands, H. B. G., van de Bor, M. & Egberts, J. (1992). Cerebral and aortic blood flow velocity patterns in preterm infants receiving prophylactic surfactant treatment. *Acta Paediatrica*, **81**, 504–10.

van de Bor, M., Ma, E. J. & Walther, F. J. (1991). Cerebral blood flow velocity after surfactant instillation in preterm infants. *Journal of Pediatrics*, **118**, 285–7.

van Daal, G-J., So, K. L , Gommers, D. et al. (1991). Intratracheal surfactant administration versus gas exchange in experimental adult respiratory distress syndrome associated with viral pneumonia. *Anesthesia and Analgesia*, **72**, 589–95.

van Daal, G-J., Bos, J. A. H., Eijking, E. P., Gommers, D., Hannappel, E. & Lachmann, B. (1992). Surfactant replacement therapy improves pulmonary mechanics in end-stage influenza A pneumonia in mice. *American Review of Respiratory Disease*, **148**, 859–63.

van Houten, J., Long, W., Mullett, M. et al. (1992). Pulmonary hemorrhage in premature infants after treatment with synthetic surfactant: an autopsy evaluation. *Journal of Pediatrics*, **120**, S40-S44.

van Iwaarden, F., Welmers, B., Verhoef, J., Haagsman, H. P. & van Golde, L. M. G. (1990). Pulmonary surfactant protein A enhances the host-defence mechanism of rat alveolar macrophages. *American Journal of Respiration and Cell Molecular Biology*, **2**, 91–8.

van Iwaarden, J. F., van Strijp, J. A. G., Ebskamp, M. J. M., Welmers, A. C., Verhoef, J. & van Golde, L. M. G. (1991). Surfactant protein A is opsonin in phagocytosis of herpes simplex virus type 1 by rat alveolar macrophages. *American Journal of Physiology* **261** (*Lung Cellular & Molecular Physiology* 5): L204-L209.

Vaucher, Y. E., Merritt, T. A., Hallman, M., Jarvenpaa, A-L., Telsey, A. M. & Jones, B. L. (1988). Neurodevelopmental and respiratory outcome in early childhood after human surfactant. *American Journal of Diseases of Children*, **142**, 927–30.

Vaucher, Y. E., Merritt, T. A. & Hallman, M. (1990). Improved outcome following rescue versus prophylactic surfactant treatment in RDS. *Pediatric Research*, **260**, A1543 (Abstract).

Verder, H., Agertoft, L., Albertsen, P. et al. (1992). Surfaktantbehandling af nyfdte med respiratory distress syndrom primaert behandlet med nasal-CPAP. En pilot-undersgelse. *Ugeskrift for Laeger*, **154**, 2136–39.

Victorin, L. H., Deverajan, L. V., Curstedt, T. & Robertson, B. (1990). Surfactant replacement in spontaneously breathing babies with hyaline membrane disease – a pilot study. *Biology of the Neonate*, **58**, 121–6.

Vidyasagar, D., Maeta, H., Raju, T. N. K. et al. (1985). Bovine surfactant (Surfactant TA) therapy in immature baboons with hyaline membrane disease. *Pediatrics*, 75, 1132–42.

Ware, J., Taeusch, H. W., Soll, R. F. & McCormick, M. C. (1990). Health and developmental outcomes of a surfactant controlled trial: follow-up at 2 years. *Pediatrics*, **85**, 1103–7.

Waring, A., Taeusch, W., Bruni, R. et al. (1989). Synthetic amphipathic sequences of surfactant protein-B mimic several physicochemical and in vivo properties of native pulmonary surfactant proteins. *Peptide Research*, **2**, 308–313.

Whitsett, J. A., Ohning, B. L., Ross, G. et al. (1986). Hydrophobic surfactant-associated protein in whole lung surfactant and its importance for biophysical activity in lung surfactant extracts used for replacement therapy. *Pediatric Research*, **20**, 460–7.

Whitsett, J. A., Hull, W. M. & Luse, S. (1991). Failure to detect surfactant protein-specific antibodies in sera of premature infants treated with Survanta, a modified bovine surfactant. *Pediatrics*, **87**, 505–10.

Wilkinson, A. R., Jenkins, P. A. & Jeffrey, J. A. (1985). Two controlled trials of dry artificial surfactant: early effects and later outcome in babies with surfactant deficiency. *Lancet*, **ii**, 287–91.

Williams, M. C., Hawgood, S. & Hamilton, R. L. (1991). Changes in lipid structure produced by surfactant proteins SP-A, SP-B and SP-C. *American Journal of Respiration and Cell Molecular Biology*, **5**, 41–50.

Yao, L. J., Richardson, C., Ford, C. et al. (1990). Expression of mature pulmonary surfactant-associated protein B (SP-B). *Biochemistry and Cell Biology*, **68**, 559–66.

13

Antenatal promotion of pulmonary function

NICHOLAS M. FISK and HEATHER JEFFERY

Introduction

Despite the success of postnatal resuscitatory, ventilatory and pharmacological strategies against respiratory disease (Chapters 11 & 14), conditions such as pulmonary hypoplasia, respiratory distress syndrome and
meconium aspiration syndrome remain associated with substantial morbidity and mortality. In some, neonatal interventions will be instituted
too late or will fail, whereas in others the pathology is already irreversible
at the time of birth. The development of antenatal strategies to facilitate
neonatal respiration has been slow due to ethical and technical restraints
on access to the human fetus. Whereas transplacental therapy to promote
surfactant release was first used 20 years ago, surgical possibilities only
arose in the late 1980s when invasive procedures and high-resolution
ultrasound combined to render direct fetal treatment practical.

Antenatal intervention may benefit the pathologies affecting lung
growth, lung maturation, and lung expansion at birth.

Strategies to promote lung growth

Background

Pulmonary hypoplasia (PH) results when any of the three prerequisites
for normal fetal lung growth (adequate intrathoracic space, normal fetal
breathing movement and presence of amniotic fluid) are deficient during
the canalicular phase, i.e. between 17 and 26 weeks (Burri, 1984). The
following aetiological conditions have been identified in clinical series
and confirmed in animal models: skeletal dysplasias affecting the thorax
(Page & Stocker, 1982; Hepworth, Seegmiller & Carey, 1990), intrathoracic space-occupying lesions (Campanale & Rowland, 1955; Harrison,
Jester & Ross, 1980), neurological deficit impairing breathing movements (Wigglesworth & Desai, 1979; Dornan, Ritchie & Meban, 1984),

and oligohydramnios secondary to fetal urinary tract pathology or amniotic fluid leakage (Perlman & Levin, 1974; Moessinger et al., 1986).

In conditions in which the underlying disorder is not relevant after birth (i.e. ruptured membranes), or is amenable to postnatal correction (i.e. urethral valves, diaphragmatic hernia), PH is the principal determinant of perinatal survival, and its prevention should permit survival at birth. In contrast, antenatal intervention to prevent PH does not have a role in lethal conditions such as renal agenesis. Accordingly, antenatal strategies have focused on two areas (i) relief of lung compression from intrathoracic space-occupying lesions, and (ii) correction of oligohydramnios in fetuses with functioning renal tissue.

Experimental basis

The scientific basis for the above interventions has been established in animal models. Compression of the developing lung by intrathoracic space-occupying lesions produces PH, whereas its relief is associated with continued lung growth. Harrison et al. (1980) showed in controlled experiments in fetal sheep (canalicular period 80–125 days) that inflating an intrathoracic balloon between 100–140 days gestation resulted in PH and fatal respiratory insufficiency at birth; deflating the balloon at 120, but not 140 days produced improved lung growth and allowed survival at birth. They (Harrison, Ross & de Lorimier, 1981) and another group (Pringle et al., 1984; Soper, Pringle & Schofield, 1984) then repaired experimentally created diaphragmatic herniae in utero before the end of the canalicular period, which improved both lung size and morphometry, and survival at birth. Although a strong causal relationship has been established between PH and oligohydramnios, the underlying mechanism of oligohydramnios-related PH remains controversial (Fisk, 1992). Chronic loss of lung liquid occurs in oligohydramnios-related PH (Adzick et al., 1984; Dickson & Harding, 1989), but the reason for this is obscure. Chest compression (Nicolini et al., 1989), at least in the resting state (Harding, Hooper & Dickson, 1990), and/or a reduction in fetal breathing movements (Dickson & Harding, 1991; Fisk et al., 1992) do not seem to be involved. Lack of understanding of the pathogenesis of oligohydramnios-related PH hampers the development of preventative/ therapeutic strategies other than simple restitution of amniotic volume. In animal fetuses with experimental bladder outlet obstruction, restoration of amniotic fluid volume before the end of the canalicular phase, either by diversion of urine or infusion of saline into the amniotic cavity, has significant beneficial effects on lung development (Harrison et al., 1982*a*; Nakayama et al., 1983) and allows survival at birth (Harrison et al., 1982*a*; Nakayama et al., 1983).

Patient selection

Our knowledge of the vulnerability of human lung development to external insults is largely based on clinical oligohydramnios series, which suggest that the likelihood of PH depends on three variables: gestation at onset, duration and severity of oligohydramnios (Harrison et al., 1982*b*; Nimrod et al., 1984; Moore et al., 1989; Rotschild et al., 1990). Virtually no amniotic fluid is found from 16 weeks in fetuses with renal agenesis (Hislop, Hey & Reid, 1979; Moore et al., 1989), which die from respiratory insufficiency, and show the most severe PH at necropsy (Reale & Esterly, 1973). In contrast, PH secondary to amniorrhexis is unlikely when membrane rupture occurs >25 weeks or lasts ≤5 weeks (Nimrod et al., 1984). Gestational age at rupture is the most important variable determining PH, the relative risk declining from 50% at 19 weeks to 15% at 24 weeks (Rotschild et al., 1990). PH is also ten times as likely after severe, compared to mild/moderate oligohydramnios (60% vs 6%) (Moore et al., 1989).

As an alternative to selection based on clinical risk, the likelihood of PH might be assessed using ultrasonic measurements of lung size, such as fetal chest circumference (Nimrod et al., 1986, Vintzileos et al., 1989), and lung length (Roberts & Mitchell, 1990). However, these parameters have not been widely adopted because of concerns about their reproducibility in severe oligohydramnios. A newer approach involves Doppler interrogation of the fetal ductus (van Eyck, van der Mooren & Wladimiroff, 1990), with reduced velocity modulation during fetal breathing predicting PH. However, longitudinal studies suggest that, in PH, progressive lag in these biophysical parameters does not occur ≥24 weeks (Songster, Gray & Crane, 1989; Roberts & Mitchell, 1990; van Eyck et al., 1990). As the canalicular phase is almost over by then, these parameters are of value only in indicating the presence of established PH, but not in selecting patients for interventions to prevent PH.

In severe PH, death occurs soon after birth, with the diagnosis based on postmortem indices of reduced lung growth (Chapter 10). In milder cases, infants survive after recovering from respiratory insufficiency characterised by high ventilatory pressures (Thibeault et al., 1985; Bhutani, Abashi & Weiner, 1986) and reduced radiographic lung size (Leonidas, Bahn & Beatty, 1982). As catch-up lung growth occurs in survivors (Thompson, Greenough & Nicolaides, 1990), preventative strategies have concentrated on those at risk of lethal PH.

Antenatal interventions to promote lung growth may be considered before the end of the canalicular period in fetuses at risk of lethal PH, in whom the aetiological condition is non-lethal. Simple interventions include ultrasound-guided needling for aspiration or drainage, whereas attempts at fetal surgery have taken one of two forms: open surgical correction at hysterotomy, or by-passing obstructive lesions by ultrasound-guided insertion of catheter shunts.

These techniques should only be contemplated in a few centres with expertise, and for conditions in which animal models have demonstrated benefit from correction in utero. Chromosomal and other structural malformations must first be excluded. Reliable antenatal predictors are needed in selecting cases, so that intervention is withheld both from those who would otherwise have a satisfactory outcome, and from those in whom the pathology is irreversible. The anecdotal and uncontrolled nature of the clinical series discussed below prevents firm conclusions being made on the benefit of these interventions.

Relief of lung compression
Drainage of pleural effusions

The 45–55% perinatal mortality rate in fetal hydrothorax is only in part due to PH secondary to lung compression (Longaker et al., 1989a; Weber & Philipson, 1992). Large effusions also cause hydrops by vena caval obstruction/cardiac compression and polyhydramnios by impaired swallowing (Petres, Redwine & Cruickshank, 1982; Benacerraf & Frigoletto, 1985). In a recent meta-analysis (Weber & Philipson, 1992), hydrops was associated with the poorest prognosis, only 31% surviving. In contrast, isolated or unilateral effusions frequently resolve in utero without sequelae.

Although one of the aims of in utero drainage is to allow lung growth to prevent respiratory embarrassment at birth, this is only relevant if the fetus does not succumb in utero from hydrops, or die from prematurity due to polyhydramnios. Thus a more immediate aim is restoration of normal haemodynamics and swallowing (Rodeck et al., 1988). Because

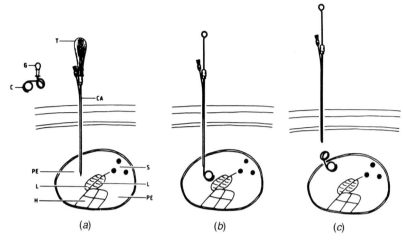

Fig. 13.1. Pleuro-amniotic shunting. The trochar (T) and cannula (CA) are inserted transamniotically into the effusion (*a*). The guidewire (G) is then straightened, the double pigtail catheter (C) inserted into the cannula, and the wire removed. A short introducer rod then deposits half the catheter within the hemithorax (*b*). The cannula is then withdrawn into the amniotic cavity, and a long introducer rod is inserted to position the other half of the shunt in the amniotic cavity (*c*). H denotes heart, S spine, L lungs. (From Rodeck et al. (1988). Reproduced with permission.)

fluid re-accumulates within 6–48 hours of a single ultrasound-guided aspiration (Petres et al., 1982; Nicolaides et al., 1985), chronic drainage is usually required; this is indicated for (i) bilateral effusions in the canalicular phase or (ii) hydrops at any gestation. A plastic double pigtail pleuro-amniotic shunt is inserted under ultrasound guidance (Fig. 13.1). Several series indicate that, providing the lungs initially re-expand (Fig. 13.2), bilateral pleuro-amniotic shunting is efficacious both in achieving long term drainage, and in 50–70% in reversing hydrops and polyhydramnios (Blott, Nicolaides & Greenough, 1988; Rodeck et al., 1988; Nicolaides & Azar, 1990). However, if the lungs fail to expand, the outcome is almost universally poor due to underlying PH (Rodeck et al., 1988; Vaughan, Fisk & Rodeck, 1992). Hypoplastic lungs seem unable to expand after fluid aspiration, and in this light intrapleural pressure remains positive after aspiration in fetuses without PH, but is negative in those subsequently shown to have PH (Vaughan et al., 1994). Published series of pleuro-amniotic shunts are small, comprising fewer than 60 cases in total; the vast majority were inserted after the canalicular phase allowing no inferences on the utility of

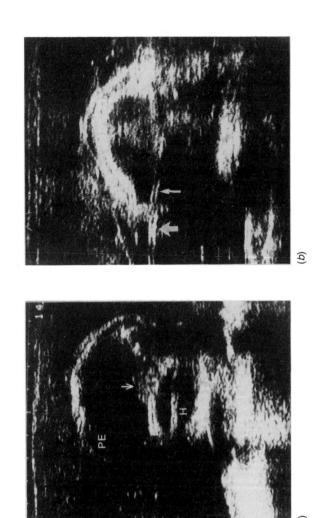

(a)

(b)

Fig. 13.2. Ultrasound cross-sectional views of the fetal chest. Panel (a) shows a large right sided pleural effusion (PE) with mediastinal shift, displacement of the heart (H), and a markedly compressed right lung (arrow). In panel (b), 24 h after shunt insertion, the effusion has drained and the lung re-expanded. Note the intrapleural (thin arrow) and extrapleural (thick arrow) portions of the catheter in situ. (From Rodeck, et al. 1988. Reproduced with permission.)

this procedure in preventing PH. The catheters are clamped at delivery to avoid pneumothoraces.

Drainage of pulmonary cysts

Congenital cystic adenomatoid malformation is a rare hamartomatous lesion of the lung which may result in PH, hydrops and perinatal death (Adzick et al., 1985a). These sequelae occur more commonly in association with the microcystic rather than macrocystic type. Nevertheless, large solitary cysts producing mediastinal shift have been drained in utero.

The cyst re-accumulated in one of two cases treated by simple aspiration (Adzick et al., 1985a,b; Nugent, Hayashi & Rubin, 1989). The shunting device discussed above may be used for chronic drainage (Clark et al., 1987; Nicolaides & Azar, 1990): in three of four shunted cases, insertion was in the mid-trimester and in none was there evidence of PH at birth.

Repair of diaphragmatic hernia

Perinatal mortality from diaphragmatic hernia diagnosed in utero has been reported to exceed 75% despite optimal postnatal care (Adzick et al., 1985b, Harrison et al., 1990a). The main determinant of outcome is the degree of PH secondary to lung compression, which has been assumed by extrapolation from animal studies to depend on the timing and volume of visceral herniation through the diaphragm. Reported adverse factors include polyhydramnios, mediastinal shift, and a large volume of viscera within the chest. Following demonstration in animal models of the benefit of in utero repair (Harrison et al., 1980; Soper et al., 1984), and the safety to the mother of fetal surgery (Adzick et al., 1986), and after a decade developing appropriate techniques, Harrison's San Francisco group have now operated in the late mid-trimester on eight human fetuses with adverse factors (Harrison et al., 1990a,b). Technical problems were encountered in the first four, when herniated liver could not be returned to the abdomen without kinking the umbilical vein. Successful repairs were accomplished in the next four: one died at 3 weeks of age from intestinal complications, one from an unrelated accident, and there were two postneonatal survivors. Thus surgical correction in utero of highly selected cases is feasible.

While this approach is being pursued in a few highly specialized centres, data are emerging which challenge many of the above assumptions. The association of polyhydramnios, mediastinal shift and intrathoracic stomach with PH has not been confirmed (Thorpe-Beeston, Gosden & Nicolaides, 1989), while perinatal mortality rates as low as 40–45% have been reported with conservative management (Thorpe-Beeston et al., 1989; Wenstrom, Weiner & Hanson, 1991). With the limited knowledge currently available, survival rates following in utero surgery appear no better than with conservative management. Despite the elegant animal models of PH in congenital diaphragmatic hernia, it remains possible that PH in this condition results from a concomitant embryological defect in the post-hepatic mesenchymal plate (Iritani, 1984), rather than intrathoracic compression. This controversy will only be resolved by a randomized controlled trial.

Resection of pulmonary lesions

Although the natural history of echogenic lung lesions is still being elucidated, large microcystic adenomatoid malformations carry a poor prognosis when associated with hydrops (Adzick et al., 1985a,b; Neilson et al., 1991). The presence of hydrops usually reflects marked mediastinal shift and a high risk of PH. Based on their experience with fetal surgery for diaphragmatic herniae, one group has resected macrocystic lesions in utero in two hydropic fetuses, with survival following resolution of hydrops in one (Harrison et al., 1990c).

Restoration of amniotic fluid volume
Cervical occlusion

In patients with preterm premature rupture of the membranes, attempts have been made to restore amniotic fluid volume by plugging the leak. Occluding the cervix with a fibrin gel does not prevent continued amniotic fluid drainage (Baumgarten & Moser, 1986) nor does fixation of a double balloon catheter (PROM-Fence) (Ogita et al., 1984) within the cervical canal. Nevertheless, normal saline can be infused continuously into the amniotic cavity via the catheter, which in ten patients maintained the mean deepest pool $\geq$ 5 cm (Imanaka, Ogita & Sugawa, 1989). The PROM-Fence has been mainly used in late pregnancy (Ogita et al., 1988), and its efficacy in preventing PH has yet to be evaluated.

Serial transabdominal amnioinfusion

Following establishment of the safety of transabdominal amnioinfusion (Gembruch & Hansmann, 1988) as a diagnostic procedure (Fisk et al.,

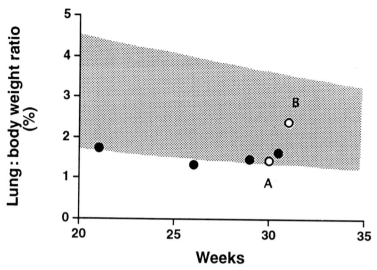

Fig. 13.3. Lung: body weight ratios in the six fetal/neonatal deaths among nine pregnancies with severe oligohydramnios that underwent serial amnioinfusions, plotted against the 95% reference range. As ventilation may artefactually elevate lung:body weight ratios, the two ventilated neonates are indicated by open circles; one of these (A) had clinical evidence of PH. (After Fisk et al. (1991), reproduced with kind permission of the American College of Obstetricians and Gynecologists.)

1991), our group conducted a pilot study of therapeutic infusions to prevent oligohydramnios sequelae. In nine women with appropriately-grown singleton fetuses in whom severe oligohydramnios had been documented ≤22 weeks, 40 infusions were performed with sufficient saline to restore normal amniotic fluid volume at weekly intervals until the end of the canalicular phase (Fisk et al., 1991). Three infants survived; one of the six perinatal deaths had a reduced lung : body weight ratio (Fig. 13.3) and another had clinical PH. Lung hypoplasia was thus found in two of nine pregnancies (22%) complicated by severe oligohydramnios diagnosed ≤22 weeks, which compares favourably to 60% reported in severe oligohydramnios diagnosed ≤28 weeks (Moore et al., 1989).

Controlled studies are now needed to evaluate any benefit from this procedure, but will need to be multicentred as only a small proportion of patients with severe mid-trimester oligohydramnios are suitable. Idiopathic oligohydramnios is rare, while the rate and degree of leakage render this approach impractical in many with ruptured membranes. If

serial amnioinfusion is confirmed as beneficial, the optimal gestation at
which to commence and cease infusions needs to be determined, as well
as the optimal fluid for, and frequency of, administration.

Decompression of urinary obstruction

In fetuses with low obstructive uropathy, the urinary tract may be
decompressed into the amniotic cavity, not only to relieve obstruction to
prevent renal dysplasia but also to restore amniotic fluid volume to
facilitate lung growth (Harrison et al., 1982*a*; Glick et al., 1984). It is
axiomatic that the latter will only be achieved in the presence of
functioning kidneys, i.e. in fetuses in which irreversible renal damage has
not yet developed.

Fetal renal function is assessed by biochemical analysis of fetal urine
obtained by ultrasound-guided aspiration. A urinary Na^+ >100 mEq/l,
Cl^- >90 mEq/l and osmolality >210 mOsm/l have been suggested as
indicative of irreversible renal damage Glick et al. (1985) but take no
account of known variation with gestational age (Wilkins et al., 1987;
Nicolini et al., 1992). A urinary sodium above the 95% reference range
for gestation seems the best predictor, yielding sensitivities and speci-
ficities of 80% for histological dysplasia (Nicolini et al., 1992). Accuracy
may be improved by serial bladder aspiration with electrolyte analysis on
'fresh' urine (Evans et al., 1991; Nicolini et al., 1992).

The standard method of decompression is by ultrasound-guided insertion of an indwelling catheter (Harrison et al., 1982*b*; Manning et al.,
1986), as for pleuro-amniotic shunting. Since some vesico-amniotic
shunts are prone to blockage or displacement (Golbus et al., 1982,
Manning et al., 1983), one group currently favours open decompression
at hysterotomy (Harrison et al., 1987). Technical problems however are
less likely with the catheters used in the UK (KCH Bladder Catheter,
Rocket of London).

The results of shunting reported to the International Registry are far
from encouraging with a perinatal loss rate among 73 fetuses of 59%, PH
being present in 27 of the 29 neonatal deaths (Manning et al., 1986).
Although patient selection was poor, these results have nevertheless
given rise to scepticism about the benefit of vesico-amniotic shunting
(Elder, Duckett & Snyder, 1987; Reuss et al., 1988). Furthermore, an
alternate embryological theory suggests that renal dysplasia is not secondary to posterior urethral valves, but a concomitant defect (Stephens,
1983). As most deaths after shunting are due to PH, restoration of
amniotic fluid volume rather than urinary decompression might be a

more important therapeutic goal, and in this light serial amnioinfusion may warrant consideration.

A multicentre randomized controlled trial of vesico-amniotic shunting has been proposed by the International Fetal Medicine & Surgery Society, but foundered on lack of consensus and recruitment. Until the value of shunting procedures is established, selection criteria should be rigorously applied to restrict them to those few fetuses who may benefit, i.e. otherwise normal euploid male fetuses with urethral valves, severe oligohydramnios, and adequate renal function. These are rarely satisfied, one centre finding only 2.5% of fetuses referred with bilateral hydronephrosis suitable (Longaker, Adzick & Harrison, 1989*b*). This is because renal function and amniotic fluid volume are interrelated, tending either both to be normal or both impaired.

Strategies to promote lung maturation

Background

Surfactant, the surface active material produced by type 2 alveolar cells, is a complex mixture of phospholipids such as saturated phosphatidylcholine, and proteins, of which three species of non-serum surfactant-associated proteins have been identified (Ballard, 1989). It is secreted into the alveoli where it forms a lipid monolayer, decreases surface tension and enhances alveolar stability. Surfactant deficiency results in respiratory distress syndrome (RDS), until recently the leading cause of neonatal death (Avery & Merritt, 1991). Both the incidence and mortality of RDS are inversely related to gestational age and increased following pre-labour Caesarean section (Usher, Allen & McLean, 1971; Hjalmarson, 1981).

Strategies to prevent RDS have been directed towards enhancing biochemical maturation of surfactant, and include (i) prolongation of gestation (ii) maternal administration of hormones and other agents to enhance fetal lung maturation. The first of these relates to standard obstetrical practice and will not be discussed here.

Experimental basis

Research on the effect of hormones on lung maturation was stimulated by the observation that dexamethasone infusion in fetal lambs allowed survival after premature delivery. Liggins (1969) noted that partial expansion of the lungs in treated lambs at 117–123 days, when the lungs were usually airless, 'strongly suggests the accelerated appearance of surfactant, possibly as a result of premature activity of enzymes involved in a biosynthetic pathway'.

Animal studies have since confirmed that glucocorticoids accelerate morphological, biochemical and physiological lung maturation both alone and in combination with other hormones. Glucocorticoids increase the synthesis of surfactant in vivo and in cultured lung explants in both animals and man (Chapter 2). This maturational effect occurs late in fetal life, recent evidence in rabbits suggesting a specific gestational time (Oulton et al., 1989), before and after which it does not occur.

A number of other hormones have been shown to influence fetal lung development in animal and human studies, including thyroid and thyroid releasing hormones, and β adrenergic agonists. The scientific basis for the action of all these agents is dealt with in Chapter 2.

Patient selection

Gestational age

Patients may be selected simply on the basis of gestation. Usher, Allen & McLean (1971) reported the incidence of RDS in vaginal births as 64% at 29–30 weeks gestation, decreasing as age increased in fortnightly increments to 35, 20, and 5% down to 0.8% at 37–38 weeks. Given the wide overlap in gestation of fetuses with mature and immature lungs, this approach is suboptimal, especially between 32–34 weeks, when although the risk of RDS is lower than at earlier gestations, the overall birth-rate is higher, accounting for substantial numbers of babies with RDS. Using this approach, some fetuses with mature lungs will be exposed unnecessarily to lung maturation strategies, which will be withheld from others with immature lungs.

Tests of fetal lung maturity

Alternatively, the likelihood of RDS can be determined by various biochemical or biophysical tests of fetal lung maturity. As surfactant is released into the alveolar lung liquid and thence flows into the amniotic cavity, tests to predict RDS are based on the amount of surfactant phospholipid in amniotic fluid. The most common tests are the lecithin to sphingomyelin (L:S) ratio (Gluck et al., 1971) and the phosphatidylglycerol (PG) concentration (Hallman et al., 1976). Lecithin increases sharply with the development of pulmonary maturity, while the sphingomyelin concentration remains relatively constant throughout gestation. The use of the ratio thus corrects for amniotic fluid volume, with the LS increasing from ≤ 1 early in the third trimester to ≥ 2 at approximately 35 weeks (Gluck et al., 1971). As the L/S ratio is dependent on thin layer chromatography and thus not available outside laboratory hours, bedside tests reflecting surfactant's biophysical properties have also been used. The shake, click, and foam stability index tests measure surface tension-lowering ability, whereas optical density and fluorescence polarization depends on other physical properties (for review see Brown & Duck-Chong, 1982; Cosmi & Di Renzo, 1989). Surfactant-associated proteins which also contribute to surfactant function, are currently under investigation (Hawgood & Clements, 1990) and rapid assays might be developed to provide a more specific test. Amniotic fluid for testing is usually obtained by amniocentesis. Vaginal fluid can be collected in those with ruptured membranes, although accuracy is often reduced owing to contamination. Blood or meconium contain other phospholipids, such as phosphatidylcholine, whereas the fetal lung is the only source of PG, making it useful in specimens collected vaginally, or contaminated with blood or meconium (Stedman et al., 1981; Whittle et al., 1982).

Several ultrasonic variables have been suggested as predictive of fetal lung maturity. Placental grade (Grannum, Berkowitz & Hobbins, 1979) is of little value prior to term (Kazzi et al., 1984; Destro, Calcagnile & Ceccarello, 1985), while there are insufficient data to evaluate the lung:liver reflectivity ratio (Sohn, Stolz & Baster, 1991).

The accuracy of lung maturity testing in published series depends on the test used, the population prevalence and diagnostic criteria for RDS, together with exclusion criteria of confounding lung pathologies. In practice, tests for the L:S ratio and PG have a 95–100% positive predictive value (a mature test correctly predicts no RDS) (Table 13.1), the principal difficulty being the high incidence of false predictions of immaturity, a common finding for both biochemical and biophysical tests of fetal lung maturity.

There are marked differences in attitude towards lung maturity testing, this practice being commonplace in the USA, but now rare in the UK (Turnbull, 1983). The argument that these tests are largely outdated (James, Tindall & Richardson, 1983) is based on (i) better dating by ultrasound reducing the need for testing before elective delivery at term (ii) better neonatal intensive care reducing the morbidity and mortality of

Table 13.1. *The accuracy of predictors of fetal lung maturity in amniotic fluid in studies of ≥100 subjects of whom ≥10 had RDS*

Reference	Number studied	No. RDS (%)	Sensitivity	Specificity	Positive predictive value	Negative predictive value
LS ratio						
Torday[a] (1979)	322	45 (14)	93	66	95	55
Sher[a] (1980)	166	27 (16)	78	81	96	41
Bent[a] (1981)	103	21 (20)	79	86	95	42
Whittle[v] (1982)	288	17 (6)	86	100	100	32
Hamilton[a] (1984)	131	10 (8)	77	100	100	26
Herbert[a] (1986)	175	13 (7)	85	85	99	31
Phosphatidyl glycerol (PG)						
Bent[a] (1981)	244	23 (9)	97	83	98	73
Whittle[v] (1982)	288	17 (6)	99	94	99	94
Kogon[a] (1986)	666	46 (7)	96	78	98	56

L/S: lecithin/spingomyelin ratio using thin layer chromatography.
PG: phosphatidylglycerol by two-dimensional thin layer chromatography.
[a]: collected abdominally.
[v]: collected vaginally.

RDS (iii) better assessment of fetal well-being facilitating decision making (delivery or not) in the individual case. The recent availability of surfactant as an effective treatment of RDS further strengthens (ii) above (Hennes et al., 1991; Avery & Merritt, 1991). Proponents of testing argue that it is (i) rarely used to decide on delivery, but more to determine whether strategies to promote lung maturation are indicated (ii) more accurate than gestational age alone in predicting RDS, thus contributing to obstetric decision making, and (iii) now a very safe procedure, following improvements in amniocentesis technique.

Glucocorticoids

Mechanism of action

Glucocorticoids, by inducing enzymes such as fatty acid synthetase (Gonzales et al., 1990), enhance synthesis of the four major phospholipids, namely phosphatidylcholine, phosphatidylethanolamine, phosphatidylinositol and phosphatidylglycerol (Chapter 2). The surfactant apoproteins, A, B, and C are also induced (Hawgood & Clements, 1990; for review see Ballard, 1989). Several studies now suggest that the beneficial effects of maternally-administered glucocorticoids on subsequent neonatal lung function are not entirely attributable to correction of surfactant deficiency. Maternal corticosteroid treatment in rabbits improves lung function in their ventilated 27 day pups, independently of change in the alveolar saturated phophatidylcholine pool size (Fiascone et al., 1987; Ikegami et al., 1987*b*; 1989*a*). A possible mechanism is decreased leakage of lung proteins into the alveolar space and increased removal (Ikegami et al., 1987*a,b*), which would reduce both surfactant inactivation (Holm, Enhorning & Notter, 1988) and proteinaceous alveolar edema, a major cause of reduced lung capacity in RDS (Jackson et al., 1990). Inducible changes in elastin and collagen may reflect increased airspace subdivision leading to more recruitable airspaces (Schellenberg et al., 1987). Prenatal glucocorticoid treatment in the rat also accelerates maturation of lung antioxidant enzymes which protect against hyperoxia-induced lung injury (Frank, Lewis & Sosenko, 1985). Furthermore, glucocorticoids induce β adrenergic receptors (Cheng et al., 1980), which increase the sensitivity of type II cells to endogenous catecholamines, which may in turn facilitate reabsorption of lung liquid (see Chapter 3). These studies support the view that RDS is not just surfactant deficiency, and that glucocorticoids act in part by mechanisms independent of the effect on surfactant.

Clinical trials

The potential benefit of antepartum glucocorticoid therapy to prematurely delivered fetuses was first demonstrated in 1972 (Liggins & Howie, 1972). These results were combined with those of their second trial, in which twice the dose of betamethasone was used (Howie & Liggins, 1982). In these double-blind randomized controlled studies, perinatal mortality and RDS were significantly lower in treated infants, with no difference in effect between the two dosage regimes. Benefit was most apparent in infants <32 weeks, but evident up to 34 weeks.

Meta-analysis of the 14 randomized controlled trials (Crowley, 1992*a*) confirms that corticosteroid treatment prior to preterm delivery significantly reduces RDS, and early neonatal mortality. Overall the reduction in the odds of neonatal respiratory morbidity is between 40–60% (Crowley, 1992*a*) (Fig. 13.4), irrespective of infant gender. The gestational age at which there is an effect ranges from 28 to 34 weeks. The effect is less predictable at <28 weeks, when lung disease may further be

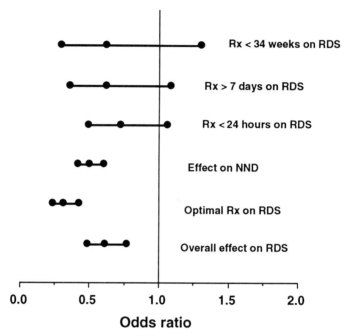

Effect of glucocorticoids
(meta-analysis of 14 RCTs)

Fig. 13.4. Graph of odds ratios with 95% confidence intervals of the overall effect in randomized controlled trials of maternal glucocorticoid treatment. (After Crowley, 1992*a*.)

influenced by alveolar immaturity, rib-cage instability, poor alveolar fluid clearance, and lung infection. Between 24–28 weeks, one uncontrolled trial reported a beneficial effect (Kwong & Egan, 1986), but this was not substantiated in a later randomized trial (Garite et al., 1991). There may be an effect after 34 weeks, but the incidence of RDS is so low that numbers larger than those in the meta-analysis would be needed to confirm this. The greatest effect is when delivery occurs >24 hours but <7 days after initiation of therapy, presumably reflecting the time course of glucocorticoid-induced protein synthesis. Controlled trials suggest some benefit for infants born outside the optimum period (Crowley, 1992a), one multicentre trial reporting an effect up to 14 days after treatment (Gamsu et al., 1989).

Glucocorticoids of established efficacy include betamethasone, dexamethasone and hydrocortisone. In the meta-analysis of 11 randomized controlled trials of preterm prelabour rupture of the membranes, steroids are just as efficacious as when used in intact membranes (Crowley, 1992b). Uncertainty prevails as to the efficacy of steroids in maternal diabetes, Rh alloimmunisation and prior to elective Caesarean, i.e. in the absence of labour. Initial concerns about fetal death in the presence of maternal hypertension (Liggins & Howie, 1972) have not been substantiated (Collaborative Group on Antenatal Steroid Therapy, 1981; Gamsu et al., 1989).

Other clinically beneficial effects include a decreased incidence of patent ductus arteriosus, periventricular haemorrhage, necrotising enterocolitis, hospital stay, respiratory complications at 18 months, and cardiac murmurs at 36 months (Collaborative Group on Antenatal Steroid Therapy, 1984; Avery, 1984; Crowley, 1992a). The incidence of maternal, fetal or neonatal infection is unchanged (Crowley, 1992a). A recent meta-analysis concludes that no further trials of steroids are necessary to establish their efficacy.

There has been concern about the possibility of long-term inhibition of growth, found after glucocorticoid administration in animals. The low level of, and brief exposure to, prenatal glucocorticoids in clinical studies, together with their safety in primate studies, has been used to argue that the growth inhibition found in animals is not applicable to human fetuses (Ballard, 1986). Human follow-up studies have shown no adverse effects on growth, neurological development, psychometric testing, lung mechanics or retrolental fibroplasia (MacArthur et al., 1981, 1982; Collaborative Group on Antenatal Steroid Therapy, 1984; Smolders-de-Haas et al., 1990).

Synergism with surfactant

The combination of antenatal glucocorticoids and postnatal surfactant in preterm rabbits results in a more pronounced improvement in lung compliance than with either therapy alone (Fiascone et al., 1987; Ikegami et al., 1987a,b, 1989b; Seidner et al., 1988). The initial report in man of synergism between antenatal corticosteroids and postnatal surfactant (Kwong, Egan & Notter, 1987) is supported by a non-randomized clinical trial of prophylactic calf surfactant and antenatal dexamethasone (Farrell et al., 1989): the incidence and severity of RDS was reduced when both were used (2 of 16 infants) compared with surfactant alone (33 of 83).

Synergism is just one reason why antenatal steroid therapy is unlikely to be replaced by postnatal surfactant therapy.

Thyroid hormones

Rationale

Antenatal corticosteroids, while efficacious and safe, have not eliminated RDS, suggesting a role for other agents. Thyroid hormones contribute to lung maturation in fetal rabbits (Wu et al., 1973) and regulate surfactant metabolism in adult rats (Redding, Douglas & Stein, 1972). In animal models, surfactant production and morphological and functional fetal lung development are enhanced by intra-amniotic administration of thyroid hormones (Wu et al., 1973; Ballard et al., 1980; Korda et al., 1984) and retarded by thyroidectomy (Erenberg et al., 1979).

In human infants with RDS, reduced cord levels of T_3 and T_4 have been reported (Redding & Pereira, 1974), although the design of this study was not optimal (Klein et al., 1981). Next, T_4 was given intra-amniotically to eight women (Mashiach et al., 1978): none of their nine neonates developed RDS when delivered between 30–36 weeks. However, in a further uncontrolled study, intra-amniotic T_3 failed to prevent RDS in 7/15 infants, although their cord T_3 concentrations were not increased suggesting inadequate absorption (Schreyer et al., 1982).

Thyrotropin releasing hormone

Because T_3 and T_4 cross the placenta poorly (Grumbach & Werner, 1956), because intra-amniotic administration necessitates invasive procedures and because fetal absorption of intra-amniotic T_3 is unpredictable (Schreyer et al., 1982), clinical interest has focused on thyrotropin releasing hormone (TRH). This hormone crosses the placenta (Roti et al., 1981; Moya et al., 1986) and has been shown in human fetuses at term to stimulate the release of fetal TSH, T_3, and T_4, as well as prolactin. In the preterm human fetus, TSH has been shown to be elevated following maternal TRH (Thorpe-Beetson et al., 1991) although, unlike the ovine and primate fetus, prolactin levels did not increase (Roti et al., 1990). The effect of maternal TRH on lung maturation has been well documented in the fetal rabbit, comprising increased surfactant secretion (Rooney et al., 1979), improved lung compliance, decreased alveolar protein leaks (Ikegami et al., 1987*b*) and enhanced morphological and functional maturation (Devaskar et al., 1987). In contrast, no consistent fetal lung response has been shown in sheep (Liggins et al., 1988*b*; Ikegami et al., 1991), although in some studies a subtle improvement in pulmonary distensibility was seen (Warburton et al., 1988). There are no clinical trials of TRH usage in isolation, with which to evaluate its effect on human fetal lung.

Synergism with glucocorticoids

Synergistic effects shown in several species both in vitro and vivo include enhanced phosphatidylcholine synthesis (Ballard, Hovey & Gonzales, 1984; Gross et al., 1984), and accelerated morphological maturation (Hitchcock, 1979). The response with combined treatment is more than additive, being greater after 24 h stimulation with both hormones than after 72 h of corticosteroids alone (Ballard et al., 1984).

In contrast to the species difference in the effect of single thyroid agents, the addition of T_3 or TRH to glucocorticoids had minimal effect on lung compliance in preterm fetal rabbits (Ikegami et al., 1987*b*; El Kady & Jobe, 1988) but major effects in preterm lambs (Schellenberg et al., 1988). The synergistic effect in lambs of cortisol, T_3 and prolactin resulted in lung function equivalent to that of a term fetus, whereas treatment with either hormone singly had no effect (Schellenberg et al., 1988). Combined corticosteroid and TRH treatment in fetal lambs produced a fivefold increase in surfactant protein A compared with control or single hormone treatment (Ikegami et al., 1991).

Mechanism of action of glucocorticoid-thyroid hormones

The mechanism proposed for the effect of TRH on lung maturation is stimulation of the fetal pituitary–thyroid axis to release TSH which stimulates T_3 and T_4 production, and prolactin. However, this has recently been challenged by the finding that DN1417, a TRH analog which inhibits TSH and prolactin release, still produced lung maturation similar to TRH-treated rabbits (Devaskar, de Mello & Ackerman, 1991), the authors suggesting a neurotransmitter rather than a neuroendocrine role for TRH.

The mechanism of glucocorticoid-thyroid synergism involves differential action on different germ cell layers: glucocorticoids on mesenchyme, to induce fibroblast pneumocyte factor (FPF) production and thyroid hormone on epithelium, to increase the response to FPF and enhance production of phosphatidylcholine. The induction of FPF in lung fibroblasts by glucocorticoids is felt to make the lungs receptive to surfactant

(Smith & Post, 1989), and may explain synergism between antenatal corticosteroid therapy and postnatal surfactant (Ikegami et al., 1987*a*). The combination of corticosteroids, TRH and postnatal surfactant (Ikegami et al., 1987*b*) seems the most effective treatment, as assessed in rabbits by ventilatory measurements and air-space protein leak.

Clinical trials

Five trials of combined corticosteroids/TRH have now been reported, the first by Liggins et al. (1988*a*) in abstract form and subsequently abstract (Jikihara et al., 1990; Althabe et al., 1991) and journal format (Morales et al., 1989; Ballard et al., 1992). Their methodology was similar, that is, randomized, controlled trials in women prior to expected preterm delivery, receiving corticosteroids, and given 4–6 doses of 400 μg TRH at 24–31 weeks (Liggins et al., 1988*a*; Ballard et al., 1992), 23–29 weeks (Jikihara et al., 1990), <34 weeks (Morales et al., 1989), whereas Althabe et al. (1991) used two 200 μg doses of TRH at 26–31 weeks. Meta-analyses of the five trials (Crowther & Grant, 1992) (Fig. 13.5) confirms that combined treatment compared with steroids alone significantly reduced the need for oxygen (Althabe et al., 1991), the incidence of bronchopulmonary dysplasia (Morales et al., 1989; Althabe et al., 1991) and the need for oxygen therapy $\geq$28 days (Morales et al., 1989; Althabe et al., 1991; Ballard et al., 1992). RDS was less common in the TRH treated group in all four trials for which data are available (Morales et al., 1989; Jikihara et al., 1990; Althabe et al., 1991; Ballard et al., 1992). Further trials are likely to confirm an overall significant, rather than the presently marginal statistical reduction in RDS. Combined treatment has not been associated with reduction in hospital mortality. Maternal side-effects were noted in 31% of TRH treated mothers and lasted for less than 20 minutes (Morales et al., 1989); they included nausea, flushing and vomiting (Ballard et al., 1992) and palpitations (Morales et al., 1989; Jikihara et al., 1990) but no clinically significant rise in blood pressure (Ballard et al., 1992).

The necessity for multiple TRH doses has been questioned (Tabor et al., 1990), since a single dose in pregnant rabbits produces similar effects on surfactant and lung compliance as multiple doses.

Caution with the clinical use of TRH has been advised by some since the stimulatory effects of dexamethasone on antioxidant enzymes (Sosenko & Frank, 1987), fetal lung glycogen and fatty acid synthesis (Rooney, Gobran & Chu, 1986), are antagonized by combined therapy

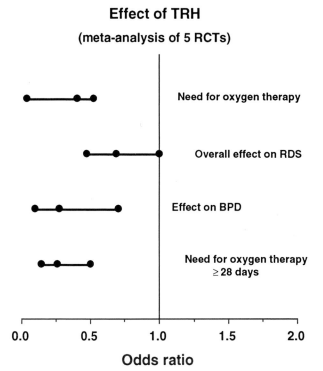

Effect of TRH

(meta-analysis of 5 RCTs)

Fig. 13.5. Graph of odds ratios with confidence intervals of the overall effect in randomized controlled trials of maternal TRH and glucocorticoid therapy compared to glucocorticoids alone. (After Crowther & Grant, 1992.)

with T_3, at least in the rat. Furthermore, the fetal response to repetitive doses of TRH has not been studied with regard to possible down-regulation of pituitary TRH receptors, which has been documented in adult rats (Banerji & Prasad, 1982). Further randomized, placebo-controlled trials of TRH are needed to provide more reliable evidence of efficacy, dosage regime and safety.

β *Adrenergic agonists*

In addition to stimulating surfactant release, β adrenergic agonists induce absorption of lung liquid (Walters & Olver, 1978; Brown et al., 1983; Warburton et al., 1987). The switch from secretion to absorption in the ovine fetal lung is normally activated by a rise in fetal plasma epinephrine, secondary to the stress of labour and delivery (Brown et al., 1983).

The maturation of this resorptive response to intravenous adrenaline increases twentyfold in the last 2 weeks of gestation (Brown et al., 1983) and can be prematurely induced by combined hydrocortisone/T3 treatment but not by either hormone alone (Barker et al., 1990). This effect may underlie the improvement in lung mechanics and tracheal phosphatidylcholine content found in fetal lambs when β agonists were added to corticosteroid and TRH infusion (Warburton et al.,1988).

The possible addition of β agonists to conventional treatments might be especially useful where delivery by Caesarean section is indicated in the absence of prior labour. There have as yet been no clinical trials of such therapy.

Other agents

Studies in animals have produced variable results for the methylxanthines, oestradiol, prolactin alone and insulin. In contrast, enhanced fetal lung maturation has been shown for the following: endogenous opioids, epidermal growth factor, prostaglandins, fibroblast pneumocyte factor and benzylamine, ambroxol (for review see Ballard, 1986; Rooney, 1985; Comer et al., 1987; Smith & Post, 1989; Moya & Gross, 1988). Epidermal growth factor is of potential clinical application, since it produces, in fetal monkeys, additional morphological effects on the lung parenchyma and conducting airways (Read & George-Nascimento, 1990), suggesting a secondary role in the prevention of chronic lung disease in preterm infants.

Strategies to facilitate neonatal resuscitation

Relief of lung compression

Aspiration of pleural effusions

In the presence of fetal hydrothoraces, thoracocentesis facilitates neonatal resuscitation if done within hours of delivery, and may be done in labour (Petres et al., 1982). Similarly, thoracocentesis has been performed prior to Caesarean section in hydropic fetuses (Schmidt, Harms & Wolf, 1985). Aspiration immediately after delivery should produce similar results, but relies on the premise that delivery be attended by adequately equipped and suitably trained staff. Aspiration just before, or during, labour avoids this uncertainty. Chronic drainage by shunting ensures preparedness for delivery at all times, but would not seem justified for this reason alone.

Aspiration of pulmonary cysts

Aspiration of large intrathoracic adenomatoid cysts would similarly be expected to facilitate lung expansion at birth.

Prevention of meconium aspiration syndrome
Pathogenesis

Meconium aspiration syndrome (MAS) is characterized by neonatal respiratory distress and a chest X-ray typical of aspiration, following meconium staining of the liquor (MSL). Whereas MSL is found relatively commonly, in over 14% of term pregnancies (Carson et al., 1976), MAS develops in only 2:1000 live births (Katz & Bowes, 1992) and respiratory distress without MAS (O_2 requirements for >6 hours) in 10 : 1 000 live births (Coughtery et al., 1991). Thus the vast majority of fetuses with MSL do not have perinatal problems, MSL being a physiological sign of fetal maturity. Suggested pathological stimuli to meconium passage include vagal activation secondary to cord compression or peristalsis and sphincter relaxation secondary to fetal hypoxaemia (Miller et al., 1975).

Although the pathogenesis of MAS has historically been largely attributed to chemical pneumonitis, there is now considerable evidence implicating mechanical, biochemical and vascular mechanisms (Katz & Bowes, 1992). In addition to inflammation, airway obstruction by meconium leads to air trapping, atelectasis and ventilation-perfusion defects. Meconium inhibits surfactant, further contributing to alveolar instability (Chen, Toung & Rogers, 1985; Clark et al., 1987; Moses et al., 1991). The chief aetiological agent, however, is asphyxia, which explains the high frequency of pulmonary vasospasm and hypertension in MAS (Hutchison & Russell, 1976). In non-acidaemic fetuses, little if any amniotic fluid enters the lungs (Adams, Desilets & Towers, 1967; Block et al., 1981; Harding, Bocking & Sigger, 1986). Fetal acidaemia causes gasping in both animal (Adams et al., 1967; Block et al., 1981) and human (Starks, 1980; Mitchell et al., 1985) studies and is necessary for aspiration of meconium into the fetal lungs. However, isolated, asphyxial gasping moves little fluid into the fetal lungs, whereas periods of rhythmical breathing of normal amplitude, associated with prolonged hypoxia, result in the ingress of large quantities of amniotic fluid (Hooper & Harding, 1990). This asphyxial prerequisite for MAS may explain why MAS is largely confined to those with thick as opposed to thin MSL (Benny et al., 1987; Rossi et al., 1989; Coughtery et al., 1991). The consistency of MSL is largely a bioassay of the amniotic fluid volume in which it is diluted (Barham, 1969). Thick meconium is therefore simply a marker for underlying oligohydramnios, which in turn is closely associated with intrapartum fetal distress (Sarno et al., 1989; Robson et al., 1992), either because oligohydramnios indicates a fetus with pre-existing compromise (Nicolaides et al., 1990) or because oligohydramnios predisposes to cord compression in labour (Gabbe et al., 1976; Moberg, Garite & Freeman, 1984).

For the past three decades, postnatal strategies have focused on preventing and/or reducing the quantity of meconium believed to be inhaled at birth (Gregory et al., 1974; Carson et al., 1976). Despite adequate neonatal resuscitation however, MAS still occurs (Davis et al., 1985; Dooley et al., 1985; Falciglia, 1988) and has been documented in stillborn infants who have never breathed air (Brown & Gleicher, 1981; Byrne & Gau, 1987). Antenatal prevention seems a more appropriate strategy.

Antepartum prevention of asphyxia

As oligohydramnios appears a sensitive index of chronic fetal compromise (Chamberlain et al., 1984; Nicolaides et al., 1990), semi-quantitative indices of amniotic fluid volume (deepest pool, amniotic fluid index) are increasingly used in fetal monitoring in late pregnancy (Chamberlain et al., 1984; Phelan et al., 1987). The combination of Doppler studies and amniotic fluid volume appears a more accurate predictor of adverse perinatal outcome than conventional monitoring (non-stress testing and fetal movement counting) (Tyrrell et al., 1990; Pearce & McParland, 1991), being associated with a reduction in perinatal morbidity in one randomized trial (Tyrrell et al., 1990). Monitoring amniotic fluid volume may allow identification of at-risk pregnancies earlier in the disease process, better obstetric decision-making and a reduction in the incidence of antepartum or intrapartum fetal acidaemia.

Intrapartum prevention of meconium staining of liquor

One intrapartum strategy to reduce the incidence of MSL is amnioinfusion, which corrects oligohydramnios (Owen, Henson & Hauth, 1990; Strong, Hetzler & Paul, 1990b). In randomized studies of women with variable decelerations and/or premature rupture of the membranes, transcervical intrapartum amnioinfusion has been shown to normalize fetal heart rate patterns and improve cord PH at delivery (Miyazaki & Nevarez, 1985; Nageotte et al., 1985). Similarly, Strong et al. (1990*a*) randomized 60 women with oligohydramnios to find significantly lower rates of MSL in the amnio-infusion group, in addition to less frequent variable decelerations, end-stage bradycardia and operative delivery for fetal distress. The mechanism for this is unclear but may involve the prevention of excessive cord compression associated with uterine contractions, improved utero-placental perfusion or both.

Intrapartum prevention of asphyxia

The prevention of asphyxia during labour is based on standard obstetric management employing continuous fetal heart rate monitoring and scalp PH measurements. Fetal blood sampling is indicated on admission or in early labour in women with thick MSL, 15% (15/101) of whom will have a scalp PH < 7.25, compared to none (0/76) with thin MSL (Starks, 1980). In the presence of MSL, operative delivery has been recommended if the scalp PH is < 7.25 (Mitchell et al., 1985).

In women with pre-existing MSL, amnioinfusion appears also to have a role. In four randomized control trials, amnioinfusion reduced the incidence of both MAS and meconium below the vocal cords. Operative delivery for fetal distress was also reduced and fetal condition at birth improved (Wenstrom & Parsons, 1989; Adam et al., 1989; for review see Hofmeyer, 1992, see Fig. 13.6; Sadovsky et al., 1989; Macri et al., 1991).

Utility of preventive strategies

The failure of the above strategies to prevent all cases of MAS suggests that attributing MAS to asphyxia in the presence of MSL may be an oversimplification. Recent evidence suggests that neonates who develop respiratory distress in association with MSL, differ from healthy newborns. Coughtery et al. (1991) found a high incidence (74%) compared with other term infants (<5%) of histological chorioamnionitis, which could not be attributed to MSL's chemical effect, but rather to amniotic fluid infection. Further, their reduced skinfold thickness indicative of relative malnutrition (Coughtery et al., 1991) may well be a reflection of the underlying aetiology for oligohydramnios. Murphy, Vawter and Reed (1984), in reporting abnormal muscularization of small intra-acinar arteries in infants with fatal MAS, suggested that persistent pulmonary

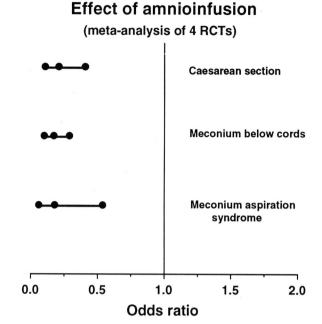

Fig. 13.6. Graph of odds ratios with confidence intervals of the overall effect in randomized controlled trials of intrapartum amnioinfusion in pregnancies with meconium stained liquor. (After Hofmeyer, 1992.)

hypertension in MAS may be the result of a structurally abnormal pulmonary circulation. Both studies thus suggest that new-borns with MAS are not entirely normal before birth or indeed before the onset of labour.

Conclusions

Antenatal strategies may improve neonatal pulmonary function in a variety of pathologies by promoting lung growth, lung maturation or lung expansion at birth. Despite encouraging animal data, experience with procedures to promote lung growth either by relieving lung compression or restoring amniotic fluid volume, is limited in human pregnancy and as yet no controlled data exist documenting any benefit. In contrast, randomized controlled trials indicate a clear role for maternal gluco-corticoid therapy in reducing the incidence and sequelae of RDS in preterm neonates. Recent clinical trials suggest a further role for TRH in combination with glucocorticoids. Prevention of fetal acidaemia is the most important strategy in reducing the incidence of meconium aspiration syndrome, in which a role is emerging for intrapartum amnioinfusion.

References

Adam, K., Cano, L. & Moise, K. J. (1989). The effect of intrapartum amnioinfusion on the outcome of the fetus with heavy meconium stained amniotic fluid. In *Proceedings of the 9th Annual Meeting of the Society of Perinatal Obstetricians*, New Orleans, Louisiana USA, Abstract 438.

Adams, F. H., Desilets, D. T. & Towers, B. (1967). Control of flow of fetal lung fluid at the laryngeal outlet. *Respiration Physiology*, **2**, 302–9.

Adzick, N. S., Harrison, M. R., Glick, P. L., Golbus, M. S. et al. (1985*a*). Fetal cystic adenomatoid malformation: prenatal diagnosis and natural history. *Journal of Pediatric Surgery*, **20**, 483–8.

Adzick, N. S., Harrison, M. R., Glick, P. L., Nakayama, D. K. & Manning, F. A. (1985*b*). Diaphragmatic hernia in the fetus: prenatal diagnosis and outcome in 94 cases. *Journal of Pediatric Surgery*, **20**, 357–61.

Adzick, N. S., Harrison, M. R., Glick, P. L. et al. (1986). Fetal surgery in the primate. III. Maternal outcome after fetal surgery. *Journal of Pediatric Surgery*, **21**, 477–80.

Adzick, N. S., Harrison, M. R., Glick, P. L., Villa, R. L. & Finkbeiner, W. (1984). Experimental pulmonary hypoplasia and oligohydramnios: relative contributions of lung fluid and fetal breathing movements. *Journal of Pediatric Surgery*, **19**, 658–65.

Althabe, F., Fustianana, C., Althabe, O. & Ceriani-Cernadas, J. M. (1991). Controlled trial of prenatal betamethasone plus TRH vs betamethasone plus placebo for prevention of RDS in preterm infants. *Pediatric Research*, **29**, 200A.

Avery, M. E. (1984). The argument for prenatal administration of dexamethasone to prevent respiratory distress syndrome. *Journal of Pediatrics*, **104**, 240.

Avery, M. E. & Merritt, T. A. (1991). Surfactant- replacement therapy. *New England Journal of Medicine*, **324**, 910–12.

Ballard, P. L. (1986). Glucocorticoid effects in vivo. In *Hormones and Lung Maturation (Monographs in Endocrinology; 28)*, ed. P. L. Ballard. pp. 56–82. Springer-Verlag: New York.

Ballard, P. L. (1989). Hormonal regulation of pulmonary surfactant. *Endocrine Reviews*, **10**, 165–81.

Ballard, R. A., Ballard, P. L., Creasy, R. K. et al. (1992). Respiratory disease in very low birthweight infants after prenatal thyrotropin releasing hormone and glucocorticoid. *Lancet*, **339**, 510–15.

Ballard, P. L., Benson, B. J., Brehier, A., & Carter, J. P. (1980). Transplacental stimulation of lung development in the fetal rabbit by 3,5-dimethyl–3-isopropyl-L- thyronine. *Journal of Clinical Investigation*, **65**, 1407–17.

Ballard, P. L., Hovey, M. L. & Gonzales, L. K. (1984). Thyroid hormone stimulation of phosphatidylcholine synthesis in cultured fetal rabbit lung. *Journal of Clinical Investigation*, **74**, 898–905.

Banerji, A. & Prasad, C. (1982). In vivo autoregulation of rat adenohypophyseal thyrotropin-releasing hormone receptor. *Life Sciences*, **30**, 2293–9.

Barham, K A. (1969). Amnioscopy, meconium and fetal well-being. *Journal of Obstetrics and Gynaecology of the British Commonwealth*, **176**, 412–18.

Barker, P. M., Markiewicz, M., Parker, K. A., Walters, D. V. & Strang, L. B. (1990). Synergistic action of triiodothyronine and hydrocortisone on epinephrine-induced reabsorption of fetal lung liquid. *Pediatric Research*, **27**, 588–91.

Baumgarten, K. & Moser, S. (1986). The technique of fibrin adhesion for premature rupture of the membranes during pregnancy. *Journal of Perinatal Medicine*, **14**, 43–9.

Benacerraf, B. R. & Frigoletto, F. D. (1985). Mid-trimester fetal thoracocentesis. *Journal of Clinical Ultrasound*, **13**, 202–4.

Benny, P. S., Malani, S., Hoby, M. A. & Hutton, J. D. (1987). Meconium aspiration: role of obstetric factors and suction. *Australian and New Zealand Journal of Obstetrics and Gynaecology*, **27**, 36–9.

Bent, A. E., Gray, J. H., Luther, E. R., Oulton, M. & Peddle, L. J. (1981). Phosphatidylglycerol determination on amniotic fluid 10, 000 x g pellet in the prediction of fetal lung maturity. *American Journal of Obstetrics and Gynaecology*, **139**, 259–63.

Bhutani, V. K., Abbashi, S. & Weiner, S. (1986). Neonatal pulmonary manifestations due to prolonged amniotic leak. *American Journal of Perinatology*, **3**, 225–30.

Block, M. F., Kallenberger, D. A., Kern, J. D. & Nepveaux, D. (1981). In utero meconium aspiration by the baboon fetus. *Obstetrics and Gynecology*, **57**, 37–40.

Blott, M., Nicolaides, K. H. & Greenough, A. (1988). Pleuro-amniotic shunting for decompression of fetal pleural effusions. *Obstetrics and Gynecology*, **71**, 798–800.

Brown, B. L. & Gleicher, N. (1981). Intrauterine meconium aspiration. *Obstetrics and Gynecology*, **57**, 26–9.

Brown, L. M. & Duck-Chong, C. G. (1982). Methods of evaluating fetal lung maturity. *CRC Critical Reviews in Clinical Laboratory Sciences*, 85–145.

Brown, M. J., Olver, R. E., Ramsden, C. A., Strang, L. B. & Walters, D. V. (1983). Effects of adrenaline and of spontaneous labour on the secretion and absorption of lung liquid in the fetal lamb. *Journal of Physiology*, **344**, 137–52.

Burri, P. H. (1984). Fetal and postnatal development of the lung. *Annual Review of Physiology*, **46**, R617–628.

Byrne, D. L. & Gau, G. (1987). In utero meconium aspiration: an unpreventable cause of neonatal death. *British Journal of Obstetrics and Gynaecology*, **94**, 813–14.

Campanale, R. P. & Rowland, R. H. (1955). Hypoplasia of the lung associated with congenital diaphragmatic hernia. *Annals of Surgery*, **142**, 176–9.

Carson, B. S., Losey, R. W., Bowes, W. A. & Simmons, M. A. (1976). Combined obstetric and pediatric approach to prevent meconium aspiration syndrome. *American Journal of Obstetrics and Gynecology*, **126**, 712–15.

Chamberlain, P. F., Manning, F. A., Morrison, I., Harman, C. R. & Lange, I. R. (1984). Ultrasound evaluation of amniotic fluid volume I.

The relationship of marginal and decreased amniotic fluid volumes to perinatal outcome. *American Journal of Obstetrics and Gynecology*, **150**, 245–49.

Chen, C. T., Toung, T. J. K. & Rogers, M. C. (1985). Effect of intra-alveolar meconium on pulmonary surface tension properties. *Critical Care Medicine*, **13**, 233–6.

Cheng, J. B., Goldfien, A., Ballard, P. L. & Roberts, J. M. (1980). Glucocorticoids increase pulmonary beta-adrenergic receptors in fetal rabbit. *Endocrinology*, **107**, 5, 1646–8.

Clark, D. A., Nieman, G. F., Thompson, J. E., Paskanik, A. M., Rokhar, J. E. & Bredenberg, C. E. (1987). Surfactant displacement by meconium free fatty acids: An alternative explanation for atelectasis in meconium aspiration syndrome. *Journal of Pediatrics*, **110**, 765–70.

Clark, S. L., Vitale, D. J., Minton, S. D., Stoddard, R. A. & Sabey, P. L. (1987). Successful fetal therapy for cystic adenomatoid malformation associated with second-trimester hydrops. *American Journal of Obstetrics and Gynecology*, **157**, 294–5.

Collaborative Group on Antenatal Steroid Therapy (1981). Effect of antenatal dexamethasone administration on the prevention of respiratory distress syndrome. *American Journal of Obstetrics and Gynecology*, **141**, 276–87.

Collaborative Group on Antenatal Steroid Therapy (1984). Effects of antenatal dexamethasone administration in the infant: long-term follow-up. *Journal of Pediatrics*, **104**, 259–67.

Comer, C. R., Grunstein, J. S., Mason, R. J., Johnston, S. C. & Grunstein, M. M. (1987). Endogenous opioids modulate fetal rabbit lung maturation. *Journal of Applied Physiology*, **62**, 2141–6.

Cosmi, E. V. & Di Renzo, G. C (1989). Assesment of foetal lung maturity. *European Respiratory Journal*, **2**, 40–9.

Coughtrey, H., Jeffery, H. E., Henderson-Smart, D. J., Storey, B. & Poulos, V. (1991). Possible causes linking asphyxia, thick meconium and respiratory distress. *Australian and New Zealand Journal of Obstetrics and Gynaecology*, **31**, 97–102.

Crowley, P. (1992*a*). Corticosteroids and preterm labour. In *Oxford Database of Perinatal Trials*, ed. I. Chalmers, Version 1. 3, Disk Issue 7, 1992, Record 6871. Oxford University Press, Oxford.

Crowley, P. (1992*b*). Corticosteroids after preterm prelabour rupture of membranes. In *Oxford Database of Perinatal Trials*, ed. I. Chalmers. Version 1. 3, Disk Issue 7, 1992, Record 4395. Oxford University Press, Oxford.

Crowther, C. A. & Grant, A. M. (1992). Antenatal thyrotropin-releasing hormone prior to preterm delivery. In *Oxford Database of Perinatal Trials*, Version 1. 2, Disk Issue 8, 1992, Record 4749. ed. I. Chalmers. Oxford University Press, Oxford.

Davis, R. O., Philips, J. B., Harris, B. A., Wilson, E. R. & Huddleston, J. F. (1985). Fatal meconium aspiration occurring despite airway management considered appropriate. *American Journal of Obstetrics and Gynecology*, **151**, 731–6.

Destro, F., Calcagnile, F. & Ceccarello, P. (1985). Placental grade and pulmonary maturity in premature fetuses. *Journal of Clinical Ultrasound*, **13**, 637–9.

Devaskar, U., Nitta, K., Szewczyk, K., Sadiq, H. F. & de Mello, D. (1987). Transplacental stimulation of functional and morphologic fetal rabbit lung maturation: Effect of thyrotropin-releasing hormone. *American Journal of Obstetrics and Gynecology*, **157**, 460–4.

Devaskar, U. P., de Mello, D. E. & Ackerman, J. (1991). Effect of maternal administration of thyrotropin-releasing hormone or DN1417 on functional and morphological fetal rabbit lung maturation and duration of survival after premature delivery. *Biology of the Neonate*, **59**, 346–51.

Dickson, K. A. & Harding, R. (1989). Decline in lung liquid volume and secretion rate during oligohydramnios in fetal sheep. *Journal of Applied Physiology*, **67**, 2401–7.

Dickson, K. A. & Harding, R. (1991). Fetal breathing and pressures in the trachea and amniotic sac during oligohydramnios in sheep. *Journal of Applied Physiology*, **70**, 293–9.

Dooley, S. L., Pesavento, D. J., Depp, R., Socol, M. L., Tamura, R. K. & Wiringa, K. S. (1985). Meconium below the vocal cords at delivery: Correlation with intrapartum events. *American Journal of Obstetrics and Gynecology*, **153**, 767–70.

Dornan, J. C., Ritchie, J. W. K. & Meban, C. (1984). Fetal breathing movements and lung maturation in the congenitally abnormal human fetus. *Journal of Developmental Physiology*, **6**, 367–75.

Elder, J. S., Duckett, J. W. & Snyder, H. M. (1987). Intervention for fetal obstructive uropathy. Has it been effective? *Lancet*, **ii**, 1007–10.

El Kady, T. & Jobe, A. (1988). Maternal treatments with corticosteroids and/or T_3 change lung volumes and rupture pressures in preterm rabbits. *Biology of the Neonate*, **54**, 203–10.

Erenberg, A., Rhodes, M. L., Weinstein, M. M. & Kennedy, R. L. (1979). The effect of fetal thyroidectomy on ovine fetal lung maturation. *Pediatric Research*, **13**, 230–5.

Evans, M. I., Sacks, A. J., Johnson, M. P., Robichaux, A. G. & Moghissi, M. M. (1991). Sequential invasive assessment of fetal renal function and the intrauterine treatment of fetal obstructive uropathies. *Obstetrics and Gynecology*, **77**, 545–50.

Falciglia, H. (1988). Failure to prevent meconium aspiration syndrome. *Obstetrics and Gynecology*, **71**, 349–53.

Farrell, E. E., Silver, R. K., Kimberlin L. V., Wolf, E. S. & Dusik, J. M. (1989). Impact of antenatal dexasmethasone administration on respiratory distress syndrome in surfactant-treated infants. *American Journal of Obstetrics and Gynecology*, **161**, 628–33.

Fiascone, J. M., Jacobs, H. C., Moya, F. R., Mercurio, M. R. & Lima, D. M. (1987). Betamethasone increases pulmonary compliance in part by surfactant-independent mechanisms in preterm rabbits. *Pediatric Research*, **22**, 730–5.

Fisk, N. M. (1992). Oligohydramnios-related pulmonary hypoplasia. *Contemporary Reviews in Obstetrics and Gynaecology*, **4**, 191–201.

Fisk, N. M., Ronderos-Dumit, D., Soliani, A., Nicolini, U., Vaughan, J. & Rodeck, C. H. (1991). Diagnostic and therapeutic transabdominal amnioinfusion in oligohydramnios. *Obstetrics and Gynecology*, **78**, 270–8.

Fisk, N. M., Talbert, D. G., Nicolini, U., Vaughan, J. & Rodeck, C. H. (1992). Fetal breathing movements in oligohydramnios are not altered by amnioinfusion. *British Journal of Obstetrics and Gynaecology*, **99**, 464–8.

Frank, L., Lewis, P. L. & Sosenko, I. R. S. (1985). Dexamethasone stimulation of fetal rat lung antioxidant enzyme activity in parallel with surfactant stimulation. *Pediatrics*, **75**, 569–74.

Gabbe, S. G., Ettinger, B. B., Freeman, R. K. & Martin, C. B. (1976). Umbilical cord compression associated with amniotomy; laboratory observations. *American Journal of Obstetrics and Gynecology*, **126**, 353–5.

Gamsu, H. R., Mullinger, B. M., Donnai, P. & Dash, C. H. (1989). Antenatal administration of betamethasone to prevent respiratory distress syndrome in preterm infants: report of a UK multicentre trial. *British Journal of Obstetrics and Gynaecology*, **96**, 401–10.

Garite, T. J., Rumney, P., Harding, J. & Briggs, G. (1991). A randomized controlled trial of betamethasone in the prevention of RDS at 24–28 weeks. *American Journal of Obstetrics and Gynecology*, **164**, 375.

Gembruch, U. & Hansmann, M. (1988). Artificial instillation of amniotic fluid as a new technique for the diagnostic evaluation of cases of oligohydramnios. *Prenatal Diagnosis*, **8**, 33–45.

Glick, P. L., Harrison, M. R., Adzick, N. S., Noall, R. A. & Villa, R. L. (1984). Correction of congenital hydronephrosis in utero. IV. In utero decompression prevents renal dysplasia. *Journal of Pediatric Surgery*, **19**, 649–57.

Glick, P. L., Harrison, M. R., Golbus, M. S. et al. (1985). Management of the fetus with congenital hydronephrosis II: Prognostic criteria and selection for treatment. *Journal of Pediatric Surgery*, **20**, 376–87.

Gluck, L., Kulovich, M., Borer, R., Brenner, P. H., Anderson, G. G. & Spellacy, W. N. (1971). Diagnosis of the respiratory distrss syndrome by amniocentesis. *American Journal of Obstetrics and Gynecology*, **109**, 440–5.

Golbus, M. S., Harrison, M. R., Filly, R. A., Callen, P. W. & Katz, M. (1982). In utero treatment of urinary tract obstruction. *American Journal of Obstetrics and Gynecology*, **142**, 383–8.

Gonzales, L. W., Ertsey, R., Ballard, P. L., Froh, D., Geoerke, J. & Gonzales, J. (1990). Glucocorticoid stimulation of fatty acid synthesis in explants of human fetal lung. *Biochimica et Biophysica Acta*, **1042**, 1–12.

Grannum, P. A. T., Berkowitz, K. L. & Hobbins, J. C. (1979). The ultrasonic changes in the maturing placenta and their relation to fetal pulmonic maturity. *American Journal of Obstetrics and Gynecology*, **133**, 915–22.

Gregory, G. A., Gooding, C. A., Phibbs, R. H. & Tooley, W. (1974). Meconium aspiration in infants – a prospective study. *Journal of Pediatrics*, **85**, 848–52.

Gross, I., Dynia, D. W., Wilson, C. M., Ingleson, L. D., Gewolb, I. H. & Rooney, S. A. (1984). Glucocorticoid–thyroid hormone interactions in fetal rat lung. *Pediatric Research*, **18**, 191–6.

Grumbach, M. M. & Werner, S. C. (1956). Transfer of thyroid hormone across the human placenta at term. *Journal of Clinical Endocrinology*, **16**, 1392–5.

Hallman, M., Kulovich, M., Kirkpatrick, E., Sugarman, R. G. & Gluck, L. (1976). Phosphatidylinositol and phosphatidylglycerol in amniotic fluid: indices of lung maturity. *American Journal of Obstetrics and Gynecology*, **125**, 613–17.

Hamilton, P. R., Hauschild, D., Broekhuizen, F. F. & Beck, R. M. (1984). Comparison of lecithin:sphingoyelin ratio, fluorescence polarisation, and phosphatidylglycerol in the amniotic fluid in the prediction of respiratory distress syndrome. *Obstetrics and Gynecology*, **63**, 52–6.

Harding, R., Bocking A. D. & Sigger, J. N. (1986). Influence of upper respiratory tract on liquid flow to and from fetal lungs. *Journal of Applied Physiology*, **61**, 68–74.

Harding, R., Hooper, S. B. & Dickson, K. A. (1990). A mechanism leading to reduced lung expansion and lung hypoplasia in fetal sheep during oligohydramnios. *American Journal of Obstetrics and Gynecology*, **163**, 1904–13.

Harrison, M. R., Adzick, N. S., Jennings, R. W. et al. (1990*c*). Antenatal intervention for congenital cystic malformation. *Lancet*, **336**: 965–7.

Harrison, M. R., Adzick, N. S., Longaker, M. T. et al. (1990*b*). Successful repair in utero of a fetal diphragmatic hernia after removal of herniated viscera from the left thorax. *New England Journal of Medicine*, **322**, 1582–4.

Harrison, M. R., Golbus, M. S., Filly, R. A. et al. (1987). Fetal hydronephrosis: selection and surgical repair. *Journal of Pediatric Surgery*, **22**, 556–8.

Harrison, M. R., Golbus, M., Filly, R. A. et al. (1982*b*). Management of the fetus with congenital hydronephrosis. *Journal of Pediatric Surgery*, **17**, 728–42.

Harrison, M. R., Jester, J. A. & Ross, N. A. (1980). Correction of congenital diaphragmatic hernia in utero. I. The model: intrathoracic balloon produces fetal pulmonary hypoplasia. *Surgery*, **88**, 174–82.

Harrison, M. R., Langer, J. C., Adzick, N. S. et al. (1990*a*). Correction of congenital diaphragmatic hernia in utero. V: Initial clinical experience. *Journal of Pediatric Surgery*, **25**, 47–57.

Harrison, M. R., Nakayama, D. K., Noall, R. & de Lorimier, A. A. (1982a). Correction of congenital hydronephrosis in utero II: decompression reverses the effects of obstruction on the fetal lung and urinary tract. *Journal of Pediatric Surgery*, **17**, 965–74.

Harrison, M. R., Ross, N. A. & de Lorimier A. A. (1981). Correction of congenital diaphragmatic hernia in utero. III. Development of a successful surgical technique using abdominoplasty to avoid compromise of umbilical blood flow. *Journal of Pediatric Surgery*, **16**, 934–42.

Hawgood, S. & Clements, J. A. (1990). Pulmonary surfactant and its apoproteins. *Journal of Clinical Investigation*, **86**, 1–6.

Hennes, H. M., Lee, M. B., Rimm, A. A. & Shapiro, D. L. (1991). Surfactant replacement therapy in respiratory distress syndrome. *American Journal of Diseases of Children*, **145**, 102–4.

Hepworth, W. B., Seegmiller, R. E. & Carey, J. C. (1990). Thoracic volume reduction as a mechanism for pulmonary hypoplasia in chondrodystrophic mice. *Pediatric Pathology*, **10**, 919–29.

Herbert, W. N. P. & Chapman, J. F. (1986). Clinical and economic considerations associated with testing for fetal lung maturity. *American Journal of Obstetrics and Gynecology*, **155**, 820–2.

Hislop, A., Hey, E. & Reid, L. (1979). The lungs in congenital bilateral renal agenesis and dysplasia. *Archives of Disease in Childhood*, **54**, 32–8.

Hitchcock, K. R. (1979). Hormones and the lung. 1. Thyroid hormones and glucocorticoids in lung development. *Anatomical Record*, **194**, 15–40.

Hjalmarson, O. (1981). Epidemiology and classification of acute, neonatal respiratory disorders. *Acta Paediatrica Scandinavica*, **70**, 773–783.

Hofmeyer, G. J. (1992). Amnioinfusion for meconium-stained liquor in labour. In *Oxford Database of Perinatal Trials*, ed. I. Chalmers. Version 1. 2 Disk issue 7, Record 5379, Oxford University Press, Oxford.

Holm, B. A., Enhorning, G. & Notter, R. H. (1988). A biophysical mechanism by which plasma proteins inhibit lung surfactant activity. *Chemistry and Physics of Lipids*, **49**, 49–55.

Hooper, S. B. & Harding, R. (1990). Changes in lung liquid dynamics induced by prolonged fetal hypoxaemia. *Journal of Applied Physiology*, **69**, 127–35.

Howie, R. N. & Liggins, G. C. (1982). The New Zealand study of antepartum glucocorticoid treatment in lung development. In *Lung Development: Biological and Clinical Perspectives*, Vol 2, ed. P. M. Farrell, pp. 255–265. Academic Press, New York.

Hutchison, A. A. & Russell, G. (1976). Effective pulmonary capillary blood flow in infants with birth asphyxia. *Acta Paediatrica Scandinavica*, **65**, 669–72.

Ikegami, M., Berry, D., El Kady, T., Pettenazzo, A., Seidner, S. & Jobe, A. (1987*a*). Corticosteroids and surfactant change lung function and protein leaks in the lungs of ventilated premature rabbits. *Journal of Clinical Investigation*, **79**, 1371–8.

Ikegami, M., Jobe, A. H., Pettenazzo, A., Seidner, S. R., Berry, D. D. & Ruffini, L. (1987*b*). Effects of maternal treatment with corticosteroids, T$_3$, TRH, and their combinations on lung function of ventilated preterm rabbits with and without surfactant treatments. *American Review of Respiratory Diseases*, **136**, 892–8.

Ikegami, M., Jobe, A. H., Yamada, T. & Seidner, S. (1989*a*). Relationship between alveolar saturated phosphatidyldoline pool sizes and compliance of preterm rabbit lungs. *American Review of Respiratory Disease*, **139**, 367–9.

Ikegami, M., Jobe, A. H., Seidner, S., & Yamada, T. (1989*b*). Gestation effects of corticosteroids and surfactant in ventilated rabbits. *Pediatric Research*, **25**, 32–7.

Ikegami, M., Polk, D., Tabor, B., Lewis, J., Yamada, T. & Jobe, A. (1991). Corticosteroid and thyrotropin-releasing hormone effects on preterm sheep lung function. *Journal of Applied Physiology*, **70**, 2268–78.

Imanaka, M., Ogita, S. & Sugawa, T. (1989). Saline solution amnioinfusion for oligohydramnios after premature rupture of the membranes. *American Journal of Obstetrics and Gynecology*, **161**, 102–6.

Iritani, I. (1984). Experimental study on embryogenesis of congenital diaphragmatic hernia. *Anatomy and Embryology*, **169**, 133–9.

Jackson, J. C., Mackenzie, A. P., Chi, E. Y. & Standaert, T. A. (1990). Mechanisms for reduced total lung capacity at birth and during hyaline membrane disease in premature newborn monkeys. *American Review of Respiratory Distress*, **142**, 413–19.

James, D. K., Tindall, V. R. & Richardson, T. (1983). Is the lecithin/spingomyelin ratio outdated? *British Journal of Obstetrics and Gynaecology*, **90**, 995–1 000.

Jikihara, H., Sawade, Y., Imai, S. et al. (1990). Maternal administration of thyrotropin-releasing hormone for prevention of neonatal respiratory distress syndrome. In *Proceedings of the 6th Congress of Federation of Asia and Oceania Perinatal Society, Perth, 1990*.

Reprinted in Oxford Database of Perinatal Trials, ed. I. Chalmers. Version 1. 2, Disk Issue 8, 1992,. Record 5912, Oxford University Press, Oxford.

Katz, V. L. & Bowes, W. A. (1992). Meconium aspiration syndrome: reflections on a murky subject. *American Journal of Obstetrics and Gynecology*, **166**, 171–83.

Kazzi, G. M., Gross, T. L., Rosen, M. G. & Jaatoul-Kazzi, N. Y. (1984). The relationship of placental grade, fetal lung maturity, and neonatal outcome in normal and complicated pregancies. *American Journal of Obstetrics and Gynecology*, **148**, 54–8.

Klein, A. H., Foley, B., Foley, T. P., Macdonald, H. M. & Fisher, D. A. (1981). Thyroid function studies in cord blood from premature infants with and without RDS. *Journal of Pediatrics*, **98**, 818–20.

Kogon, D. P., Oulton, M., Gray, J. H. et al. (1986). Amniotic fluid phosphatidylglycerol and phosphatidylcholine phosphorus as predictors of fetal lung maturity. *American Journal of Obstetrics & Gynecology*, **154**, 226–30.

Korda, A. R., Fleming, S. F., Senior, C. et al. (1984). The effect of intra-amniotic injection of triiodothyronine on pulmonary maturity in lambs at 130 days gestation. *Pediatric Research*, **18**, 932–5.

Kwong, M. S. & Egan, E. A. (1986). Reduced incidence of hyaline membrane disease in extremely premature infants following delay of delivery in mother with preterm labor: use of ritodrine and betamethasone. *Pediatrics*, **78**, 767–74.

Kwong, M. S., Egan, E. & Notter, R. (1987). Synergistic response of antenatal bethamethasone and tracheal instillation of calf lung surfactant extract (CLSE) at birth. *Paediatric Research*, **21**, 458A.

Leonidas, J. C., Bahn, I. & Beatty, E. C. (1982). Radiographic chest contour and pulmonary air leaks in oligohydramnios related pulmonary hypoplasia. *Investigative Radiology*, **17**, 6–10.

Liggins, G. C. (1969) Premature delivery of foetal lambs infused with glucocorticoids. *Journal of Endocrinology,* **45**, 515–23.

Liggins, G. C. & Howie, R. N. (1972). A controlled trial of antepartum glucocorticoid treatment for prevention of the respiratory distress syndrome in premature infants. *Pediatrics*, **50**, 515–25.

Liggins, G. C., Knight, D. B., Wealthall, S. R., & Howie, R. N. (1988*a*). A randomized, double-blind trial of antepartum TRH and steroids in the prevention of neonatal respiratory disease. In *Clinical Reproductive Medicine – The Liggins Years*, Auckland, New Zealand, July, 1988.

Liggins, G. C., Schellenberg, J., Manzai, M., Kitterman, J. A. & Lee, C. H. (1988*b*). Synergism of cortisol and thyrotropinc-releasing hormone in lung maturation in fetal sheep. *Journal of Applied Physiology*, **65**, 1880–4.

Longaker, M. T., Laberge, J. M., Dansareau, J. et al. (1989*a*). Primary fetal hydrothorax: natural history and management. *Journal of Pediatric Surgery*, **24**, 573–6.

Longaker, M. T., Adzick, N. S. & Harrison, M. R. (1989*b*). Fetal obstructive uropathy. *British Medical Journal*, **299**, 325–6.

MacArthur, B. A., Howie, R. N., Dezoete J. A. & Elkins, J. (1981). Cognitive and psychosocial development of four-year-old children whose mothers were treated antenatally with betamethasone. *Pediatrics*, **68**, 638–43.

MacArthur, B. A., Howie, R. N., Dezoete, J. A. & Elkins, J. (1982). School progress and cognitive development of 6-year-old children whose mothers were treated antenatally with betamethasone. *Pediatrics*, **70**, 99–105.

Macri, C. J., Schrimmer, D. B., Leung, A., Greenspoon, J. S. & Paul, R. H. (1991). Amnioinfusion improves outcome in labor complicated by meconium and oligohydramnios. *American Journal of Obstetrics and Gynecology*, **164**, Suppl., 252.

Manning, F. A., Harman, C. R., Lange, I. R., Brown, R., Deter, A. & MacDonald, N. (1983). Antepartum chronic fetal vesicoamniotic shunts for obstructive uropathy: a report of two cases. *American Journal of Obstetrics and Gynecology*, **145**, 819–22.

Manning, F. A., Harrison, M. R., Rodeck, C. H. & members of the International Fetal Medicine and Surgery Society. (1986). Catheter shunts for fetal hydronephrosis and hydrocephalus. *New England Journal of Medicine*, **315**, 336–40.

Mashiach, S., Barkai, G., Sack, J. et al. (1978). Enhancement of fetal lung maturity by intra-amniotic administration of thyroid hormone. *American Journal of Obstetrics and Gynecology*, **130**, 289–93.

Miller, F. C., Sacks, D. A., Yeh, S. et al. (1975). Significance of meconium during labor. *American Journal of Obstetrics and Gynecology*, **122**, 573–80.

Mitchell, J., Schulman, H., Fleischer, A., Farmakides, G. & Nadeau, D. (1985). Meconium aspiration and fetal acidosis. *Obstetrics and Gynecology*, **65**, 352–5.

Miyazaki, F. S. & Nevarez, F. (1985). Saline amnioinfusion for relief of repetitive variable decelerations: A prospective randomized study. *American Journal of Obstetrics and Gynecology*, **153**, 301–6.

Moberg, L. J., Garite, T. J. & Freeman, R. K. (1984). Fetal heart rate patterns and fetal distress in patients with preterm premature rupture of membranes. *Obstetrics and Gynecology*, **64**, 60–4.

Moessinger, A. C., Collins, M. H., Blanc, W. A., Rey, H. R. & James, L. S. (1986). Oligohydramnios-induced lung hypoplasia: the influence of timing and duration in gestation. *Pediatric Research*, **20**, 951–4.

Moore, T. R., Longo, J., Leopold, G. R., Casola, G. & Gosink, B. B. (1989). The reliability and predictive value of an amniotic fluid scoring system in severe second trimester oligohydramnios. *Obstetrics and Gynecology*, **73**, 739–42.

Morales, W. J., O'Brien, W. F., Angel, J. L., Knuppel, R. A. & Sawai, S. (1989). Fetal lung maturation: The combined use of corticosteroids and thyrotropin-releasing hormone. *Obstetrics and Gynecology*, **73**, 111–15.

Moses, D., Holm, B. A., Spitale, P., Liu, M. & Enhorning, G. (1991). Inhibition of pulmonary surfactant function by meconium. *American Journal of Obstetrics and Gynecology*, **164**, 477–81.

Moya, F. R. & Gross, I. (1988). Prevention of respiratory distress syndrome. *Seminars in Perinatology*, **12**, 348–58.

Moya, F., Mena, P., Heusser, F. et al. (1986). Response of the maternal, fetal, and neonatal pituitary–thyroid axis to thyrotropin-releasing hormone. *Pediatric Research*, **20**, 982–6.

Murphy, J. D., Vawter, G. F. & Reid, L. M. (1984) Pulmonary vascular disease in fatal meconium aspiration. *Journal of Pediatrics,* **104**, 758–62.

Nageotte, M. P., Freeman, R. K., Garite, T. J. & Dorchester W. (1985). Prophylactic intrapartum amnioinfusion in patients with preterm premature rupture of membranes. *American Journal of Obstetrics and Gynecology,* **153**, 557–62.

Nakayama, D. K., Glick, P. L., Harrison, M. R., Villia, R. L. & Noall R. (1983). Experimental pulmonary hypoplasia due to oligohydramnios and its reversal by relieving thoracic compression. *Journal of Pediatric Surgery,* **18**, 347–53.

Neilson, I. R., Russo, P., Laberge, J-M., Filiatrault, D., Nguyen, L. T., Collin, P. P. & Guttmen, F. M. (1991). Congenital adenomatoid malformation of the lung: current management and prognosis. *Journal of Pediatric Surgery*, **26**, 975–81.

Nicolaides, K. H. & Azar, G. B. (1990). Thoraco-amniotic shunting. *Fetal Diagnosis and Therapy,* **5**, 153–64.

Nicolaides, K. H., Rodeck, C. H., Lange et al. (1985). Fetoscopy in the assessment of unexplained fetal hydrops. *British Journal of Obstetrics and Gynaecology,* **92**, 671–9.

Nicolaides, K. H., Peters, M. T., Vyas, S., Rabinowitz, R., Rosen, D. J. & Campbell, S. (1990). Relation of rate of urine production to oxygen tension in small-for-gestational-age fetuses. *American Journal of Obstetrics and Gynecology,* **162**, 387–91.

Nicolini, U., Fisk, N. M., Beacham, J. & Rodeck, C. H. (1992). Fetal urine biochemistry: an index of renal maturation and dysfunction. *British Journal of Obstetrics and Gynaecology,* **99**, 46–50.

Nicolini, U., Fisk, N. M., Rodeck, C. H., Talbert, D. G. & Wigglesworth, J. S. (1989). Low amniotic pressure in oligohydramnios – is this the cause of pulmonary hypoplasia? *American Journal of Obstetrics and Gynecology,* **161**, 1098–101.

Nimrod, C., Varela-Gittings, F., Machin, G., Campbell, D. & Wesenberg, R. (1984). The effect of very prolonged membrane rupture on fetal development. *American Journal of Obstetrics and Gynecology,* **148**, 540–3.

Nimrod, C., Davies, D., Iwanicki, S., Harder, J., Persaud, D. & Nicholson, S. (1986). Ultrasound prediction of pulmonary hypoplasia. *Obstetrics and Gynecology,* **68**, 495–7.

Nugent, C. E., Hayashi, R. H. & Rubin, J. (1989). Prenatal treatment of Type I congenital cystic malformation by intrauterine fetal thoracocentesis. *Journal of Clinical Ultrasound*, **17**, 675–7.

Ogita, S., Imanaka, M., Matsumoto, M. & Hatanaka, K. (1984). Premature rupture of the membranes managed with a new cervical catheter. *Lancet,* **i**, 1330–1.

Ogita, S., Mizuno, M., Takeda, Y. et al. (1988). Clinical effectiveness of a new cervical indwelling catheter in the management of premature rupture of the membranes: a Japanese collaborative study. *American Journal of Obstetrics and Gynecology,* **159**, 336–41.

Oulton, M., Rasmusson, M. G., Yoon, R. Y. & Fraser, M. (1989). Gestation-dependent effects of the combined treatment of glucocorticoids and thyrotropin-releasing hormone on surfactant production by fetal rabbit lung. *American Journal of Obstetrics and Gynecology,* **160**, 961–7.

Owen, J., Henson, B. V. & Hauth, J. C. (1990). A prospective randomized study of saline solution amnioinfusion. *American Journal of Obstetrics and Gynecology,* **162**, 1146–9.

Page, D. V. & Stocker, J. T. (1982). Anomalies associated with pulmonary hypoplasia. *American Review of Respiratory Disease,* **125**, 216–21.

Pearce, J. M. & McParland, P. J. (1991). A comparison of doppler flow velocity waveforms, amniotic fluid columns and the nonstress test as a a means of monitoring post-dates pregnancies. *Obstetrics and Gynecology,* **77**, 204–8.

Perlman, M. & Levin, M. (1974). Fetal pulmonary hypoplasia, anuria and oligohydramnios: clinicopathologic observations and review of the literature. *American Journal of Obstetrics and Gynecology,* **118**, 1119–23.

Petres, R. E., Redwine, F. O. & Cruickshank, D. P. (1982). Congenital bilateral hydrothorax: antepartum diagnosis and successful intrauterine surgical management. *Journal of the American Medical Association,* **248**, 1360–61.

Phelan J. P., Smith C. V., Broussard P. & Small, M. (1987). Amniotic fluid volume assessment with the four-quadrant technique at 36–42 weeks gestation. *Journal of Reproductive Medicine,* **32**, 540–2.

Pringle, K. C., Turner, J. W., Schofield, J. C. & Soper, R. T. (1984). Creation and repair of diaphragmatic hernia in the fetal lamb: lung development and morphology. *Journal of Pediatric Surgery,* **19**, 131–40.

Read, L. C. & George-Nascimento, C. (1990). Epidermal growth factor: physiological roles and therapeutic applications. *Biotechnology Therapeutics,* **1**, 237–72.

Reale, F. R. & Esterly, J. R. (1973). Pulmonary hypoplasia: a morphometric study of the lungs of infants with diaphragmatic hernia, anencephaly, and renal malformations. *Pediatrics,* **51**, 91–6.

Redding, R. A., Douglas, W. H. J. & Stein, M. (1972). Thyroid hormone influence upon lung surfactant metabolism. *Science,* **175**, 994–6.

Redding, R. A. & Pereira, C. (1974). Thyroid function in respiratory distress syndrome (RDS) of the newborn. *Pediatrics,* **54**, 423–8.

Reuss, A., Wladimiroff, J. W., Stewart, P. A. & Scholtmeijer, R. J. (1988). Non-invasive management of fetal obstructive uropathy. *Lancet,* **ii**, 949–51.

Roberts, A. B. & Mitchell, J. M. (1990). Direct ultrasonographic measurement of fetal lung length in normal pregnancies and pregnancies complicated by prolonged rupture of membranes. *American Journal of Obstetrics and Gynecology,* **163**, 1560–6.

Robson, S. C., Crawford, R. A., Spencer, J. A. D. & Lee, A. (1992). Intrapartum amniotic fluid index and its relationship to fetal distress. *American Journal of Obstetrics and Gynecology,* **166**, 78–82.

Rodeck, C. H., Fisk, N. M., Fraser, D. I. & Nicolini, U. (1988). Long-term in utero drainage of fetal hydrothorax. *New England Journal of Medicine,* **319**, 1135–8.

Rooney, S. A. (1985). The surfactant system and lung phospholipid biochemistry. *American Review of Respiratory Disease,* **131**, 439–60.

Rooney, S. A., Marino, P. A., Gobran, L. I., Gross, I. & Warshaw, J. B. (1979). Thyrotropin-releasing hormone increases the amount of surfactant in lung lavage from fetal rabbits. *Pediatric Research,* **13**, 623–5.

Rooney, S. A., Gobran, L. I. & Chu, A. J. (1986). Thyroid hormone opposes some glucocorticoid effects on glycogen content and lipid synthesis in developing fetal rat lung. *Pediatric Research,* **20**, 545–50.

Rossi, E. M., Philipson, E. H., Williams, T. G. & Kalhan, S. C. (1989). Meconium aspiration syndrome: intrapartum and neonatal attributes. *American Journal of Obstetrics and Gynecology,* **161**, 1106–10.

Roti, E., Gardini, E., Minelli, R., Alboni, A. & Braverman, L. E. (1990). Thyrotropin releasing hormone does not stimulate prolactin release in the preterm human fetus. *Acta Endocrinologica,* **122**, 462–6.

Roti, E., Gnudi, A., Braverman, L. E. et al. (1981). Human cord blood concentration of thyrotropin, thyroglobulin, and iodothyronines after maternal administration of thyrotropin-releasing hormone. *Journal of Clinical Endocrinology and Metabolism,* **53**, 813–17.

Rotschild, A., Ling, E. W., Puterman, M. L. & Farquharson, D. (1990). Neonatal outcome after prolonged preterm rupture of the membranes. *American Journal of Obstetrics and Gynecology,* **162**, 46–52.

Sadovsky, Y., Amon, E., Bade, M. E. & Petrie, R. H. (1989). Prophylactic amnioinfusion during labor complicated by meconium: a preliminary report. *American Journal of Obstetrics and Gynecology,* **161**, 613–17.

Sarno, A. P., Ahn, M. O., Brar, H. S., Phelan, J. P. & Platt, L. D. (1989). Intrapartum Doppler velocimetry, amniotic fluid volume, and fetal heart rate as predictors of subsequent fetal distress. 1. An initial report. *American Journal of Obstetrics and Gynecology,* **161**, 1508–14.

Schellenberg, J., Liggins, G. C., Kitterman, J. A. & Lee, C. H. (1987). Elastin and collagen in the fetal sheep lung. II. Relationship to mechanical properties of the lung. *Pediatric Research,* **22**, 339–43.

Schellenberg, J., Liggins, G. C., Manzai, M., Kitterman, J. A. & Lee C. H. (1988). Synergistic hormonal effects on lung maturation in fetal sheep. *Journal of Applied Physiology,* **65**, 94–100.

Schmidt, W., Harms, E. & Wolf, D. (1985). Successful prenatal treatment of non-immune hydrops fetalis due to congenital chylothorax. *British Journal of Obstetrics and Gynaecology,* **92**, 671–9.

Schreyer, P., Caspi, E., Letko, Y., Ron-El, R., Pinto, N. & Zeidman, J. L. (1982). Intraamniotic triidothyronine instillation for prevention of respiratory distress syndrome in pregnancies complicated by hypertension. *Journal of Perinatal Medicine,* **10**, 27–33.

Seidner, S., Pettenazzo, A., Ikegami, M. & Jobe A. (1988). Corticosteroid potentiation of surfactant dose repsone in preterm rabbits. *Journal of Applied Physiology,* **64**, 2366–71.

Sher, G., Statland, B. E. & Freer, D. E. (1980). Clinical evaluation of the quantitative foam stability index test. *Obstetrics and Gynecology,* **55**, 617–20.

Smith, B. T. & Post, M. (1989). Fibroblast-pneumonocyte factor. *American Journal of Physiology,* **257**, 174–8.

Smolders-de-Haas, H., Neuvel, J., Schmand, B., Treffers, P. E., Koppe, J. G. & Hoeks, J. (1990). Physical development and medical history of children who were treated antenatally with corticosteroids to prevent respiratory distress syndrome: a 10 to 12 year follow-up. *Pediatrics,* **85**, 65–70.

Sohn, C. H., Stolz, W. & Bastert, G. (1991). Diagnosis of fetal lung maturity by ultrasound: a new method and first results. *Ultrasound in Obstetrics and Gynecology*, **1**, 345–8.

Songster, G. S., Gray, D. L. & Crane, J. P. (1989). Prenatal prediction of lethal pulmonary hypoplasia using ultrasonic fetal chest circumference. *Obstetrics and Gynecology*, **73**, 261–6.

Soper, R. T., Pringle K. C. & Schofield, J. C. (1984). Creation and repair of diaphragmatic hernia in the fetal lamb: techniques and survival. *Journal of Pediatric Surgery*, **19**, 33–40.

Sosenko, I. R. S. & Frank, L. (1987). Thyroid hormone depresses antioxidant enzyme maturation in fetal rat lung. *American Journal of Physiology*, **22**, 592–8.

Starks, G. C. (1980). Correlation of meconium-stained amniotic fluid, early intrapartum fetal pH, and Apgar scores as predictors of perinatal outcome. *Obstetrics and Gynecology*, **56**, 604–9.

Stedman, C. M., Crawford, S., Staten, E. & Cherny, W. B. (1981). Management of preterm premature rupture of membranes: Assessing amniotic fluid in the vagina for phosphatidylglycerol. *American Journal of Obstetrics and Gynaecology*, **140**, 34–8.

Stephens, F. D. (1983). *Congenital Malformations of the Urinary Tract*, 1st edn. Praeger, New York.

Strong, T. H., Hetzler, G. & Paul, R. H. (1990*b*). Amniotic fluid volume increase after amnioinfusion of a fixed volume. *American Journal of Obstetrics and Gynecology*, **162**, 746–8.

Strong, T. H., Hetzler, G., Sarno, A. P. & Paul, R. H. (1990*a*). Prophylactic intrapartum amnioinfusion: A randomized clinical trial. *American Journal of Obstetrics and Gynecology*, **162**, 1370–5.

Tabor, B. L., Ikegami, M., Jobe, A. H., Yamada, T. & Oetomo, S. B. (1990). Dose response of thyrotropin-releasing hormone on pulmonary maturation in corticosteroid-treated preterm rabbits. *American Journal of Obstetrics and Gynecology*, **163**, 669–76.

Thibeault, D. W., Beatty, E. C., Hall, R. T., Bowen, S. K. & O'Neill, D. H. (1985). Neonatal pulmonary hypoplasia with premature rupture of fetal membranes and oligohydramnios. *Journal of Pediatrics*, **107**, 273–7.

Thompson, P. J., Greenough, A. & Nicolaides, K. (1990). Chronic respiratory morbidity after prolonged premature rupture of membranes. *Archives of Disease in Childhood*, **65**, 878–80.

Thorpe-Beeston, J. G., Gosden, C. M. & Nicolaides, K. H. (1989). Prenatal diagnosis of congenital diaphragmatic hernia: associated malformations and chromosomal defects. *Fetal Therapy*, **4**, 21–8.

Thorpe-Beeston, J. G., Nicolaides, K. H., Snijders R. J. M., Butler, J. & McGregor, A. M. (1991). Fetal thyroid-stimulating hormone response to maternal administration of thyrotropin-releasing hormone. *American Journal of Obstetrics and Gynaecology*, **164**, 1244–5.

Torday, J., Carson, L. & Lawson, E. E. (1979). Saturated phosphatidylcholine in amniotic fluid and prediction of the respiratory-distress syndrome. *New England Journal of Medicine*, **301**, 1013–18.

Turnbull, A. C. (1983). The lecithin/sphingomyelin ratio in decline. *British Journal of Obstetrics and Gynaecology*, **90**, 993–4.

Tyrrell, S. N., Lilford, R. J., Macdonald, H. N., Nelson, E. J., Porter, J. & Gupta, J. K. (1990). Randomized comparison of routine versus highly selective use of Doppler ultrasound and biophysical scoring to investigate high risk pregnancies. *British Journal of Obstetrics and Gynaecology,* **97**, 909–16.

Usher, R. H., Allen, A. C. & McLean, F. (1971). Risk of respiratory distress syndrome related to gestational age, route of delivery, and maternal diabetes. *American Journal of Obstetrics and Gynecology,* **11**, 826–32.

van Eyck, J., van der Mooren, K. & Wladimiroff, J. W. (1990). Ductus arteriosus flow velocity modulation by fetal breathing movements as a measure of fetal lung development. *American Journal of Obstetrics and Gynecology,* **163**, 558–66.

Vaughan, J. I., Fisk, N. M. & Rodeck, C. H. (1994). Investigation and management of fetal pleural effusions. In *Invasive Fetal Testing and Treatment,* ed. C. R. Harman. Blackwell Scientific, Massachusetts (in press).

Vintzileos, A. M., Campbell, W. A., Rodis J. F., Nochimson, D. J., Pinette, M. G. & Petrikovsky, B. M. (1989). Comparison of six different ultrasonographic methods for predicting lethal fetal pulmonary hypoplasia. *American Journal of Obstetrics and Gynecology,* **161**, 606–12.

Walters, D. V. & Olver, R. E. (1978). The role of catecholamines in lung liquid absorption at birth. *Pediatric Research,* **12**, 239–42.

Warburton, D., Parton, L., Buckley, S., Cosico, L. & Saluna, T. (1987). Effects of beta–2 agonist on tracheal fluid flow, surfactant and pulmonary mechanics in the fetal lamb. *Journal of Pharmacology and Experimental Therapeutics,* **242**, 394–8.

Warburton, D., Parton L., Buckley, S., Cosico, L., Enns, G. & Saluna, T. (1988). Combined effects of corticosteroid, thyroid hormones and β-agonist on surfactant, pulmonary mechanics, and β-receptor binding in fetal lamb lung. *Pediatric Research,* **24**, 166–70.

Weber A. M. & Philipson, E. H. (1992). Fetal pleural effusion: a review and meta-analysis for prognostic indicators. *Obstetrics and Gynecology,* **79**, 281–6.

Wenstrom, K. D. & Parsons, M. T. (1989). The prevention of meconium aspitration in labour using amnioinfusion. *Obstetrics and Gynecology,* **73**, 647–51.

Wenstrom, K. D., Weiner, C. P. & Hanson, J. W. (1991). A five-year statewide experience with congenital diaphragmatic hernia. *American Journal of Obstetrics and Gynecology,* **165**, 838–42.

Whittle, M. J., Wilson, A. I., Witfield, C. R., Paton, R. D., & Logan, R. W. (1982). Amniotic fluid phosphatidylglycerol and the lecithin/spingomyelin ratio in the assessment of fetal lung maturity. *British Journal of Obstetrics and Gynaecology,* **89**, 727–32.

Wigglesworth, J. S. & Desai, R. (1979). Effects on lung growth of cervical cord section in the rabbit fetus. *Early Human Development,* **3**, 51–65.

Wilkins, I. A., Chitkara, U., Lynch, L., Goldberg, J. D., Mehalek, K. E. & Berkowitz, R. L. (1987). The non-predictive value of fetal urinary electrolytes: preliminary report of outcomes and correlations with pathological diagnosis. *American Journal of Obstetrics and Gynecology,* **157**, 694–8.

Wu, B., Kikkawa, Y., Orzalesi, M. M. et al. (1973). The effect of thyroxine on the maturation of fetal rabbit lungs. *Biology of the Neonate,* **22**, 161–8.

14

Non-invasive cardiorespiratory monitoring at home and in hospital

PAUL JOHNSON and DAVID C. ANDREWS

Introduction

The extensive sequence of changes in organization of sleep during postnatal development (see Chapter 8), the length of time spent in sleep, and the fact that pathophysiology of many respiratory and affective disorders in infancy are sleep-related, clearly indicates the need for measurement and recording methods that take them into account. It follows that non-laboratory (rather than laboratory) techniques must play an increasing role simply to meet the demand and varied locations of most of these infants.

Background: developmental physiology

The fact that sleep state organization is a marker of neurodevelopment as well as a major influence on systemic functions such as breathing and heart rate, is central to the measurement techniques that have to be used. Postnatal adaptation, especially to accomplish independent thermoregulation and growth, has major effects on neurobehaviour and cardiorespiratory function even under basal conditions. Basal metabolic rate (BMR) rises, and is directly related to thyroid and brown adipose tissue activity. Heart rate and breathing frequency increase to meet this demand as well as that of independent nutrition and growth. The rise and subsequent fall in BMR, T_3, heart and breathing rates are directly related, in the lamb reaching a peak at 14 days or so (Johnson & Andrews, 1992) and in man at 6 to 10 weeks (Azaz et al., 1992), which reflects the differences in rates of maturation and growth.

Antenatal as well as postnatal factors greatly influence the magnitude and time course of these changes. Undernutrition, as in growth retardation (Hull & Hull, 1982), and malnutrition, as in selective protein deprivation (Conradi et al., 1984) have substantial effects on the time course of postnatal adaptation. Both significantly decrease thermometabolic set points, such that a lower environmental temperature is sought by the newborn for many days after birth than in later life. Possible cardiorespiratory and other neurobehavioural consequences were not measured in these studies. Shearing the pregnant ewe 14 days before birth, whilst also on partial diet restriction, has no obvious effects on the lamb at birth. However, it does have profound effects on thermoregulatory mechanisms, breathing and heart rates of the newborn for several days after birth, suggesting that antenatal processes have had profound effects which persist into the neonatal period. Effects on expiratory pattern of breathing even persist beyond 30 days of age (Symonds et al., 1993), possibly due to an effect on lung and airway development.

Modest changes in ambient temperature, such as those used to define the thermoneutral range in early postnatal life, have large effects on sleep pattern. In the lamb at the lower critical ambient temperature limit (i.e. where thermogenesis starts to increase) rapid eye movement (REM) sleep is decreased (Andrews et al., 1990), whereas in the human infant it increases (Azaz et al., 1992). BMR is also increased in REM sleep compared to quiet sleep in human infants but decreased in most other mammals including the lamb. Modest changes beyond the upper and lower critical temperatures normally lead to arousal in both species. The two species are finely tuned to switch to their optimal thermoregulatory behavioural states. Differences in brain size between species may be a critical factor. Metabolic rates are known to be higher in most parts of the brain in REM and the brain of the human infant is much larger than that of the lamb (30% of body weight versus 2%).

These observations serve to indicate the influences on cardiorespiratory development which are closely integrated with neurobehaviour in postnatal life. Thus any method for cardiorespiratory monitoring must take these facts into account. Merely using instruments which identify apnoeas of an arbitrary length, with or without hypoxaemia, or bradycardia, have proven to be of little value either in the assessment of infants with known disorders or those considered at risk of apnoea or SIDS.

Development of monitoring methods

Antenatal

The interdependence of heart rate, breathing and neurobehaviour in fetal medicine is now accepted and increasingly used in the assessment of normal development of the fetus – the so-called biophysical profile. This is somewhat paradoxical, because the use of continuous recording of multiple fetal measurements antepartum is more advanced than those used after birth, despite their derivation from more detailed measurements in infants during sleep after birth (Prechtl, 1974; Visser et al., 1982), following the discovery of active sleep in infants in 1955 (Aserinsky & Kleitman, 1955). Disorders of fetal development can now be detected, where the primary intention is to distinguish life- and permanent health-threatening compromise from normal developmental.

While accurate prediction of sudden fetal death, or stillbirth, has not been achieved, disturbed behaviour, expressed as changes in body movements, breathing and heart rate activity patterns have been recognized by automatic analysis in fetal life (e.g. in intrauterine growth retarded fetuses, oligohydramnios) (Swarties et al., 1987; Arduini et al., 1989), leading to selective intervention. Recently, such techniques have been developed, and preferred, for home use and are suitable for a large proportion of high risk fetuses (Reece et al., 1992). Fetal heart rate measurement is one of the most reliable indices of early change, even in labour (Spencer & Johnson, 1986) being directly influenced by body movements, arousal state, breathing, thermovasomotor control and blood pressure. However, 90 minutes or more are required to define fetal sleep cycles, as opposed to a 'reactive' trace, where changes in fetal heart rate are seen, often in only 30 minutes of recording.

Non-laboratory monitoring of the at-risk fetus is becoming established, whereas comparable continuous monitoring of the infant population is rare. The clinical logic of linking antenatal to similar postnatal surveillance must become a reality. It has been suggested that many of the respiratory disorders that are studied postnatally have their origin in disturbances in fetal life. Apparently 'normally' grown fetuses may be at increased risk (Patterson & Pouliot, 1987) and may have suffered intrauterine insult (Hinchcliffe et al., 1993).

Postnatal

It has been shown that changes in cardiorespiratory rates and variability are reliable indices of wakefulness, quiet and active sleep in healthy infants when compared to full (i.e. EEG montage) polysomnography, and that this can be detected automatically (Harper, Schectman & Kluge, 1987; Johnson & Andrews, 1992) from heart rate and breathing pattern. Subtle but clear indications of abnormalities of development, even the ability to distinguish differences in rhythm before SIDS (note: these were not apnoeas) have been claimed from continuous breathing and heart rate recording during sleep cycles (Schectman et al., 1990). It has recently been suggested that early abnormality of quiet sleep epochs measured from breathing pattern relates to subsequent adverse neurodevelopmental assessment at 6 months of age (Thoman & Freudigman, 1991). Neurobehaviour and cardiorespiratory control are both influenced by environmental factors such as temperature, hypoxaemia and airway obstruction. Monitoring methods must also take this into account.

A paediatric subgroup of the non-laboratory monitoring (NLM) working group of the European Community on the sleep wake continuum recently agreed a basis for the investigation of sleep disorders in infants and young children. Briefly, non laboratory monitoring was a readily accepted description of a system that combined a number of sensors with an acquisition (recording) system that facilitated appropriate data reduction and analysis, but with all original data retrievable.

The use of a combination of measurements, without recourse to an EEG sleep montage, gives a good insight into sleep state (but not stage) in many instances, as well as cardiorespiratory abnormality, and could be used as a basic system with expansion to a full sleep montage recording for specific infant problems. The lack of training in developmental sleep medicine in perinatal medicine, especially neonatology, is a drawback. Significantly, all the listed abnormalities should include cardiorespiratory measurements as a part of the NLM. Repeat studies are usually required to distinguish normal developmental patterns from abnormality as well as those related to changes in disease state.

Basic diagnostic NLM for infants

A portable system which could display and record the following measurements should form the baseline diagnostic system for infants and children (up to pre-school age). Some adjustment for age would be necessary mainly because of changes in mobility. There is a need for a system for unsupervised monitoring in the home. Effective means of data handling (e.g. sample rate, rapid review, and analysis) would make such a system practical for the wider application that was needed to address sleep related problems in early life.

1. ECG/heart rate: essential for continuous accurate heart rate for the measurement of heart rate variability.
2. Breathing: individual; chest and abdominal excursion measurement was the favoured method, because of the ability to examine details of abdominal/thoracic asynchrony (rather than amplitude of breathing/

tidal volume). Inductance plethysmography (cross-sectional) was the technique of choice, although unnecessarily expensive.

A single sensor that reflects 'global' breathing movements such that frequency and qualitative amplitude change can be derived for breathing pattern recognition, may prove to be acceptable in some circumstances. The non-contact feature of a mattress sensor was an obvious advantage for the more mobile child (as well as for long-term monitoring, see below).

3. Sound/microphone: sited at the bedhead to detect noisy breathing during obstruction.
4. Activity: measurements of body/limb movements is an important guide to arousal state as well as for identifying artefact on other sensor signals. A mattress breathing sensor has the advantage of measuring all body movements.
5. Oxygen measurement: (a) Oxygen saturation (pulse oximetry) was considered to be the first line technology, although a series of deficiencies in the commercially available systems have to be recognized. Among these were motion artefact, inability to discriminate arterial from venous pulsatile signals (note ECG gating does nothing to correct for this), and a wide variety of algorithms which modify lagtime and response time (differentially for desaturation and resaturation). The magnitude of these errors varies greatly between instruments, is not generally known to the users nor easily quantified, and greatly influences accuracy of automated event detection. The pulse plethysmograph signal contains useful physiological information on changes in blood flow that assist in artefact detection and obstructed breathing, if it can be visualized and analysed in its unfiltered state. (b) Transcutaneous PO_2 can be an important adjunct where artefact errors in pulse oximetry exist. This technique itself has many limitations which have been well documented; a transcutaneous reading below 25 torr should be verified by arterialized capillary/arterial blood gas measurement, if the value is to be clinically relied upon.
6. Temperature: Temperature control during infancy (up to 9 months) is not only of specific clinical importance but directly influences other physiological variables being measured. Reliable 'deep tissue' temperatures measured from skin surface probes are needed.

The need to consider carefully the limits of individual sensors and optimize the function of others (as above) is important. The demand for validation studies has to be tempered by the fact that there is no adequate 'gold' standard in existence for these measurements.

Data review and analysis can be economically and efficiently handled by portable computers if the sample rates are set at sensible values (e.g. sampling at 177 Hz for 12 hours gives a total of 7.56 Mbytes, or 2.0 Mbytes compressed). Such systems with appropriate analysis should be commercially viable at under £5000.

Patients for whom basic NLMs should be used

Many infants in modern ITUs, while having many of these parameters measured, do not have adequate recording (namely sample rates) for analysis of sleep-related disorder to be undertaken. Systems measuring the six parameters listed above should ideally be the base system, with additional measurement as indicated in Table 14.1.

Any infant/child who is still oxygen dependent should have $TcPCO_2$ or alveolar PCO_2 measured at the first study. (If the $TcPCO_2$ is > than 60 torr, arterial PCO_2 measurement should be undertaken).

EEG

Continuous EEG analysis such as with the use of neural networks is urgently required. The possibility of accurate second by second sleep staging from the mature EEG alone has been demonstrated. The advantage (indeed necessity) for analysing fragmented or disturbed sleep is clear. The application to ontogenetic aspects of EEG development has yet to be reported.

Home monitoring – special considerations

Routine continuous monitoring for apnoea/SIDS risk generally uses impedance systems for ECG/heart rate and breathing. In Europe many simple contact and non-contact (pad or mattress) breathing monitors are used. Newer systems offer event capture and on- or off-line modem telephone transmission. None has been adequately validated or proven. They are unnecessarily expensive. Any review of monitoring in SIDS shows the wide disparity in current opinion; yet parental demand is increasing.

The scientific and clinical advantage of recording and analysing continuous data is imperative and, with appropriate use of selective sampling frequencies, this is now economically achievable. Because the methods used require even more care in the unsupervised (unobserved) situation, the basic system described above is still not practical (unless clinical

Table 14.1. *Patients for whom basic NLMs should be used*

	Additional second measures
Preterm healthy	
Chronic lung diseases	
Persistent oxygen dependence	
Birth asphyxia	+ EEG
Apnoea	+ pH (oesophageal)
Seizure/epilepsy	+ EEG
Reflux	+ pH (oesophageal)
Congenital abnormalities	
Metabolic disorders	
Small airways disease	+ pH (oesophageal)
Neuromuscular disorder	
Sleep disorder	
Movement/behaviour disorder	
Tonsil/adenoid hypertrophy	
Risk for SIDS	

evidence directly indicates the need), because of infant mobility and the training being beyond everyday use by most parents. In the meantime, continuous measurement from non-contact devices (e.g. mattress sensors) could be highly informative, e.g. for sleep/breathing patterns, and should be validated.

The use of video, especially as techniques now exist to merge video and other sensor signals via a PC board for display and analysis, should be actively considered. Advances in data compression techniques (such as fractal compression) mean that such systems can be used for remote (modem) monitoring.

The use of an hierarchical system that steps up the level of measurement from a non-contact system, to the basic system, and then to any additional special measurements (i.e. expansion from screening to diagnostic investigation) is desirable.

Definitions of cardiorespiratory abnormality

Most current criteria such as excessive periodic breathing, hypoxaemia, tachycardia, bradycardia have not been validated and await data from a substantial data base. Event capture of such isolated cardiorespiratory events are not interpretable without the basal or intervening data. Some important analyses can only be performed on continuously recorded data (e.g. heart rate variability, activity cycles), and this should be the requirement of future systems.

An incremental computer aided system for remote monitoring

This system uses a software program (CARDAS) that records from any sensor combination at individually selectable sample frequencies (1–100 Hz), displays and analyses on a PC which means that sensors require patient isolation and minimal conditioning before connection to memory, modem or PC. The sensors and combinations, very similar to those recommended above, have been extensively tested against invasive clinical measurements (ITU) and in animal studies.

In our studies on healthy infants in the home we added body movement detection, oximetry and ambient temperature measurement to chest and abdominal excursion, and heart rate in sequential once-a-month overnight studies at home (Fig. 14.1). The chest and abdominal phase angle was helpful in distinguishing active from quiet sleep (and both from obstruction (Fig. 14.4(b)). The variation in environmental conditions at home, especially the range of ambient temperature and clothing used, exceeded previously ethically approved laboratory investigation. The effects on breathing pattern in particular exceeded those in laboratory based studies (Carse et al., 1981). Nonetheless a clear pattern of development in sleep organization and related heart rate and breathing patterns was observed (Fig. 14.2). The initial high mean heart and breathing rates at 1 and 2 months are contributed to by frequent awakening for feeding, whereas at 4 months onward most infants slept through the night. It can

---

Fig. 14.1. (a) A 12-hour review display of an overnight recording from a 4-month old infant at home (via modem). SaO_2, heart rate, HR (ECG) and pulse rate, PR (plethysmograph) on same scale, chest abdomen phase angle, respiratory frequency Rf, body movements and microphone (bed head), and computer-derived sleep state (awake, quiet and active sleep: thick line) are displayed from above downward. Wakefulness at the beginning and end are obvious on all channels , as are the quiet and active sleep cycles in between. Note SaO_2, HR, PR and Rf decline over the first two hours although HR and Rf are more variable and elevated in active sleep. Phase angle is increased in active sleep as can be seen in Fig. 14.1(b) where 60 s 'windows' show typical quiet and active sleep segments respectively. Note the change from in-phase thoraco-abdominal breathing in active sleep. The dotted line separates the non-contact NCM-derived data from that from body sensors, and forms the basis for NCM screening system (see other figures). 14.1(c) shows a typical pattern of periodic breathing over 10-minute and 2-minute 'windows', respectively, from a healthy infant. Clearly seen is the 'fixed' oscillatory cycle with intervening apnoea length related to the amplitude of breathing.

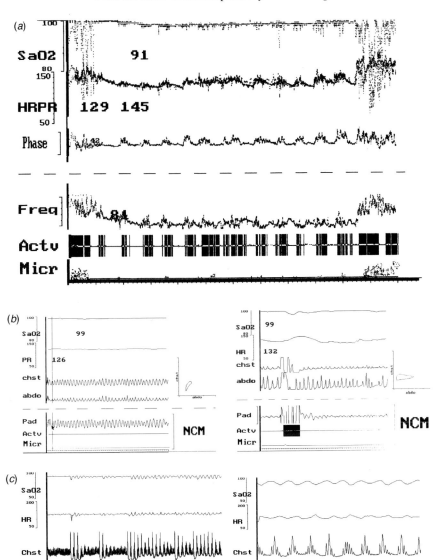

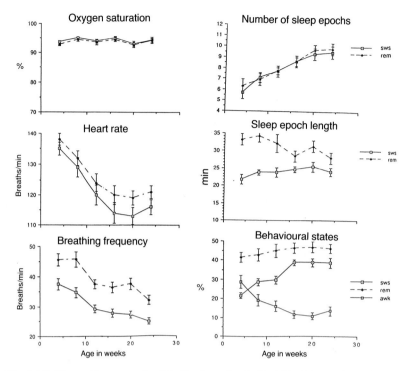

Fig. 14.2. Shows the mean (and 1sd) values for SaO_2, PR, Rf, number of sleep epochs, epoch length and percent time in quiet, active (and awake) in 30 healthy infants studied once a month at home up to 6 months of age. Note: the level of wakefulness (feeding) in the younger infants which contributes to their higher PR and Rf.

be seen in Fig. 14.1(*a*) that heart rate and breathing frequency are still falling after 2 hours of sleep and two active/quiet sleep cycles. Thus stable cardiorespiratory values are seldom a feature of sleep in infancy even though sleep cycles become relatively stable.

The important cardiorespiratory differences between quiet and active sleep can be observed and quantified by the expected chest and abdominal asynchrony (Andersson, Gennser & Johnson, 1986) in REM, also seen in the chest/abdominal lissajous loop (Fig. 14.1(*b*), Fig. 14.3(*b*)), from which changes in phase angle can be calculated and used in the objective assessment of upper airway obstruction (Fig. 14.4(*b*), Fig. 14.5(*b*)(*c*)) (Sivan, Deakers & Newth, 1990; Sirvan et al., 1991) (see below). The non-contact measurements (mattress, breathing patterns and body movement, and microphone) provide a quantifiable indication of breathing pattern during rest activity cycles.

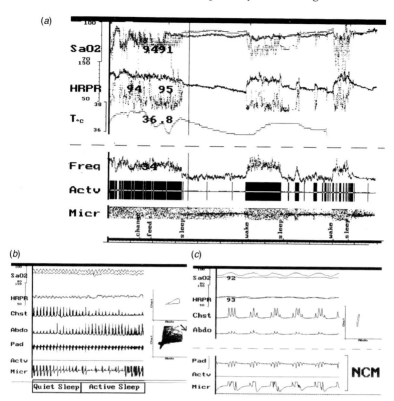

Fig. 14.3. (*a*) 12 hour review display from a 14 month old retarded infant with excessive night-time wakefulness and noisy breathing during sleep. It is extensively described in the text. Note the extensive variation in SaO_2 and PR (compared with ECG-HR). Body temperature (To_C) and HR and their large fall with sleep are seen. Note the annotation keyed by the mother. (*b*) is a 10 minute expansion in the middle of sleep as the infant switches from quiet to active sleep as judged by Ch/Ab asynchrony – the sequential phase angles increased (arrow). PB and noisy breathing continue through sleep. (*c*) is a 70 second expansion in quiet sleep (note the phase loop position), where the repetitive PB cycle is clearly seen with no movements but noisy inspiratory breathing, and was a feature of all sleep time. The NCM channels are highly informative.

Periodic breathing (PB), appropriately defined by cycle length and amplitude, and not a hybrid definition of three or more apnoeas of greater than 3 seconds separated by less than 20 seconds of breathing (Kelly & Shannon, 1979), was very common (Johnson et al., 1990). It was increased by warm ambient temperatures, between 1 and 4 months, in female infants, those of lower weight, but decreased in infants of mothers who smoked. PB cycle length was remarkably constant between 12 and 14 seconds and apnoea length, which increased as amplitude of breathing

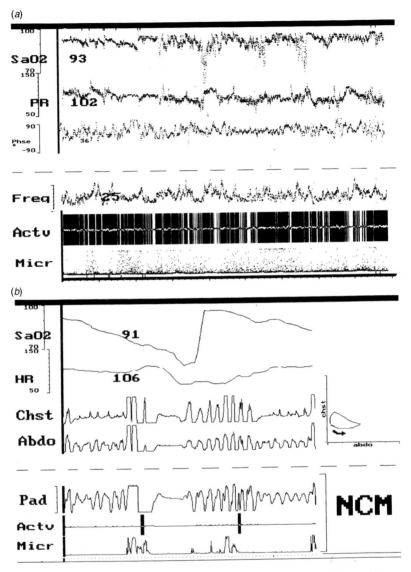

Fig. 14.4. (*a*) A nine hour review display from an 11 month infant with acute inflammatory upper airway obstruction (tonsillar hypertrophy). All channels indicate continuous disturbance with no active–quiet sleep structure apparent. (*b*) is a 60 second window typical of the recurrent obstructive apnoea. The NCM channels are diagnostic.

increased (Fig. 14.1(*c*)), did not exceed 10 seconds. This latter pattern could then fit the definition above and would be described as being excessive periodic breathing (i.e. more than 5% of sleep time) indicating risk for SIDS and the need for home monitoring and treatment with a respiratory stimulant such as theophylline. These and our earlier studies have shown that many of the cardiorespiratory indices used to categorize risk for SIDs are seen in healthy infants when observed sequentially and in their 'natural' environment.

Isolated central apnoeas greater than 11 seconds were not seen in over 3 000 hours of recording in 67 infants born after 37 weeks of GA. Obstructive apnoea, as evidenced by complete asynchrony of the chest and abdominal excursion for 3 breaths or more was not observed.

Sleep staging into awake, active, and quiet was automatically analysed but user-verified (Fig. 14.1) and used to automatically calculate, tabulate or graph the state-related data (Fig. 14.6).

The need for, and performance of such systems is demonstrated in the investigation of a selection of cardiorespiratory and neurological disorders. The first example is from a study of a 14 month old infant known to be severely retarded, but admitted for the investigation of excessive wakefulness at night and noisy breathing when asleep. A routine oximetry study on the ward had been interpreted as showing sleep hypoxaemia. However, it can be seen from the review (Fig. 14.3(*a*)), that the SaO_2 measured with two oximeters (which differ both when recording correctly and artefactually, see legend) is in the normal range when asleep but is artefactually low when awake, as can be seen by the difference between HR (ECG) darker line, and the pulse rate (PR) derived from the plethysmograph. During sleep they coincide and the SaO_2 is valid. The pattern of arousal over-night was clearly different from that observed in healthy infants (Fig. 14.1), 3.5 hours of constant activity followed by 2.5 hours of sleep (all annotated by the mother into the recording) with only two movements but continuous noisy breathing, when it can be seen that heart rate and body temperature falls progressively from 96 to 73, and 37.4 °C to 35.7 °C respectively at the end of sleep.

These changes during sleep exceeded those seen even in younger healthy infants (above). In an expanded view (Fig. 14.3(*c*)) during sleep breathing is periodic at 5 cycles per minute, noisy with no body movements and a low variability heart rate. PB persisted throughout the whole sleep period including an active sleep period seen in Fig. 14.3(*b*) where the chest amplitude decreases as the abdomen increases. The cycle lengthened as body temperature and heart rate fell, before the infant aroused when both rose abruptly. It was concluded from the trend and

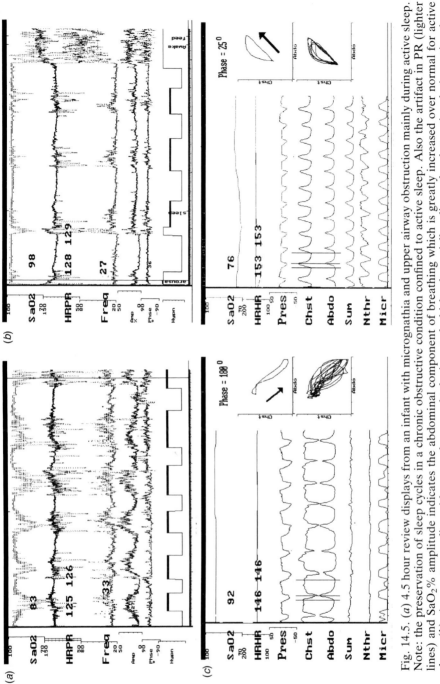

Fig. 14.5. (a) 4.5 hour review displays from an infant with micrognathia and upper airway obstruction mainly during active sleep. Note: the preservation of sleep cycles in a chronic obstructive condition confined to active sleep. Also the artifact in PR (lighter lines) and SaO₂% amplitude indicates the abdominal component of breathing which is greatly increased over normal for active sleep. (b). A repeat recording with a nasopharyngeal tube inserted which substantially relieves the obstruction during active sleep. (c). These are 30 second 'windows' before and after inserting a nasopharyngeal tube. Oesophageal pressure, nasal airflow and microphone all confirm the benefit of reducing upper airway respiratory obstruction. However, the phase loops are equally effective in quantifying this change.

```
Events captured from file : UL
 #   Start     Finish    Channel   Lo/Hi  Length  Area  Extrem      true
 1 22:05:58   22:06:16   11-SaO2    low    18s     25   83   %      YES
 2 00:16:54   00:17:26   11-SaO2    low    33s    281   74   %      YES
 3 00:22:24   00:22:52   11-SaO2    low    29s    153   77   %      YES
 4 00:24:14   00:24:46   11-SaO2    low    33s    225   75   %      YES
 5 00:35:00   00:35:16   11-SaO2    low    17s     65   88   %      YES
 6 00:39:12   00:39:30   11-SaO2    low    19s    162   79   %      YES
 7 00:39:10   00:39:44   11-SaO2    low    35s    225   75   %      YES
 8 00:42:40   00:42:56   11-SaO2    low    17s     53   81   %      YES
 9 00:43:46   00:44:08   11-SaO2    low    23s    103   79   %      YES
10 00:45:34   00:45:58   11-SaO2    low    25s    129   78   %      YES

            Summary of events      Channel   Lo/Hi  Length  Extrem
        162  Events on channel    11-SaO2    low     37s      75
```

Statistics from file : KHR
Over period - 18:51 to 05:35 on 03JUN92

	_PR		HR		SaO2		Freq		Phse		Amp		Chs%	
	bpm		bpm		%		br/m		°		%		%	
	Mean	SD	Mean	SD	Mean	SD	Mean	SD	Mean	SD	Mean	SD	Mean	SD
User verified:															
All Stdy	114	29.5	133	16.0	92	6.6	29	14.4	32	56.6	21	16.3	51	27.4
Awake	76	37.1	156	17.6	87	6.5	42	39.1	44	78.8	27	20.7	40	24.3
All slp	120	22.5	129	11.4	93	6.3	28	11.2	30	53.0	20	15.0	52	27.5
Actv slp	116	27.9	131	13.8	90	7.4	28	13.2	24	47.1	26	16.7	43	24.3
Quiet sl	125	10.0	127	6.2	96	2.1	27	8.6	37	58.4	12	7.2	61	27.6
Unkwn sl	0	0.0	0	0.0	0	0.0	0	0.0	-242	0.0	0	0.0	0	0.0
Computerised:															
Actv slp	111	29.4	130	15.3	89	7.9	28	13.8	22	48.1	27	17.7	43	23.4
Quiet sl	126	11.6	129	7.3	95	2.7	27	9.1	35	55.5	15	10.1	58	28.3
Unkwn sl	122	25.4	130	10.0	93	5.2	29	10.7	33	49.5	19	12.8	44	25.9

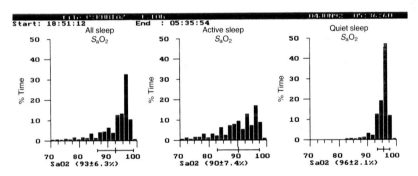

Fig. 14.6. Illustrates some selected automatic data displays as events, mean for sleep states, and as histograms. Note: the user verified data compared with automatically derived data.

analysis of the sleep portions of the recording that temperature regulation was deficient and hypothalamic dysfunction was a part of galaxy of CNS disorders. The lower three, non-contact measurements, breathing pattern, body activity and microphone were highly informative of such a neurological lesion which included a thermovasomotor PB pattern similar to that observed in many young infants especially when warm.

Another review from a previously healthy infant (Fig. 14.4(*a*)), contrasts a continuously disturbed pattern in all parameters overnight with no rest activity cycle apparent. On expansion (Fig. 14.4(*b*)) this can be seen to be repetitive obstructive apnoea relieved transiently by arousal seen clearly on breathing pattern, activity and the microphone traces (i.e. non-contact). This infant had acute inflammatory upper airway disease (tonsillitis) which resolved with antibiotic treatment.

Review recordings from another infant with micrognathia (Fig. 14.5(*a*)) showed a well-preserved quiet/active sleep pattern accentuated because of the upper airway obstruction being more marked in REM sleep. Automatic sleep state identification was effective and could be used to quantify the improvement in REM sleep caused by nasopharyngeal intubation (Fig. 14.5(*b*)). Another infant with micrognathia and chronic lung disease causing persistent hypoxaemia benefited from nasopharyngeal intubation inserted between recordings in Fig. 14.5(*c*). The addition of intra-oesophageal pressure measurement and oro-nasal thermistor confirmed the change in pattern observed on the chest abdomen distortion (phase angle), breathing frequency and pattern. Additional inspired oxygen therapy was removed between first and second panels in Fig. 14.5(*c*), explaining the fall in SaO_2. The management of this infant was complex because of the balance between providing a bypass for upper airway obstruction and increasing inspiratory resistance, and thus adding to already compromised respiratory function from chronic lung disease (the latter being variably affected by recurrent infection). Repeated overnight studies, again annotated by the mother, were necessary to vary management between NP tube, CPAP and oxygen therapy.

Finally, illustrations of apnoea patterns typical of ex-preterm infants with bronchiolitis (Fig. 14.7(*a*)) show that recurrent apnoea, either central (Fig. 14.7(*b*)), or central followed by obstruction (so call 'mixed') (Fig. 14.7(*c*)), are apparently promoted by the increased oxygen administration. Note the delay in desaturation from 100% (indicative of hyperoxia) and bradycardia. This observation coincides with that seen when apnoea induced by laryngeal mucosal stimulation in lambs is also prolonged by hyperoxia (Johnson, 1988). The recent observation in neonatal kittens that very mild levels of hypoxia inhibit hypoglossal motoneurones (which supply the genioglossus and other upper airway muscles) provides an intriguing parallel as the fall in PaO_2 caused by the central apnoea may compromise upper airway stability and lead to obstruction (Smith et al., 1993*a,b,c*; Noble, personal communication).

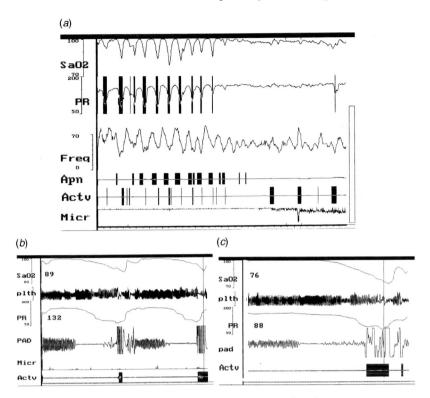

Fig. 14.7. (*a*) is a 30 minute 'window' during a recording from an ex-preterm infant with bronchiolitis breathing 40% oxygen. Periodic apnoea with the SaO_2 falling from 100% is seen associated with bradycardia (flagged as events – also apnoeas and movements on the NCM channels). The microphone channel has a continuous high signal due to oxygen flow in the headbox which was reduced after 25 minutes. (*b*) Is a 3 minute window showing the late fall in SaO_2 and bradycardia followed by arousal. (*c*) Is a 90 second window also with a late desaturation and bradycardia, but with evidence of obstructed breathing occurring before arousal terminates the apnoea.

Summary

Appropriate use of the methods described in this chapter, can give objective insight into changes of central and peripheral respiratory control and airway mechanics and are more than a supplement to laboratory investigation of cardiorespiratory function. It is our contention that computer-aided non-laboratory monitoring is the platform for most laboratory function tests. In many instances, the sedation and limited time scale of laboratory testing gives an entirely misleading

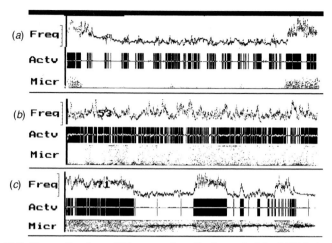

Fig. 14.8. Shows the three 12 hour review displays of of the NCM channels from the three infants (Figs. 14.1, 4 and 3 above), from which the patterns of sleep and breathing and the differing characteristics of their disruption are clearly seen using continuous recording from these simple measurements.

picture of the nature and cause of the prevailing dysfunction(s). Arousal state and its disturbance is a major dynamic influence together with substantial developmental changes extending throughout infancy and early childhood, of a magnitude which is not seen in adult life.

It is of interest, however, that a recent review of institutionalized polysomnography (which is expensive) versus portable pulse oximetry (which is relatively cheap) for diagnosing cardiorespiratory sleep disorders in the adult found neither to be effective. Simple measurement of breathing pattern, body movements and breath sounds (microphone) were found to be the fundamental measurements needed (Douglas, Thomas & Jan, 1992). The same measures provide clear insight into the nature and stability of the disorder in infants and children, where the advantages (both cost and practicality) are obvious (Fig. 14.8).

An effective incremental strategy for the investigation and management of sleep disorders which accompany many illnesses during development is described. It is clear that event recording, unless it encompasses the data from an entire night (or 24 hours in infants) or several nights with careful selection of sensors and awareness of their limitations, is very limited and often misleading. Undoubtedly advances in powerful inexpensive computing which assist display and analysis and in telecommunications provide a unique opportunity to operate an effective strategy for investigation, clinical management and much-needed research.

A standardized approach to measurement, particularly sample rates, and digital storage (much more economic and clinically useful than paper traces or averaged trend displays or printouts) can also be used to build clinical databases. Only with these will clinical audit and objective criteria be attained.

The future – telemedicine

Advances that make telemedicine for the remote investigation and management of many illnesses of this type a reality, now mean that primary care and specialist centres can be effectively linked by automated telemetry networks. Fusion of continuous medical monitoring with video over such networks (even the standard telephone) is now possible taking advantage of spectacular advances in data compression (e.g. fractal compression) and capacity of storage media. This unprecedented opportunity for an international effort against developmental disorders requires that standards for measurement and data acquisition are set now. Telemedicine is a unique tool for research as well as a practical clinical advance.

References

Andersson, D., Gennser, G. A. & Johnson, P. (1986). The effect of carbon dioxide inhalation on phase characteristics of breathing movements in healthy newborn infants. *Journal of Developmental Physiology*, **8**, 147–57.

Andrews, D. C., Ball, N. J., Symonds, M. E., Vojeck, L. & Johnson, P. (1990). The effect of ambient temperature and age on sleep state in developing lambs. In *Sleep '90*, ed. J. Horne. pp. 115–118. Pontenagael Press, Bochum.

Arduini, D., Rizzo, G., Caforio, L., Boccolini, R., Romannini, R. & Mancuso, S. (1989). Behavioural state transitions in healthy and growth retarded fetuses. *Early Human Development*, **19**, 155–65.

Aserinsky, E. & Kleitman, N. (1955). A motility cycle in sleeping infants as manifested by ocular and gross bodily activity. *Journal of Applied Physiology*, **8**, 11–18.

Azaz, Y., Fleming, P. J., Levine, M., McCabe, R., Stewart, A. & Johnson, P. (1992). The relationship between environmental temperature, metabolic rate, sleep state and evaporative water loss in infants from birth to three months. *Pediatric Research*, **32**, 417–23.

Carse, E. A., Wilkinson, A. R., Whyte, P. L., Henderson-Smart, D.S. & Johnson, P. (1981). Oxygen and carbon dioxide tensions, breathing and heart rate in normal infants during the first six months of life. *Journal of Developmental Physiology*, **3**, 85–100.

Conradi, N. G., Muntzing, K., Sourander, P. & Hamberger, A. (1984). Effect of ambient temperature on rectal temperature in normal and malnourished rats during early and postnatal development. *Acta Physiologica Scandinavica*, **121**, 147–53.

Douglas, N. J., Thomas, S. & Jan, M.A. (1992). Clinical value of polysomnography. *Lancet*, **339**, 347–50.

Harper, R. M., Schectman, V. L. & Kluge, K. A. (1987). Machine classification of infant sleep states using cardiorespiratory measures. *Electroencephalography and Clinical Neurophysiology*, **67**, 379–87.

Hinchcliffe, S. A., Howard, C. V, Lynch, M. R. J., Sargent, P. H., Judd, B. A. & van Velzen, R. (1993). Renal development arrest in sudden infant death syndrome. *Pediatric Pathology*, **13**, 333–4.

Hull, J. & Hull, D. (1982). Behavioural thermoregulation in newborn rabbits. *Journal of Comparative Physiology and Pschology*, **96**, 143–47.

Johnson, P., Head, J., Hughes, M. & Sands, P. (1990). Periodic breathing in healthy infants monitored at home. *American Review of Respiratory Disease*, **141**(4), 1108.

Johnson, P. (1988). Airway reflexes and the control of breathing in postnatal life. In *Sudden Infant Death Syndrome*, ed. P.J. Schwartz, D.P. Southall, M. Valdes Dapena. pp. 262–275. New York Academy of Sciences, New York.

Johnson, P. & Andrews, D. C. (1992). Thermometabolism and cardiorespiratory control during the perinatal period. In *Respiratory Control Disorders in Infants and Children*, ed. R. C. Beckerman, R. T. Brouilette & C. E. Hunt. pp. 76–88. Williams and Wilkins, Baltimore.

Kelly, D. H. & Shannon, D. (1979). Periodic breathing in infants with near-miss sudden infant death syndrome. *Pediatrics*, **63**, 355–9.

Patterson, R. M. & Pouliot, R. N. (1987). Neonatal morphometrics and perinatal outcome: who is growth retarded? *American Journal of Obstetris and Gynecology*, **157**, 691–3.

Prechtl, H. F. R. (1974). The behavioural states of the newborn infant (a review). *Brain Research*, **76**, 185–212.

Reece, E. A., Hagay, Z. Garafolo, J. & Hobbins, J. C. (1992). A controlled trial of self-nonstress test versus assisted nonstress test in the evaluation of fetal well-being. *American Journal of Obstetrics and Gynecology*, **166**, 489–92.

Schectman, V. L., Harper, R. M., Kluge, K. A. & Wilson, A. J. (1990). Correlations between cardiorespiratory measures in normal infants and victims of sudden infant death syndrome. *Sleep*, **13**, 304–7.

Sirvan, Y., Davidson Ward, S., Deakers, T., Keens, T. G. & Newth, C. J. L. (1991). Rib cage to abdominal asynchrony in children undergoing polygraphic sleep studies. *Pediatric Pulmonology*, **11**, 141–6.

Sirvan, Y., Deakers, T. W. & Newth, C. J. L. (1990). Thoraco abdominal asynchrony in acute upper airway obstruction in small children. *American Review of Respiratory Disease*, **142**, 540–4.

Smith, J. A., Li, F. & Noble, R. (1993*a*). The effect of mild hypoxia on discharge frequency of hypoglossal motoneurones in anaesthetized neonatal kittens. *Journal of Physiology*, **459**, 143P.

Smith, J. A., Li, F. & Noble, R. (1993*b*). Effect of isocapnic hypoxia on membrane potentials of hypoglossal motoneurones recorded in anaesthetized neonatal kittens. *Journal of Physiology*, **459**, 335P.

Smith, J. A., Li, F. & Noble, R. (1993*c*). Evidence for inhibitory mechanisms mediating hypoglossal motoneurone response to mild hypoxia in anaesthetized neonatal kittens. *Journal of Physiology*, **473**, 62P.

Spencer, J. A. D. & Johnson, P. (1986). Fetal heart rate variability changes and fetal behavioural cycles during labour. *British Journal of Obstetrics and Gynaecology*, **93**, 314–21.

Swarties, J. M., Van Geijn, H. P., Caron, F. J. M. & Van Woerden, E. E. (1987). Automated analysis of fetal behavioural states and state transitions. In *The Fetus as a Patient*, ed. K Maeda. pp. 39–48. Elsevier Science Publishers, Amsterdam.

Symonds, M. E., Lomax, M. A., Kenwood, M. L., Andrews, D. C. & Johnson, P. (1993). Effect of the prenatal maternal environment on the control of breathing during non-rapid eye movement sleep in the developing lamb. *Journal of Developmental Physiology*, **19**, 43–50.

Thoman, E. B. & Freudigman, K. A. (1991). Non-intrusive monitoring of sleep in newborns: delivery mode, sex differences and prediction of later development. *Sleep Research*, **8**, 217.

Visser, G. H. A., Carse, E. A., Goodman, J. D. S. & Johnson, P. (1982). A comparison of episodic heart rate patterns in the fetus and newborn. *British Journal of Obstetrics and Gynaecology*, **89**, 50–5.

15

Respiratory resuscitation and ventilation of the neonate

C. ANDREW RAMSDEN

In this chapter, techniques of respiratory resuscitation and artificial ventilation of newborn infants are reviewed. Particular consideration is given to the interrelation between the mechanical properties of the lung and positive pressure ventilation. The argument is developed that strategies of respiratory support should be sensitive to the wide range of mechanical properties exhibited by the lungs of newborn infants.

Respiratory resuscitation at birth

Physiological considerations

Mechanical properties of the lungs at birth

At the time of birth the respiratory system possesses remarkable mechanical properties, quite unlike those found at any other time of life. These are almost entirely attributable to the future airspace of the lung being filled with liquid (see Chapter 3). Substantial forces must be overcome for this liquid to be displaced by gas. When inflation commences, inertial and flow resistive forces are maximal (Agostoni et al., 1958) but rapidly diminish as the liquid moves distally and the total cross-sectional area of the airways increases. As gas reaches the terminal airways, viscous forces are overshadowed by surface forces whose magnitude is determined by the Laplace equation, $P = 2T/r$ (where P is the distending pressure, T is the surface tension and r is the radius of curvature of the air–liquid interface). The distending pressure required to advance gas further then depends on r and reaches a maximum, the opening pressure, as r reaches a minimum at the point of transition between the conducting airways and terminal air spaces. Classical observations of the first breath (Karlberg et al., 1962) and later measurements during neonatal resuscitation (Boon, Milner & Hopkin, 1979*a,b*) indicate that opening pressures normally lie around 20–25 cm H_2O, and agree well with predictions from the Laplace equation (Avery & Mead, 1959). Although some infants have been reported to inflate their lungs without generating opening pressures (Karlberg et al., 1962; Milner & Saunders, 1977) this confusing observation probably results from underestimation of the true distending pressure and phase effects related to the prolonged time constant of the liquid-filled lung (Milner, 1991).

For respiration to commence efficiently, newly expanded lung units must remain open in expiration and thereby establish functional residual capacity (FRC), without which opening pressures would need to be repeatedly generated. Surfactant plays an essential role. Dynamic compression of the surfactant film in expiration causes surface tension to fall to extremely low values (<10 dynes/cm) and diminishes elastic recoil of the lung to the point at which it can be balanced by an equal and opposite recoil of the chest wall.

Respiratory efforts at birth

The first inspiratory effort is singularly forceful. It generates a negative pleural pressure that averages -50 cm H_2O and may exceed -100 cm H_2O and gives rise to an inspired volume that is correspondingly large, averaging about 40 ml (Mortola et al., 1982a; Vyas et al., 1986). The first expiration is usually very prolonged. Typically, it lasts about 4 s and is characterized by glottic closure – a strategy that may help to maintain FRC, clear alveolar liquid and improve lung compliance (Mortola et al., 1982*a*).

An FRC of about 15 ml is normally established during the first breath. Its volume correlates with the volume of gas inspired (Mortola et al., 1982a; Vyas et al., 1986) and with measures of inspiratory effort such as the product of inspiratory pressure and time (Vyas et al., 1986). In subsequent breaths FRC progressively increases to reach an average of 42 ml after 15 breaths (Mortola et al., 1982*b*) and close to its final volume of about 100 ml by 1 hour (Geubelle, 1959).

Clinical applications

Despite the manifest importance of effective resuscitation techniques, remarkably little attempt has been made to evaluate clinically the various methods that are employed. In the absence of data from clinical trials, inferences drawn from physiological measurements have had special influence on clinical practice.

Care of the airway at birth

Suctioning of the nose and oropharynx immediately after birth is a routine and long-established practice in many centres. Yet what little evidence is available indicates that this doubtful exercise may be detrimental unless the airway is contaminated with meconium. Typically, suctioning of the airway causes a fall in arterial oxygen saturation which may be accentuated, in those infants with respiratory problems, by removal of supplemental oxygen while the procedure is performed (Sendak, Harris & Donham, 1986). Prolonged and overzealous suctioning at best delays more effective resuscitative measures and at worst may trigger reflex vagal bradycardia (Cordero & Hon, 1971), laryngospasm and apnoea.

The delivery room management of infants born in the presence of meconium-stained liquor has been the subject of some clinical investigation. Early reports suggested that if the trachea was routinely suctioned after birth, the incidence and severity of meconium aspiration was reduced (Gregory et al., 1974; Ting & Brady, 1975). These were soon followed by evidence (based on historical controls) that the need for tracheal suction could be almost entirely eliminated if the nose and oropharynx were carefully suctioned as the head delivered (Carson et al., 1976). Almost two decades later the role of routine tracheal suction remains unresolved (Katz & Bowes, 1992). In its favour, further retrospective evidence shows apparent benefit (Wiswell, Tuggle & Turner, 1990; Wiswell & Henley, 1992). However, evidence that diligent suctioning fails to prevent all cases of meconium aspiration (Davis et al., 1985) and that death from meconium aspiration is associated with abnormalities of the pulmonary vasculature that are established well before birth (Murphy, Vawter & Reid, 1984) has led others to favour a more selective approach (Cunningham et al., 1990). Remarkably, only one clinical trial has addressed the role of tracheal suction (Linder et al., 1988) and it found no benefit in infants that are vigorous at birth (1 minute Apgar score >8). Until further trials are performed consensus favours thorough pharyngeal suctioning as the head delivers, followed by a selective policy of tracheal suction for those infants that are born through thick meconium and are depressed at birth (Cunningham et al., 1990).

Indications for resuscitation at birth

While the majority of newborn infants commence breathing without assistance, a minority suffering from the effects of asphyxia, maternal drugs or prematurity, require help if death or damaging delay is to be avoided. Of all births, about 5% fail to establish regular respiration within the first 3 minutes (Chamberlain et al., 1975) and 1–2% are deemed to need resuscitation by endotracheal intubation (MacDonald et al., 1980).

Guidelines for the initiation and conduct of resuscitation abound and vary considerably in their complexity. However, the more complex protocols based on Apgar scores offer no obvious advantage over simpler schemes based on just two parameters – heart rate and respiratory effort (Milner, 1991). If the infant is apnoeic but has a heart rate of >80–100/min, stimulation and provision of oxygen is usually sufficient to establish respiration. However, if the heart rate is <80–100/min or stimulation fails to induce adequate breathing within a reasonable time (probably about 1 min or so) then artificial ventilation should be commenced without further delay (Milner, 1991).

Ventilation parameters for neonatal resuscitation

Observations made during the normal onset of breathing and in the course of resuscitation indicate that both pressure and time are important in aerating previously unexpanded lung (Vyas et al., 1981; Vyas et al., 1986). Although we may predict from physiological measurements that a distending pressure of around 25 cm H_2O should be sufficient to overcome opening pressures in the lung, observations made during resuscitation of term infants indicate that a pressure of 30 cm H_2O sustained for 1 s gives rise to a relatively small inspired volume for the first inflation, averaging only 19 ml (Boon et al., 1979*b*). Furthermore, only 25% of these infants established an FRC with the first inflation and when they did its volume averaged only 7 ml. Larger volumes are achieved only when the lung is exposed to a higher distending pressure, which may arise from summation between the applied pressure and spontaneous inspiratory activity (Boon et al., 1979*b*; Hoskyns, Milner & Hopkin, 1987), or when the inflation pressure is sustained for a longer period of time (Vyas et al., 1981). Employing an inspiratory pressure of 30 cm H_2O and an inspiratory time of up to 5 s for the first inflation, Vyas and colleagues (1981) achieved an inspired volume and an FRC that more closely approximate a spontaneous first breath, being 34 ml and 16 ml respectively. FRC subsequently rose to 54 ml over the first 30 s.

The choice between endotracheal and mask ventilation

Endotracheal intubation gives greatest control of the airway and the inflation pressure and time. However, the procedure requires considerable skill and, even when performed well, causes significant physiological disturbance (Marshall et al., 1984). Performed badly it can result in considerable trauma.

Ventilation by face mask may be an effective alternative for some infants. A round silicone rubber mask, such as the Laerdal, is preferable, being easy to use and giving a good seal. Moulded masks such as the Rendell-Baker are hopeless (Palme, Nystrom & Tunnel, 1985). Although gastric distension is a potential risk, gas apparently only enters the stomach if the inflation pressure is allowed to exceed 35 cm H_2O (Vyas, Milner & Hopkin, 1983). The main shortcoming of mask ventilation lies in the tidal volume delivered which is often insufficient to maintain adequate alveolar ventilation. Success appears to depend instead on stimulating the infant's own respiratory efforts (Milner, Vyas & Hopkin, 1984). Thus for the severely asphyxiated or very immature infant, in whom respiratory activity may be minimal, face mask ventilation may prove ineffective.

Connection of the face mask, through a T-piece, to the oxygen supply of a conventional resuscitaire appears to be the most effective method of delivering positive pressure ventilation (Hoskyns, Milner & Hopkin, 1987a). With this method the mask can be pressurized simply by occluding the gas outlet at the 'T'. Use of a self-inflating bag is more problematic. Oxygen delivery and pressure blow-off valves are often unreliable (Finer et al., 1986) and optimal inspiratory pressures and times hard to achieve (Field, Milner & Hopkin, 1986). An anaesthetic bag can allow more control but requires much more skill in its use (Kanter, 1987).

Resuscitation of the preterm infant

Whereas less than 1% of term infants need a period of positive pressure ventilation at birth as many as 30% of preterm infants (≤32 weeks) require resuscitation (MacDonald et al., 1980). Routine intubation and ventilation of all infants weighing <1500 g has been claimed to be associated with fewer deaths (23% versus 49%) than a more selective policy (Drew, 1982) but interpretation of this trial is difficult as the skill of the resuscitators apparently differed between groups (Tyson, 1992).

Until better data is available, routine intubation of very low birthweight infants, who breathe well at birth, seems unwarranted.

The preterm infant whose lung is surfactant deficient may require higher inflation pressures to be used. Hoskyns et al. (1987*b*) examined infants resuscitated with a peak inspiratory pressure of 30 cm H_2O and found that preterm infants were less likely to achieve an 'adequate' tidal volume (defined as >4.4 ml/kg) than their term counterparts. Failure to establish an FRC was also more common in the preterm infant and, not surprisingly, was strongly associated with the development of hyaline membrane disease (Upton & Milner, 1991).

Conclusions

When pulmonary gas exchange must be established without delay, as, for example, in severe asphyxia, endotracheal intubation and positive pressure ventilation is the method of choice. The first inflation should be at a pressure of about 25–30cm H_2O and should probably be sustained for 2–3 seconds. Once lung expansion has been achieved lower pressures (around 20 cm H_2O) and shorter inspiratory times (0.5–1.0 s) usually suffice. Higher pressures may occasionally be required to expand the lung when surfactant deficiency or pulmonary hypoplasia are present. Mask ventilation may be the preferred technique if an immediate response is not essential and if some respiratory effort is present.

Whatever technique is employed careful inspection of the movement of the chest provides an invaluable guide to the adequacy of the ventilation achieved.

Assisted ventilation of the newborn infant

Despite many years of clinical and laboratory investigation, considerable controversy still surrounds the optimal methods of mechanical ventilation of the newborn (Ramsden & Reynolds, 1987). In the remainder of this chapter the principles underlying mechanical ventilation of the newborn and strategies of ventilator management will be reviewed focusing in particular on current areas of debate.

Equipment for conventional ventilation
Conventional mechanical ventilators

Mechanical ventilators for neonatal use are mostly pressure-limited, time-cycled devices in which gas flows continuously into the ventilator circuit and is cyclically pressurised by a variable resistor in the expiratory limb. The operator selects the pressure to be applied in inspiration and expiration and the duration of both the inspiratory and expiratory phases. Some (usually limited) control may also be exerted over the pressure waveform which normally resembles a square-wave that is somewhat rounded in inspiration. By increasing gas flow rate, the ventilator circuit is pressurised more rapidly in inspiration and a waveform that more closely approximates to a square-wave is usually achieved. Measures that diminish circuit compliance have a similar effect. The tidal volume delivered by pressure-limited devices depends on the inspiratory pressure and time, and on the mechanical properties of the infant's lungs (see below). Net alveolar ventilation depends also on the infant's own inspiratory efforts which, through the continuous supply of fresh gas, are able to contribute usefully to net ventilation.

Volume-cycled ventilators require the operator to choose a tidal volume and a frequency with which that volume is to be delivered. Although conceptually simple, these devices are problematic in neonatal use. Of the chosen tidal volume, a variable and unpredictable proportion is lost as leak around the (uncuffed) endotracheal tube and is taken up in pressurizing the ventilator circuit. The proportion lost to the circuit may be particularly large if the compliance of the infant's lung is low relative to that of the humidifier and ventilator tubing.

Humidifiers

During mechanical ventilation the gas conditioning that is normally provided by the upper airway is bypassed and in its place the inspired gas needs to be artificially warmed and humidified. This simple objective is made complex by uncertainty regarding the 'ideal' conditions of temperature and humidity that should be aimed for (Chatburn & Primiano, 1987). Although it is often assumed that a temperature of 37°C and relative humidity of 100% are optimal, such conditions may in fact be quite unphysiological. As yet there are no data for the human infant but in the adult, quietly breathing room air, gas enters the trachea at a temperature of around 32°C and is warmed to 35.5°C by the subsegmental bronchi (McFadden et al., 1985). Relative humidity in the trachea is probably close to 100% (Chatburn & Primiano, 1987).

While the optimal condition of the inspired gas remains unclear, available evidence indicates that too much or too little humidity may be harmful. Too little decreases cilial beating (Toremalm, 1961), dries secretions and risks airway obstruction (Lomholt, Cooke & Lundig,

1968) whereas too much may inactivate surfactant (Tsuda et al., 1977) and reduce lung compliance (Noguchi, Takumi & Aochi, 1973). The significance of gas conditioning in the clinical setting has been highlighted more recently by retrospective evidence that an inspired gas temperature of <36.5°C is associated with more air leaks and chronic lung disease than an inspired gas temperature of >36.5°C (Tarnow-Mordi et al., 1989). Unfortunately, humidity was not measured. Further studies are needed of this important but relatively neglected aspect of mechanical ventilation.

Principles underlying mechanical ventilator settings

The discussion below refers to pressure-limited ventilators though many of the principles outlined can also be applied to volume-cycled ventilation.

Inspiratory and expiratory pressures

During pressure-limited mechanical ventilation of the lungs the pressure at the airway opening (P_{ao}) is regularly cycled between peak inspiratory pressure (PIP) and end-expiratory pressure (EEP). The latter is generally maintained positive and is usually referred to as PEEP. Flow of gas into or out of the lung is driven by the difference between P_{ao} and alveolar pressure (P_A) and continues until P_A has equilibrated with P_{ao}. In inspiration, gas flows into the lung until P_A has risen to equal PIP or the inspiratory phase is terminated. In expiration, gas exits from the lung as long as P_A exceeds PEEP. The tidal volume depends therefore on the change in pressure at the airway opening (ΔP_{ao}) between PIP and PEEP, the compliance of the respiratory system, and the provision of sufficient time for P_A and P_{ao} to equilibrate (see below).

Peak inspiratory pressure. Increases in PIP increase tidal volume and thereby elevate alveolar ventilation and lower $PaCO_2$. Under circumstances where lung units are collapsed, of which hyaline membrane disease is the classic example, an increase in PIP may also re-expand collapsed lung as opening pressures are exceeded. As lung units open, intrapulmonary R–L shunting decreases and oxygenation improves (Herman & Reynolds, 1973). However, high levels of PIP increase the risk of barotrauma and chronic lung disease (Taghizadeh & Reynolds, 1976) and, when inappropriately high, may overdistend the lung, compress the pulmonary circulation and induce R–L shunting with adverse effects on oxygenation.

End-expiratory pressure. During expiration, a 'physiological' level of PEEP (about 2 cm H_2O) is required to simulate the small positive pressure that is normally maintained by laryngeal resistance during spontaneous breathing. Increases in PEEP increase FRC (Saunders, Milner & Hopkin, 1976) and in the presence of surfactant deficiency may improve oxygenation by deterring collapse of unstable lung units in expiration (Herman & Reynolds, 1973). Elevation of PEEP may at the same time decrease tidal volume and increase $PaCO_2$ (Herman & Reynolds, 1973; Greenough, Chan & Hird, 1992) by diminishing the pressure difference, ΔP_{ao} between inspiration and expiration and by reducing lung compliance. Compliance is reduced when tidal exchange is displaced to a higher and flatter part of the pressure–volume curve. High levels of PEEP may overdistend the lung and have adverse effects on gas exchange and cardiac output and increase the danger of pulmonary barotrauma. These effects have been thoroughly reviewed by Tyler (1983) and are a particular risk when compliance is relatively normal or the underlying lung disease is not homogeneously distributed.

Inspiratory and expiratory times

Inspiratory and expiratory times (T_I and T_E) together determine ventilator rate and thereby influence minute ventilation and $PaCO_2$. Under particular circumstances that are discussed below, variations in T_I and T_E may also have other critical effects on tidal volume, gas trapping and intrapulmonary R–L shunting.

Tidal volume and gas trapping. Time is required in inspiration and expiration for P_A to equilibrate with P_{ao}. If the duration of either T_I or T_E is insufficient for equilibration to occur, tidal volume will be diminished. When tidal volume is limited by T_E, expiration becomes incomplete and gas trapping occurs. The circumstances under which this limitation occurs are intimately dependent on the mechanical properties of the lung. If we consider the inspiratory or expiratory phase of mechanical ventilation to result in a step change in P_{ao} (in the absence of spontaneous respiratory effort) the change in lung volume over time can be shown to depend on the compliance (C) and resistance (R) of the respiratory system according to the equation,

$$V/V_0 = 1 - e^{-t/RC} \qquad (1)$$

where, V is the change in lung volume that has occurred by time t after the pressure change occurred, V_0 is the total change in lung volume when P_A has equilibrated with P_{ao} and gas flow has ceased, and e is a constant with

Table 15.1. *Estimates of the compliance, expiratory resistance and expiratory time constant for infants with normal lungs, hyaline membrane disease and chronic lung disease*

	Compliance (ml/cm H_2O)	Expiratory resistance (cm H_2O/ml/s)	Expiratory time constant (s)
Normal lungs	3–5	0.05–0.10	0.15–0.25
Hyaline membrane disease	0.25–1.0	0.05–0.10	0.02–0.05
Chronic lung disease	1.0–2.5	0.15–0.20	0.2–0.5

the value 2.718. The product of R and C has units of time and is commonly known as the time constant of the respiratory system (τ_{rs}). Solving the equation for values of t equal to one, two and three times τ_{rs} we find the ratio of V/V_0 equals 0.63, 0.86 and 0.95, respectively. Thus the change in lung volume approaches completion (to within 95%) only after a period of time equal to at least 3 times τ_{rs} has passed.

The values of T_I or T_E that will limit tidal volume are thus dependent on τ_{rs}. This relationship is of fundamental importance in mechanical ventilation of the newborn in whom the value of τ_{rs} may vary by an order of magnitude or more between different respiratory disorders (Mortola et al., 1982b; Edberg et al., 1991; Grunstein & Inscore, 1986). Reasonable estimates of τ_{rs} in expiration are presented in Table 15.1.

Because the inspiratory resistance during positive pressure ventilation may be as much as 4 fold less than expiratory (Perez Fontan et al., 1986) a smaller value of τ_{rs} generally applies in inspiration than expiration. Thus, whereas limitation of inspiration by T_I is unusual unless a particularly short T_I (<0.4 s) is employed (Field, Milner & Hopkin, 1985a), limitation of expiration may be much more common (Simbruner, 1986). If a T_E is employed that is less than three times τ_{rs}, expiration will be incomplete and P_A will remain in excess of PEEP at end-expiration, giving rise to 'inadvertent PEEP' and gas trapping. In a random selection of infants ventilated with a T_E of not less than 0.8 s, Simbruner (1986) found inadvertent PEEP of up to 7 cm H_2O to be present.

The effects of inadvertent PEEP are equivalent to applied PEEP but, because it is unseen, the potential adverse effects on gas exchange, lung volume and pulmonary blood flow are a particular hazard. Furthermore, if T_E is short, spontaneous changes in τ_{rs} due, for example, to improvement of the lung disease (increasing C) or accumulation of secretions (increasing R), may result in marked changes in inadvertent PEEP that are well beyond the operator's control.

Intrapulmonary R–L shunting. Independently of any effects on tidal exchange, an increase in the ratio of T_I/T_E (I:E Ratio) in infants with hyaline membrane disease may decrease intrapulmonary R–L shunting and improve PaO_2 (Herman & Reynolds, 1973). A similar effect can be demonstrated in adult respiratory distress syndrome where reversal of the I:E ratio is gaining increasing popularity as a strategy for improving oxygenation in severe disease (Tharratt, Allen & Albertson, 1988). The mechanism of this effect remains unknown but probably depends on two factors; firstly, re-expansion of otherwise collapsed lung units by providing more time for viscous forces to be overcome and secondly, holding unstable lung units open for a greater proportion of the respiratory cycle. Excessive prolongation of T_I in a relatively compliant and stable lung may compress pulmonary and systemic vessels with adverse effects on PaO_2 and cardiac output, and increase the risk of pulmonary air leak (Primhak, 1983).

Alterations in T_I and T_E may also have independent effects on the infant's spontaneous respiratory activity which are discussed below.

Mean airway pressure

Mean airway pressure, $P_{\overline{ao}}$ is the average pressure applied at the airway opening over time. Mean P_A approximates to $P_{\overline{ao}}$ but may exceed it under circumstances where expiratory resistance exceeds that during inspiration or where inadvertent PEEP is present (Marini & Ravenscroft, 1992). If the pressure waveform were perfectly square, $P_{\overline{ao}}$ could be estimated from the equation:

$$P_{\overline{ao}} = (PIP–PEEP) \times (T_I/[T_E + T_I]) + PEEP \qquad (2)$$

In practice, the shape is usually complex and $P_{\overline{ao}}$ is best measured by integration of the area under the curve of P_{ao} on time.

The significance of $P_{\overline{ao}}$ as an independent determinant of gas exchange is currently unclear. Several authors have reported an apparently linear relationship between $P_{\overline{ao}}$ and oxygenation in hyaline membrane disease (Herman & Reynolds, 1973; Boros, 1979) and have suggested that $P_{\overline{ao}}$ may be the common denominator of oxygen exchange in this condition. Intuitively, it would seem surprising, however, if a direct relationship were to exist. PEEP, PIP and I:E ratio are each determinants of $P_{\overline{ao}}$ but, although each may improve oxygenation in hyaline membrane disease they are believed to do so through quite independent means, which have been discussed above.

More recent evidence indicates that the relationship may be accidental and breaks down under more rigorous scrutiny. Thus Stewart, Finer and Peters (1981) have shown that, for a given change in $P\overline{ao}$, changes in PEEP or PIP have a greater effect on oxygenation than a change in I : E ratio. Likewise, when $P\overline{ao}$ is changed by altering PEEP alone the relationship between $P\overline{ao}$ and oxygenation is non-linear (Fox et al., 1977); at low PEEP, changes in $P\overline{ao}$ have a greater effect than at high PEEP. A more plausible relationship may be one between lung volume and oxygenation in hyaline membrane disease. Evidence to support this is provided by comparisons between conventional ventilation and high frequency oscillation (Kolton et al., 1986). At a given $P\overline{ao}$, high frequency oscillation is associated with a higher PaO_2 than conventional ventilation, but at the same mean lung volume (and different $P\overline{ao}$) oxygenation is the same with the two techniques.

Selection of ventilator settings

The appropriate settings for PIP, PEEP, T_I and T_E depend, therefore, on the nature and severity of the underlying lung disease. In the individual infant the benefits gained from strategies designed to change tidal volume, FRC or intrapulmonary shunting, must be weighed against the potential adverse effects those changes may have on cardiac output and pulmonary barotrauma. When in doubt, careful observation of the rate and extent of chest movement provides a useful visual clue to lung compliance and the duration of τ_{rs} and may help to avoid gas trapping and inadvertent PEEP.

Strategies of conventional mechanical ventilation

Continuous positive airways pressure (CPAP)

Many reports in the early 1970s indicated that a continuous distending pressure enhanced oxygenation in hyaline membrane disease, whether it was given as CPAP (Gregory et al., 1971) or as a continuous negative pressure to the chest (Chernick & Vidyasagar, 1972). The effect of CPAP, like PEEP, is the result of an increase in FRC (Saunders, Milner & Hopkin, 1976) and decrease in intrapulmonary $R–L$ shunting consequent upon recruitment of otherwise collapsed lung units, aided over the longer term perhaps by conservation of surfactant (Wyszogrodski et al., 1975) and greater regularity of respiratory rhythm (Spiedel & Dunn, 1975).

By improving oxygenation, CPAP offered a welcome and widely-employed method of avoiding, or at least delaying, mechanical ventilation in hyaline membrane disease (Fanaroff et al., 1973; Belenky et al., 1976) which at the time carried a mortality in excess of 50%. Despite early enthusiasm, interest in CPAP as a prelude to mechanical ventilation waned as survival rates improved. However, nasal CPAP in particular has continued to play an important role in weaning from mechanical ventilation (Higgins, Richter & Davis, 1991) and in the management of apnoea.

Recently, however, interest in the early use of nasal CPAP in hyaline membrane disease has been rekindled by a survey examining respiratory management and chronic lung disease in eight North American tertiary centres (Avery et al., 1987). The incidence of chronic lung disease was much lower in one, Columbia, where the early use of nasal CPAP in hyaline membrane disease was one of several notable features of their respiratory management. Subsequently, a retrospective report from Denmark (Kamper & Ringsted, 1990) has described similar results. A small controlled trial of prophylactic CPAP for all infants of <32 weeks gestation appeared to confer no benefit, however (Han et al., 1987), even amongst those infants who subsequently developed hyaline membrane disease. The role of early nasal CPAP now needs to be tested more rigorously in trials that are large enough to detect important differences in clinical outcome.

Ventilator rate

The extremely poor survival of infants with severe hyaline membrane disease in the early 1970s led Reynolds (Reynolds, 1971; Herman & Reynolds, 1973) and others (Smith, Schach & Daly, 1972) to perform experiments designed to determine the effects of changing mechanical ventilator settings on gas exchange. The results indicated that slow (30–40/min) ventilator rates gave better oxygenation than fast (60–80/min) and that oxygenation could be improved by increasing PIP, PEEP or I:E ratio each of which increased $P\overline{\text{ao}}$. These observations led Reynolds to recommend a strategy (Reynolds, 1975) for the management of severe hyaline membrane disease that was characterized by a slow rate (30–40/min) and when necessary a prolonged T_i (I:E ratio $\geq$1:1) to avoid excessively high peak pressures (>25 cm H_2O) which, at autopsy, seemed to be the major determinant of bronchopulmonary dysplasia (Taghizadeh & Reynolds, 1976). Historical comparisons suggested that mortality fell when this strategy was introduced (Reynolds & Taghizadeh, 1974) but their interpretation is obscured by coincident changes in ventilator design that made PEEP and continuous flow ventilation possible.

Although this strategy became widely accepted in the late 1970s some centres experienced an excess of pneumothoraces that seemed to be associated with the use of a long T_I (Primhak, 1983). Others (Heicher, Kasting & Harrod, 1981) experimented with strategies that employed a faster rate (60+/min) and shorter T_I (–0.5 s). They argued that a more rapid rate would allow the same level of alveolar ventilation (and therefore $PaCO_2$) to be achieved at a lower PIP, and they hypothesized that this would be associated with less barotrauma.

Several trials have now compared strategies based on fast versus slow ventilator rates (Spahr et al., 1980; Heicher et al., 1981; OCTAVE Study Group, 1991; Pohlandt et al., 1992). In each, the faster rate appeared to be associated with less pneumothoraces but conferred no benefit in mortality or chronic lung disease. Interpretation is confounded however, by the inclusion of infants with other respiratory problems (Heicher et al., 1981; Pohlandt et al., 1992) or mild/recovering hyaline membrane disease (Spahr et al., 1980) for whom a long T_I might be predicted to confer no benefit and increase the risk of adverse effects.

The OCTAVE trial also enrolled infants without regard to their underlying disease (excluding only those with meconium aspiration) but was analysed, at least in part, on a more disease-specific basis. For the OCTAVE population as a whole, the incidence of pneumothorax, chronic lung disease or death was not statistically different when fast rates (60/min and $T_I \leq 0.5$ s) were compared with slow (30–40/min, and $T_I = 0.75 - 1.0$ s). However, for the subgroup with hyaline membrane disease less pneumothoraces (18% vs 33%) occurred at higher ventilator rates.

Thus we may conclude that if we were to use just one strategy in the management of hyaline membrane disease, a strategy based on a fast ventilator rate may be 'safer' (with respect to pneumothoraces) than a slow rate. However, the search for a single strategy of ventilation, which characterizes these trials, may be both inappropriate and futile. Inappropriate, because benefits in one group of infants may be submerged by ill-effects in others (especially when different diseases are studied together) and futile, because the enormous range of mechanical properties displayed by the newborn infant makes it improbable that a single strategy could be ideal for all. Interestingly, neither strategy in the OCTAVE trial appeared to suit all infants – the study protocol had to be relaxed in 30% of infants in both groups, usually because of failing gas exchange.

If, on the other hand, we accept that more than one strategy may have a valuable role to play, then the results of the OCTAVE trial may not be in conflict with those of Reynolds. The infants studied in the OCTAVE trial were mostly smaller, treated earlier and had less severe disease than those of Reynolds. It remains entirely possible that strategies based on a slow rate and relatively long inspiratory time may be preferable for large infants with severe disease, similar to those studied by Reynolds (though such infants are now few in number since the advent of surfactant replacement). Indeed, the OCTAVE Study Group noted that adequate oxygenation could not be achieved with an I : E ratio of 1 : 2 in infants with more severe disease without resorting to peak pressures in excess of 30 cm H_2O.

For infants with other respiratory problems, the OCTAVE trial gives no support to the indiscriminate use of fast ventilator rates. We can calculate, in fact, that such infants showed a trend towards excess pneumothoraces (21% vs 13%) when ventilated at a fast rate, though the numbers are too small to achieve statistical significance. This observation is entirely in keeping with overdistension of the lung from inadvertent PEEP that can be readily predicted when a short T_E is employed in infants whose τ_{rs} is likely to be relatively long.

Relatively fast ventilator rates may, however, be beneficial in selected infants with pulmonary hypertension, pulmonary interstitial emphysema or meconium aspiration. In pulmonary hypertension an increase in rate may lower $PaCO_2$ and cause a dramatic decrease in extrapulmonary shunting. In pulmonary interstitial emphysema and meconium aspiration a very short T_I may result in preferential ventilation of the more normal areas of lung in which τ_{rs} is relatively short (Reynolds, 1979).

Asynchronous breathing

Infants often continue to make respiratory efforts during mechanical ventilation and several studies indicate that this activity may increase the risk of pneumothorax (Greenough et al., 1983) and intracranial haemorrhage (Perlman et al., 1985). A variety of patterns of interaction have been described of which one in particular, so-called 'active expiration', has been argued by Greenough to be closely associated with the development of pneumothoraces (Greenough, Morley & Davis, 1983). Doubt remains, however, about the nature of this interaction and the mechanism by which the risk of pneumothorax is increased (Ramsden, 1986). In a very small number of infants showing active expiration Greenough and her colleagues (Greenough et al., 1983) reported that muscle relaxation with pancuronium almost completely prevented pneumothorax whereas this complication occurred in 100% of controls.

Manipulation of ventilator timing has been examined by various investigators as an alternative to muscle relaxation for those infants who interact adversely with mechanical ventilation. Several reports indicate that faster rates (in the range 60–120/min) are associated with greater synchrony between infant and ventilator (Field, Milner & Hopkin, 1984; Greenough, Morley & Pool, 1986; Greenough, Greenall & Gamsu, 1987) and less active expiration (Field, Milner & Hopkin, 1985b). This effect has been postulated to underlie the difference in incidence of pneumothorax when fast and slow rates are compared (OCTAVE Study Group, 1991).

Other investigators have attempted to achieve synchrony by measuring the infant's spontaneous T_I and T_E during brief periods of CPAP and then matching those times in the mechanical ventilator settings (South & Morley, 1986; Amitay et al., 1993). This approach appears to induce reliably a period of synchrony, but the studies were brief and it is unclear for how long synchrony is maintained.

At present, the extent to which T_I and T_E are independent determinants of the pattern of interaction between baby and ventilator remains uncertain. Interpretation of these studies is confused since they make no attempt to keep respiratory drive constant. Thus, when the ventilator settings have been changed, the component of net alveolar ventilation delivered by the ventilator and the $PaCO_2$ may change and result in alterations in respiratory behaviour that are quite independent of the precise values T_I and T_E.

Patient triggered ventilation

Theoretically patient triggered ventilation circumvents the problem of harmonising baby and ventilator by using the baby's own inspiratory effort to trigger ventilator inflation and force the ventilator into synchrony with the baby. PIP, PEEP and T_I continue to be controlled by the operator but T_E is determined by the baby, though upper and lower limits may be set to prevent excessively high or low frequencies being generated. This principle has been employed in older patients for many years but until recently application to neonatal practice has met with no success.

Newborn infants present several technical obstacles. To keep pace with the rapid respiratory rate of the neonate, the trigger system must respond swiftly to the onset of inspiration. Epstein argued, some years ago (1971) that the response time should not exceed 10% of the spontaneous inspiratory time, thus no more than 30–40 ms in the neonate. The problem of achieving a speedy response is compounded by the need for high sensitivity to detect small changes in pressure or flow that are easily submerged in artefact.

The first report of success in newborns came from Mehta and colleagues (Mehta et al., 1986) who found a novel solution to the problem of sensitivity. They used a pneumatic capsule (Graseby MR10 respiration monitor) taped beneath the xiphisternum to detect changes in abdominal contour (relatively large in the neonate) to trigger a conventional ventilator (SLE Newborn 250). Subsequently, others had less success with the same method and reported airway pressure (Greenough, Hird & Chan, 1991) or flow (Hird & Greenough, 1991a) to be preferable trigger signals. These reports indicate that patient triggered ventilation maintains gas exchange at lower ventilator pressures (though not necessarily lower transpulmonary pressures) and is associated with less pneumothoraces when compared with historical controls (Clifford, Whincup & Thomas, 1988). Predictably, limitations occur in small or sick infants in whom apnoea or inadequate inspiratory effort causes irregular triggering (Mitchell, Greenough & Hird, 1989).

However, response times have remained a problem. Typical delays of early systems were 200–250 ms for those triggered by airway pressure and 300–550 ms for the Graseby MR10 (Hird & Greenough, 1991c). Tested in vitro with a lung model such delays may cause ventilator firing to be as much as 90 degrees out of phase (Wright, Baker & Rosenthal, 1990). New purpose-built devices such as the SLE 2000, or Draeger Babylog 8000 have a faster response time of 80–100 ms (Greenough et al., 1991) and may give better results (de Boer et al., 1993).

As yet, only one very small controlled trial (Hird & Greenough, 1991b) has compared patient triggered ventilation (SLE newborn triggered by airway pressure) with fast rate ventilation (at 60–120 breaths/min). This study found that triggered ventilation failed to achieve adequate ventilation more commonly than fast rate ventilation. However, only two measures of failure were used, asynchrony and 'apnoea causing inadequate triggering'. As immature infants (≥ 27 weeks gestation) were enrolled in whom apnoea was likely, and as apnoea was an indicator of failure only in the triggered group, a result favouring high frequency ventilation seems inevitable.

As the technology of patient triggered ventilation improves, it is probable that this technique will find an important place in managing large infants interacting chaotically with their ventilator as well as in weaning from mechanical ventilation. Randomized trials are now required which are large enough to test clinically relevant hypotheses about mortality, barotrauma and weaning in populations of infants in whom triggered ventilation may reasonably be expected to be of value.

High frequency ventilation

The most novel advance in mechanical ventilation of the newborn has been the development of high frequency ventilation. Devices for high frequency ventilation include high frequency jet ventilators, high frequency flow interrupters and high frequency oscillators. These devices induce small tidal oscillations of gas that are propelled into the airway at high frequency (generally around 15 Hz) and high velocity. In so doing they enhance gas transport by eliciting several unusual mechanisms of intrapulmonary gas dispersion of which a lucid account is given by Chang (1984). Gas mixing in the lung is so enhanced that alveolar ventilation can be maintained by exceptionally small tidal volumes that are close to the anatomical dead space of the lung.

During conventional mechanical ventilation adequate tidal volumes can often be attained only by exposing the periphery of the lung to large phasic pressure changes. By contrast, during high frequency ventilation swings in alveolar pressure (Gerstmann et al., 1990) are extremely small (about 1 cm H_2O). Thus, alveolar ventilation is achieved at a relatively constant lung volume and theoretically pulmonary barotrauma should be reduced. Evidence to support this hypothesis is now accumulating in a baboon model of hyaline membrane disease (de Lemos et al., 1987). Of the three techniques of high frequency ventilation, high frequency oscillation has been the subject of most evaluation in the human infant, and the remainder of this discussion will be confined to results obtained with that technique. Uncontrolled reports indicate that high frequency oscillation may have a valuable role in 'rescue' of infants with pulmonary interstitial emphysema (Clark et al., 1986) or meconium aspiration who cannot be adequately ventilated by more conventional means. Its role in the management of hyaline membrane disease is more uncertain. In a large multicentre trial, high frequency oscillation was associated with no pulmonary advantage and a poorer neurological outcome than conventional mechanical ventilation (HIFI study group, 1989). These disappointing results have been argued to result, at least in part, from failure in some centres to follow the intended 'high lung volume' strategy in which the maintenance of alveolar expansion is given a higher priority than minimization of the applied pressure (Bryan & Froese, 1991). Two small studies have attempted to re-examine the role of high frequency oscillation in hyaline membrane disease and have given more encouraging results (Clark et al., 1992; Ogawa et al., 1993). Both trials employed higher mean airway pressures during high frequency oscillation than conventional ventilation and found high frequency oscillation to give at least as good results as more conventional methods. Importantly, both trials showed trends towards less chronic lung disease with high frequency oscillation, though the difference achieved statistical significance only in one (Clark et al., 1992).

Although high frequency oscillation is hardly the panacea that had once been hoped, it may yet have an important place in the management of neonatal respiratory failure.

References

Agostoni, E., Taglietti, A., Agostoni, A. F., & Setnikar, I. (1958). Mechanical aspects of the first breath. *Journal of Applied Physiology*, **13**, 344–8.

Amitay, M., Etches, P. C., Finer, N. N. & Maidens J. M. (1993). Synchronous mechanical ventilation of the neonate with respiratory disease. *Critical Care Medicine,* **21**, 118–24.

Avery, M. E. & Mead, J. (1959). Surface properties in relation to atelectasis and hyaline membrane disease. *American Journal of Diseases of Children,* **97**, 517–23.

Avery, M. E., Tooley, W. H., Keller, J. B. et al. (1987). Is chronic lung disease in low birth weight infants preventable? A survey of eight centres. *Pediatrics*, **79**, 26–30.

Belenky, D. A., Orr, R. J., Woodrum, D. E. & Hodson, W. A. (1976). Is continuous transpulmonary pressure better than conventional respiratory management of hyaline membrane disease? A controlled study. *Pediatrics,* **58**, 800–8.

Boon, A. W., Milner, A. D. & Hopkin, I. E. (1979a). Physiological responses of the newborn infant to resuscitation. *Archives of Disease in Childhood,* **54**, 492–8.

Boon, A. W., Milner, A. D. & Hopkin, I. E. (1979b). Lung expansion, tidal exchange, and formation of the functional residual capacity during resuscitation of asphyxiated neonates. *Journal of Pediatrics,* **95**, 1031–6.

Boros, S. J. (1979). Variations in inspiratory : expiratory ratio and airway pressure waveform during mechanical ventilation. The significance of mean airway pressure. *Journal of Pediatrics,* **94**, 114–7.

Bryan, A. C. & Froese, A. B. (1991). Reflections on the HIFI trial. *Pediatrics,* **87**, 565–7.

Carson, B. S., Losey, R. W., Bowes, W. A. & Simmons, M. A. (1976). Combined obstetric and pediatric approach to prevent meconium aspiration syndrome. *American Journal of Obstetrics and Gynecology*, **126**, 712–5.

Chamberlain, R., Chamberlain, G., Howlett, B. & Claireaux, A. (1975). *British Births 1970, Vol I. The First Week of Life.* Heinemann, London.

Chang, H. K. (1984). Mechanisms of gas transport during ventilation by high-frequency oscillation. *Journal of Applied Physiology*, **56**, 553–63.

Chatburn, R. L. & Primiano, F. P. (1987). A rational basis for humidity therapy. *Respiratory Care*, **32**, 249–54.

Chernick, V. & Vidyasagar, D. (1972). Continuous negative chest wall pressure in hyaline membrane disease: one year experience. *Pediatrics*, **49**, 753–60.

Clark, R. H., Gerstman, D. R. Null, D. M. & Yoder, B. A. (1986). Pulmonary interstitial emphysema treated by high frequency oscillatory ventilation. *Critical Care Medicine*, **14**, 926–30.

Clark, R. H., Gerstman, D. R. Null, D. M. & deLemos, R. A. (1992). Prospective randomized comparison of high-frequency oscillatory and conventional ventilation in the treatment of respiratory distress syndrome. *Pediatrics*, **89** 5–12.

Clifford, R. D., Whincup, G. & Thomas, R. (1988). Patient-triggered ventilation prevents pneumothorax in premature babies. *Lancet,* i, 529–30.

Cordero, L. Jr., & Hon, E. H. (1971). Neonatal bradycardia following nasopharyngeal stimulation. *Journal of Pediatrics*, **78**, 441–66.

Cunningham, A. S., Lawson, E. E., Martin R. J. & Pildes R. S. (1990). Tracheal suction and meconium: a proposed standard of care. *Journal of Pediatrics*, **116**, 153–4.

Davis, R., Philips, J. P., Harris, B. A., Wilson, E. R. & Huddleston, J. F. (1985). Fatal meconium aspiration syndrome occurring despite airway management considered appropriate. *American Journal of Obstetrics and Gynecology*, **151**, 731–6.

deBoer, R. C., Jones, A., Ward, P. S. & Baumer J. H. (1993). Long term trigger ventilation in neonatal respiratory distress syndrome. *Archives of Disease in Childhood*, **68**, 308–11.

de Lemos, R. A., Coalson, J. J., Gerstmann, D. R., Null, D. M. et al.,. (1987). Ventilatory management of infant baboons with hyaline membrane disease: the use of high frequency ventilation. *Pediatric Research,* **21**, 594–602.

Drew, J. (1982). Immediate intubation at birth of the very-low-birth-weight infant. *American Journal of Diseases in Childhood*, **136**, 207–210.

Edberg K. E., Sandberg K., Silbereberg, A., Ekstrom-Jodal, B. & Hjalmarson O. (1991). Lung volume, gas-mixing, and mechanics of breathing in mechanically ventilated very low birth weight infants with idiopathic respiratory distress syndrome. *Pediatric Research,* **30**, 496–500.

Epstein, R. A. (1971). The sensitivities and response times of ventilatory assists. *Anesthesiology* **34**, 321–6.

Fanaroff, A. A., Cha, C. C., Sosa, R., Crumrine, R. S. & Klaus, M. H. (1973). Controlled trial of continuous negative extrenal pressure in the treatment of severe respiratory distress syndrome. *Journal of Pediatrics*, **83**, 921–8.

Field, D., Milner, A. D. & Hopkin, I. E. (1984). High and conventional rates of positive pressure ventilation. *Archives of Disease in Childhood*, **59**, 1151–4.

Field, D., Milner, A. D. & Hopkin, I. E. (1985*a*). Inspiratory time and tidal volume during intermittent positive pressure ventilation. *Archives of Disease in Childhood*, **60**, 259–61.

Field, D., Milner, A. D. & Hopkin, I. E. (1985*b*). Manipulation of ventilator settings to prevent active expiration against positive pressure inflation. *Archives of Disease in Childhood*, **60**, 1036–40.

Field, D., Milner, A. D. & Hopkin, I. E. (1986). Efficiency of manual resuscitators at birth. *Archives of Disease in Childhood*, **61**, 300–2.

Finer, N. N, Barrington, K. J., Al Fadley, F. & Peters, K. L. (1986). Limitations of self-inflating resuscitators. *Pediatrics*, **77**, 417–20.

Fox, W. W., Gewitz, M. H., Berman, L. S., Peckham, G. I. & Downes J. J. (1977). The PaO$_2$ response to changes in end expiratory pressure in the newborn respiratory distress syndrome. *Critical Care Medicine* **5**, 226–9.

Gerstmann, D. R., Fouke, J. M., Winter, D. C., Taylor, A. F. & deLemos R. A. (1990) Proximal tracheal and alveolar pressures during high-frequency oscillatory ventilation in a normal rabbit model. *Pediatric Research* **28**, 367–73.

Geubelle, F., Karlberg, P., Koch, G., Lind, J., Wallgren, G. & Wegelius, C. (1959). L'Aération du poumon chez le nouveau-né. *Biologia Neonatorum*, **1**, 169–210.

Greenough, A., Chan, V. & Hird, M. F. (1992). Positive end expiratory pressure in acute and chronic respiratory distress. *Archives of Disease in Childhood*, **67**, 320–3.

Greenough, A., Greenall, F. & Gamsu H. (1987). Synchronous respiration: which ventilator rate is best? *Acta Paediatrica Scandinavica*, **76**, 713–8.

Greenough, A., Hird, M. F. & Chan, V. (1991). Airway pressure triggered ventilation for preterm neonates. *Journal of Perinatal Medicine*, **19**, 471–6.

Greenough, A., Morley C. & Davis, J. (1983*a*). Interaction of spontaneous respiration with artificial ventilation in preterm babies. *Journal of Pediatrics*, **103**, 769–73.

Greenough, A., Wood, S., Morley C. J. & Davis, J. A. (1983*b*). Pancuronium prevents pneumothoraces in ventilated premature babies who actively expire against positive pressure inflation. *Lancet* **i**, 1–3.

Greenough, A., Morley C. & Pool, J. (1986). Fighting the ventilator – are fast rates an effective alternative to paralysis? *Early Human Development*, **13**, 189–94.

Gregory, G. A, Gooding, C. A., Phibbs, R. H. & Tooley, W. H. (1974). Meconium aspiration in infants – a prospective study. *Journal of Pediatrics*, **85**, 848–52.

Gregory, G. A., Kitterman, J. A., Phibbs, R. H., Tooley, W. H. & Hamilton, W. K. (1971). Treatment of idiopathic respiratory distress syndrome with continuous positive airways pressure. *New England Journal of Medicine*, **284**, 1333–40.

Grunstein, M. M. & Inscore, S. C. (1986) A new method to assess respiratory mechanics in infants with pulmonary disease. *Pediatric Research*, **20**, 472A.

Han, V. K. M., Beverley, D. W., Clarson, C. et al. (1987). Randomized controlled trial of very early continuous distending pressure in the management of preterm infants. *Early Human Development*, **15**, 21–32.

Heicher, D. A., Kasting, D. S. & Harrod, J. R. (1981). Prospective clinical comparison of two methods for mechanical ventilation of neonates: rapid rate and short inspiratory time versus slow rate and long inspiratory time. *Journal of Pediatrics*, **98**, 957–61.

Herman, S. & Reynolds, E. O. R. (1973). Methods for improving oxygenation in infants mechanically ventilated for severe hyaline membrane disease. *Archives of Disease in Childhood*, **48**, 612–7.

HIFI Study Group (1989). High-frequency oscillatory ventilation compared with conventional mechanical ventilation in the treatment of respiratory failure in preterm infants. *New England Journal of Medicine*, **320**, 88–93.

Higgins, R. D., Richter, S. E. & Davis, J. M. (1991). Nasal continuous positive airways pressure facilitates extubation of very low birth weight neonates. *Pediatrics*, **88**, 999–1002.

Hird, M. F. & Greenough, A. (1991*a*). Patient triggered ventilation using a flow triggered system. *Archives of Disease in Childhood*, **66**, 1140–2.

Hird, M. F. & Greenough, A. (1991*b*). Randomised trial of patient triggered ventilation versus high frequency positive pressure ventilation in acute respiratory distress. *Journal of Perinatal Medicine*, **19**, 379–84.

Hird, M. F. & Greenough, A. (1991*c*). Comparison of triggering systems for neonatal patient triggered ventilation. *Archives of Disease in Childhood*, **66**, 426–8.

Hoskyns, E. W., Milner, A. D., Boon, A. W., Vyas, H. & Hopkin, I. E. (1987*a*). Endotracheal resuscitation of preterm infants at birth. *Archives of Disease in Childhood*, **62**, 663–6.

Hoskyns, E. W., Milner, A. D. & Hopkin, I. E. (1987*b*). A simple method of face mask resuscitation at birth. *Archives of Disease in Childhood*, **62**, 376–8.

Kamper, J. & Ringsted, C. (1990). Early treatment of idiopathic respiratory distress syndrome using binasal continuous positive airway pressure. *Acta Paediatrica Scandinavica*, **79**, 581–6.

Kanter, R. K. (1987). Evaluation of mask-bag ventilation in resuscitation of infants. *American Journal of Diseases of Children*, **141**, 761–3.

Karlberg, P., Cherry, R. B., Escardo, F. E. & Koch, G. (1962). Respiratory studies on newborn infants. II. Pulmonary ventilation and mechanics of breathing in the first minutes of life, including the onset of respiration. *Acta Paediatrica*, **51**: 121–36.

Katz, V. L., & Bowes, W. A. (1992). Meconium aspiration syndrome: reflections on a murky subject. *American Journal of Obstetrics and Gynecology*, **166**, 171–83.

Kolton, M., Cattran, C. B., Kent, G., Volgyesi, G., Froese, A. B. & Bryan, A. C. (1982). Oxygenation during high-frequency ventilation compared with conventional mechanical ventilation in two models of lung injury. *Anesthesia and Analgesia*, **61**, 323–32.

Linder, N., Aranda, J. V., Tsur, M., Atoth, I., Yatsiv, I. & Mandelberg, H. (1988). Need for endotracheal intubation and suction in meconium-stained neonates. *Journal of Pediatrics*, **122**, 613–15.

Lomholt, N., Cooke, R., & Lundig, M. (1968). A method of humidification in ventilator treatment of neonates. *British Journal of Anaesthesia*, **40**, 335–40.

McFadden, E. R., Pichurko, B. M., Bowman, H. F. et al. (1985). Thermal mapping of the airways in humans. *Journal of Applied Physiology*, **2**, 564–70.

MacDonald, H. M., Mulligan, J. C., Allen, A. C. & Taylor, P. M. (1980). Neonatal asphyxia. I: Relationship of obstetric and neonatal complications to neonatal mortality in 38,405 consecutive deliveries. *Journal of Pediatrics*, **96**, 899–902.

Marini, J. J. & Ravenscroft, S. A. (1992). Mean airway pressure: Physiological determinants and clinical importance – Part 2: Clinical implications. *Critical Care Medicine*, **20**, 1604–16.

Marshall, T. A., Deeder R., Pai, S., Berkowitz, G. P. & Austin T. L. (1984). Physiologic changes associated with endotracheal intubation in preterm infants. *Critical Care Medicine*, **12**, 501–3.

Mehta, A., Callan, K., Wright, B. M. & Stacey, T. E. (1986). Patient-triggered ventilation in the newborn. *Lancet*, ii, 17–19.

Milner, A. D. (1991). Resuscitation of the newborn. *Archives of Disease in Childhood*, **66**, 66–9.

Milner, A. D. & Saunders, R. A. (1977). Pressure and volume changes during the first breath of human neonates. *Archives of Disease in Childhood*, **52**, 918–24.

Milner, A. D., Vyas, H. & Hopkin, I. E. (1984). Efficacy of facemask resuscitation at birth. *British Medical Journal*, **289**, 1563–5.

Mitchell, A., Greenough, A. & Hird, M. (1989). Limitations of patient triggered ventilation in neonates. *Archives of Disease in Childhood*, **64**, 924–9.

Mortola, J. P., Fisher, J. T., Smith, J. B., Fox, G. S., Weeks, S. & Willis, D. (1982a). Onset of respiration in infants delivered by Caesarean section. *Journal of Applied Physiology*, **52**, 716–24.

Mortola, J. P., Fisher, J. T., Smith, J. B., Fox, G. S. & Weeks, S. (1982b). Dynamics of breathing in infants. *Journal of Applied Physiology*, **52**, 1209–15.

Murphy, J. D., Vawter, G. F. & Reid, L. M. (1984). Pulmonary vascular disease in fatal meconium aspiration. *Journal of Pediatrics* **104**, 758–62.

Noguchi, H., Takumi, Y. & Aochi, O. (1973). A study of humidification on tracheostomized dogs. *British Journal of Anaesthesia*, **45**, 844–8.

OCTAVE Study Group. (1991). Multicentre randomised controlled trial of high against low frequency positive pressure ventilation. *Archives of Disease in Childhood*, **66**, 770–5.

Ogawa, Y., Miyasaka, K., Kawano, T. et al. (1993). A multicentre randomized trial of high frequency oscillatory mechanical ventilation in preterm infants with respiratory failure. *Early Human Development*, **32**, 1–10.

Palme, C., Nystrom, B. & Tunnel, R. (1985). An evaluation of face masks in the resuscitation of newborn infants. *Lancet*, **i**, 207–10.

Perez Fontan, J. J., Heldt, G. P., Targett, R. C. Willis, M. M. & Gregory, G. A. (1986). Dynamics of expiration and gas trapping in rabbits during mechanical ventilation at rapid rates. *Critical Care Medicine*, **14**, 39–47.

Perlman, J. M., Goodman, S., Kreusser, K. L. & Volpe, J. J. (1985). Reduction in intraventricular haemorrhage by elimination of fluctuating cerebral blood-flow velocity in preterm infants with respiratory distress syndrome. *New England Journal of Medicine* **312**, 1353–7.

Pohlandt F., Saule, H., Schroder, H., Leonhardt, A. et al. (1992). Decreased incidence of extra-alveolar air leakage or death prior to air leakage in high versus low rate positive pressure ventilation: results of a randomised seven-centre trial in preterm infants. *European Journal of Pediatrics*, **151**, 904–9.

Primhak, R. A. (1983). Factors associated with air leak in premature infants receiving mechanical ventilation. *Journal of Pediatrics,* **102**, 764–8.

Ramsden, C. A. (1986). Active expiration or synchrony. *Archives of Disease in Childhood*, **61**, 820.

Ramsden, C. A. & Reynolds, E. O. R. (1987). Ventilator settings for newborn infants. *Archives of Disease in Childhood*, **62**, 529–38.

Reynolds, E. O. R. (1971). Effects of alteration in mechanical ventilator settings on pulmonary gas exchange in hyaline membrane disease. *Archives of Disease in Childhood*, **46**, 152–9.

Reynolds, E. O. R. (1975). Management of hyaline membrane disease. *British Medical Bulletin*, **31**, 81–4.

Reynolds, E. O. R. & Taghizadeh, E. O. R. (1974). Improved prognosis for infants mechanically ventilated for hyaline membrane disease. *Archives of Disease in Childhood*, **49**, 505–15.

Reynolds, O. (1979). Ventilator therapy. In *Neonatal Pulmonary Care.* ed. D. W. Thibeault, G. A. Gregory. pp. 217–36. Addison-Wesley, Menlo Park.

Saunders, R. A., Milner, A. D. & Hopkin, E. I. (1976). The effects of continuous positive airways pressure on lung mechanics and lung volumes in the neonate. *Biology of the Neonate*, **29**, 178–86.

Sendak, M. J., Harris, A. P. & Donham, R. T. (1986). Use of pulse oximetry to assess arterial oxygen saturation during newborn resuscitation. *Pediatric Research*, **14**, 739.

Simbruner, G. (1986). Inadvertent positive end-expiratory pressure in mechanically ventilated newborn infants: detection and effect on lung mechanics and gas exchange. *Journal of Pediatrics*, **108**, 589–95.

Smith, P. C., Schach, M. S., & Daly, W. J. R. (1972). Mechanical ventilation of newborn infants: II. Effects of independent variation of rate and pressure on arterial oxygenation of infants with respiratory distress syndrome. *Anesthesiology,* **37**, 498–502.

South, M. & Morley, C. J. (1986). Synchronous mechanical ventilation of the neonate. *Archives of Disease in Childhood*, **61**, 1190–5.

Spahr, R. C., Klein A. M., Brown, D. R., MacDonald, H. M. & Holzman, I. R. (1980). Hyaline membrane disease: a controlled study of inspiratory to expiratory ratio in its management by ventilator. *American Journal of Diseases of Children*, **134**, 373–6.

Spiedel, B. D. & Dunn, P. M. (1975). Effect of continuous positive airway pressure on breathing pattern of infants with respiratory distress syndrome. *Lancet*, **i**, 302–4.

Stewart, A. R, Finer, N. N. & Peters, K. L. (1981). Effects of alterations of inspiratory and expiratory pressures and inspiratory/expiratory ratios on mean airway pressure, blood gases, and intracranial pressure. *Pediatrics* **67**, 474–81.

Taghizadeh, A. & Reynolds, E. O. R. (1976). Pathogenesis of bronchopulmonary dysplasia following hyaline membrane disease. *American Journal of Pathology*, **82**, 241–58.

Tarnow-Mordi, W. O., Reid, E., Griffiths, P. & Wilkinson, A. R. (1989). Low inspired gas temperature and respiratory complications in very low birthweight infants. *Journal of Pediatrics*, **114**, 438–42.

Tharratt, R. S., Allen, R. J. & Albertson, T. E. (1988). Pressure controlled inverse ratio ventilation in severe adult respiratory failure. *Chest,* **94**, 755–62.

Ting, P. & Brady, J. P. (1975). Tracheal suction in meconium aspiration. *American Journal of Obstetrics and Gynecology*, **122**, 767–71.

Toremalm, N. G. (1961). Airflow patterns and ciliary activity in the trachea after tracheotomy. *Acta Otolaryngologica*, **53**, 442–54.

Tsuda T., Noguchi, H., Takumi, Y. & Aochi, O. (1977). Optimum humidification of air administered to a tracheostomy in dogs. *British Journal of Anaesthesia*, **49**, 965–76.

Tyler, D. C. (1983). Positive-end-expiratory pressure: a review. *Critical Care Medicine,* **11**, 300–8.

Tyson, J. E. (1992) Immediate care of the newborn infant. In *Effective Care of the Newborn Infant*. ed. J. C. Sinclair, M. B. Bracker. pp. 22–39. Oxford University Press, New York.

Upton, C. J. & Milner, A. D. (1991). Endotracheal resuscitation of neonates using a rebreathing bag. *Archives of Disease in Childhood*, **66**, 39–42.

Vyas, H., Field, D., Milner, A. D. & Hopkin, I. E. (1986) Determinants of the first inspiratory volume and functional residual capacity at birth. *Pediatric Pulmonology*, **2**, 189–93.

Vyas, H., Milner, A. D., Hopkin, I. E. & Boon, A. W. (1981). Physiologic responses to prolonged and slow-rise inflation in the resuscitation of the asphyxiated newborn infant. *Journal of Pediatrics*, **99**, 635–39.

Vyas, H., Milner, A. D., & Hopkin, I. E. (1983). Face mask resuscitation: does it lead to gastric distension? *Archives of Disease in Childhood*, **58**, 373–75.

Wiswell, T. E. & Henley, M. A. (1992). Intratracheal suctioning, systemic infection, and the meconium aspiration syndrome. *Pediatrics*, **89**, 203–6.

Wiswell, T. E., Tuggle, J. M. & Turner, B. S. (1990). Meconium aspiration syndrome: have we made a difference? *Pediatrics*, **85**, 715–21.

Wright, B. M., Baker, J. A. & Rosenthal, M. (1990). Airways-pressure triggered (APT) ventilation in the newborn. *Journal of Physiology,* 426, 6P.

Wyszogrodski, I., Kyei-Aboagye, K., Taeusch, H. W. & Avery, M. E. (1975). Surfactant inactivation by hyperventilation; conservation by end-expiratory pressure. *Journal of Applied Physiology*, **38**, 461-6.

Index